# Cough: Causes, Mechanisms and Therapy

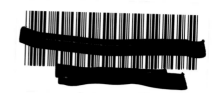

# Cough: Causes, Mechanisms and Therapy

Edited by

## Kian Fan Chung

MD DSc FRCP
National Heart and Lung Institute
Imperial College and Royal Brompton & Harefield NHS Trust
London
UK

## John G. Widdicombe

MA DPhil DM FRCP
University of London and
116 Pepys Road
London
UK

## Homer A. Boushey

MD
Department of Medicine
University of California San Francisco
San Francisco
California
USA

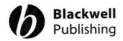

**Blackwell**
Publishing

First published 2003

Reprinted 2005

Library of Congress Cataloging-in-Publication Data

Cough : causes, mechanisms, and therapy / edited by Kian Fan Chung, John G. Widdicombe,
Homer A. Boushey.
       p. ; cm.
Includes bibliographical references and index.
  ISBN 1-4051-1634-X
1. Cough.
  [DNLM: 1. Cough. WF 143 C854 2003] I. Chung, K. Fan, 1951– II. Widdicombe,
John G. III. Boushey, Homer A.

  RC741.5.C68   2003
  616.2—dc21
                                                  2003011068

ISBN 1-4051-1634-X

A catalogue record for this title is available from the British Library

Set in 9/11 1/2 pt Sabon by SNP Best-set Typesetter Ltd., Hong Kong
Printed and bound in Great Britain by Marston Book Services Limited, Oxford

Commissioning Editor: Maria Khan
Managing Editor: Rupal Malde
Production Editor: Nick Morgan
Production Controller: Kate Charman

For further information on Blackwell Publishing, visit our website:
http://www.blackwellpublishing.com

# Contents

# Contributors

**Nisar Ahmed**
Academic Palliative Medicine Unit, Division of
Clinical Sciences, Royal Hallamshire Hospital,
Glossop Road, Sheffield S10 2JF, UK

**Sam H. Ahmedzai**
Academic Palliative Medicine Unit, Division of
Clinical Sciences, Royal Hallamshire Hospital,
Glossop Road, Sheffield S10 2JF, UK

**Elisabeth Araujo**
Otorhinolaryngology and Respiratory Diseases,
Universidade Federal do Rio Grande do Sul, 90020-
090 Porto Alegre, RS Brazil

**David M. Baekey**
Department of Physiology and Biophysics, College of
Medicine, University of South Florida, Tampa, FL
33612, USA

**Maria G. Belvisi**
Respiratory Pharmacology Group, Cardiothoracic
Surgery, National Heart & Lung Institute, Faculty of
Medicine, Imperial College of Science, Technology
and Medicine, London SW3 6LY, UK

**Donald C. Bolser**
Department of Physiological Sciences, College of
Veterinary Medicine, University of Florida, PO Box
100144, Gainesville, FL 32610-0144, USA

**Homer A. Boushey**
Professor of Medicine, Department of Medicine,
University of California San Francisco, 505 Parnassus
Avenue, San Francisco, CA 94143, USA

**Peter M.A. Calverley**
Department of Medicine, University of Liverpool, and
University Hospital Aintree, Liverpool, UK

**Brendan J. Canning**
Johns Hopkins Asthma and Allergy Center, 5501
Hopkins Bayview Circle, Baltimore, MD 21224,
USA

**Anne B. Chang**
Paediatric Respiratory Consultant, Department of
Respiratory Medicine, Royal Children's Hospital
Foundation, Herston, and Associate Professor of
Paediatrics, University of Queensland, Queensland
4029, Australia

**Kian Fan Chung**
National Heart & Lung Institute, Imperial College
and Royal Brompton & Harefield NHS Trust,
Dovehouse Street, London SW3 6LY, UK

**Paul W. Davenport**
Department of Physiological Sciences, College of
Veterinary Medicine, University of Florida,
Gainesville, FL 32610, USA

**Peter V. Dicpinigaitis**
Associate Professor of Clinical Medicine, Albert
Einstein College of Medicine, and Director, Intensive
Care Unit, Jack D. Weiler Hospital of the Albert
Einstein College of Medicine, Bronx, New York, NY
10461, USA

**Ronald Eccles**
Common Cold Centre, Cardiff School of Biosciences,
Cardiff University, Cardiff CF10 3US, UK

**Kenneth E. Fletcher**
Associate Professor of Psychiatry and the Graduate
School of Nursing, University of Massachusetts
Medical School, 55 Lake Avenue North, Worcester,
MA 01655, USA

## Giovanni A. Fontana
Dipartimento di Area Critica Medico Chirurgica, Unità Funzionale di Medicina Respiratoria, Università degli Studi di Firenze, Firenze, Italy

## W. Michael Foster
Pulmonary and Critical Care Medicine, MSRB Room #275, Research Drive, Duke University Medical Center, Durham, NC 27710, USA

## Cynthia T. French
University of Massachusetts Memorial Health Care, 55 Lake Avenue North, Worcester, MA 01655, USA

## Rick W. Fuller
Director of Science Funding, The Wellcome Trust, 183 Euston Road, London NW1 2BE, UK

## Francis J. Golder
Department of Physiological Sciences, College of Veterinary Medicine, University of Florida, Gainesville, FL 32610, USA

## David J. Hele
Respiratory Pharmacology Group, Cardiothoracic Surgery, National Heart & Lung Institute, Faculty of Medicine, Imperial College of Science, Technology and Medicine, London SW3 6LY, UK

## Alvin J. Ing
Thoracic Physician, Clinical Senior Lecturer, University of Sydney, Concord Hospital, Concord, NSW 2139, Australia

## Richard S. Irwin
Professor of Medicine, University of Massachusetts Medical School, 55 Lake Avenue North, Worcester, MA 01655-0330, USA

## Marian Kollarik
Johns Hopkins Asthma and Allergy Center, 5501 Hopkins Bayview Circle, Baltimore, MD 21224, USA

## Bruce G. Lindsey
Department of Physiology and Biophysics, College of Medicine, University of South Florida, Tampa, FL 33612, USA

## Stuart B. Mazzone
Howard Florey Institute of Experimental Physiology and Medicine, University of Melbourne, Melbourne, Victoria 3010, Australia

## Lorcan P.A. McGarvey
Senior Lecturer/Consultant Physician, Department of Medicine, The Queen's University of Belfast, Belfast, Northern Ireland

## Alyn H. Morice
Head of Academic Department of Medicine, Castle Hill Hospital, Castle Road, Cottingham, East Yorkshire HU16 5JQ, UK

## Kendall F. Morris
Department of Physiology and Biophysics, College of Medicine, University of South Florida, Tampa, FL 33612, USA

## Paul M. O'Byrne
Firestone Institute for Respiratory Health, St Joseph's Hospital, 50 Charlton Avenue East, Hamilton, Ontario L8N 4A6, Canada

## Clive P. Page
The Sackler Institute of Pulmonary Pharmacology, 5th Floor Hodgkin Building, GKT School of Biomedical Sciences, Guy's Campus, King's College London, London SE1 1UL, UK

## Bruno C. Palombini
Pavilhao Pereira Filho, Irmandade da Santa Casa de Misericordia de Porto Alegre, Universidade Federal do Rio Grande do Sul, Rua Prof. Annes Dias 285, 90020-090 Porto Alegre, RS Brazil

## Wee-Yang Pek
Visiting Postgraduate Fellow in Pulmonary and Allergy/Immunology, Department of Medicine, University of California San Francisco, 505 Parnassus Avenue, San Francisco, CA, 94143, USA

## Sandra M. Reynolds
The Sackler Institute of Pulmonary Pharmacology, 5th Floor Hodgkin Building, GKT School of Biomedical Sciences, Guy's Campus, King's College London, London SE1 1UL, UK

## Bruce K. Rubin
Professor and Vice-Chair of Pediatrics, Professor of Biomedical Engineering, Physiology and Pharmacology, Department of Pediatrics, Wake Forest University School of Medicine, Medical Center Boulevard, Winston-Salem, NC 27157-1081, USA

## Roger Shannon
Department of Physiology and Biophysics, College of Medicine, University of South Florida, Tampa, FL 33612, USA

## Domenico Spina
The Sackler Institute of Pulmonary Pharmacology, 5th Floor Hodgkin Building, GKT School of Biomedical Sciences, Guy's Campus, King's College London, London SE1 1UL, UK

## Kazuo Takahama
Department of Environmental and Molecular Health Sciences, Graduate School of Pharmaceutical Sciences, Kumamoto University, 5-1 Oe-honmachi, Kumamoto 862-0973, Japan

## Bradley J. Undem
Johns Hopkins Asthma and Allergy Center, 5501 Hopkins Bayview Circle, Baltimore, MD 21224, USA

## John G. Widdicombe
University of London and 116 Pepys Road, London SW20 8NY, UK

## Robert Wilson
Consultant Physician, Royal Brompton Hospital, and Reader, National Heart & Lung Institute at Imperial College of Science, Technology and Medicine, Sydney Street, London SW3 6NP, UK

# Preface

Cough is the most common symptom of airway and lung disease. More money is spent at the pharmacy on 'coughs and colds' than on any other symptom except perhaps 'aches and pains'. It can be a presenting symptom of more than 100 clinical conditions of the respiratory system. At international meetings of, for example, the American Thoracic Society and the European Respiratory Society, cough is one of the most frequent items listed in the Proceedings' indices. Surprisingly, it has seldom been comprehensively reviewed, although most textbooks of respiratory medicine contain a short chapter on the subject, as do texts on respiratory pharmacology and therapeutics. Physiology textbooks largely ignore it.

In 1970, Salem and Aviado published a three-volume text on *Antitussive Agents* [1] which has become a classic that, while of limited scope, badly needs updating. In 1974, Korpas and Tomori published *Cough and Other Respiratory Reflexes* [2], a valuable text dealing mainly with animal studies from distinguished research centres in Eastern Europe. There is an excellent short book (published in 2001 but in Italian!) *La Tosse Fisiopatologia e Clinica* by Fontana, Lavorini, Pantaleo and Pistolesi [3]. There have been a number of published symposium proceedings dedicated to cough [4–9]. All these publications are somewhat restricted in their approach and most need to be brought up to date. Two of the symposia [7,8], based on the 1st and 2nd International Symposia on Cough held in London in 1996 and 2001, attracted much support and interest; this response was in large part the stimulus to the present book.

We therefore believe that this book is the first comprehensive review, by internationally distinguished authors, of a subject of great importance to respiratory basic science and medicine, and to health care. We have tried to make it inclusive, but are aware that there may be gaps. We have particularly tried to review the significance of cough in the wider context of clinical medicine, a subject which has seen impressive advances in understanding in recent years; and in the basic physiological mechanisms of cough. Understanding of the latter has been transformed recently by studies of the plasticity of cough mechanisms at peripheral and central nervous levels, research that has important relevance to what happens in acute, subacute and chronic airways' disease. Basic pharmacological studies are also having a significant impact on the therapy of cough, an influence which is likely to be dramatically extended in the near future. With such an approach and coverage, we hope that our book will be helpful to a wide readership of clinicians (particularly general practitioners), respiratory and paediatric physicians, respiratory physiologists and scientists interested in cough and lung reflexes, and pharmacologists in search of better treatments for cough.

In compiling this volume, we have ourselves learnt a lot more but have also realized that there are large gaps both at the clinical and basic level of understanding and treatment of this common symptom. We hope that the readers will be similarly challenged.

We are grateful for the cooperation, diligence and expertise of our many contributors; for the valuable advice and support of our colleague Tim Higenbottam at AstraZeneca UK; and for the skill and efficiency of our publishers, Blackwell Publishing, in particular Maria Khan, Rupal Malde and Nick Morgan.

Fan Chung
John Widdicombe
Homer Boushey

## References

1 Salem H, Aviado DM, eds. *Antitussive Agents. International Encyclopedia of Pharmacology and Therapeutics*, section 27, Volumes I–III. Oxford: Pergamon Press, 1970.
2 Korpas J, Tomori Z. Cough and other respiratory reflexes. In: *Progress in Respiratory Research*, Vol. 12. Basel: Karger, 1978.
3 Fontana GA, Lavorini F, Pantaleo T *et al.*, eds. *La Tosse Fisiopatologia e Clinica*. Pisa: Primula, 2001.
4 Berglund E, Nilsson BS, Mossberg B *et al.* Cough and expectoration. *Eur J Respir Dis* 1980; 61 (Suppl. 110): 1–262.
5 Widdicombe JG, Korpas J, Salat D, eds. The cough reflex. *Bull Eur Physiopath Respir* 1987; 23 (Suppl. 10): 11S–76S.

6 Korpas J, Widdicombe JG, eds. Cough and related phenomena. *Respir Med* 1991; **85** (Suppl. A):1–68.
7 Widdicombe J, ed. Cough: methods and measurements. *Pulm Pharmacol* 1996; **9**: 261–392.
8 Widdicombe J, Chung F, eds. Cough: pharmacology and therapeutics. *Pulm Pharmacol Ther* 2002; **15**: 185–338.
9 Korpas J, Widdicombe JG, eds. Cough: recent advances in understanding. *Eur Respir Rev* 2002; **85**: 221–82.

# Introduction

# 1 The clinical and pathophysiological challenge of cough

*Kian Fan Chung*

## Introduction

Cough is a symptom that has been experienced by every human and is an essential protective and defensive act whose action secures the removal of mucus, noxious substances and infections from the larynx, trachea and larger bronchi. Coughing is the most efficient mechanism for clearing the upper airways, and can be considered to be an innate inbuilt defence mechanism. Impairment or absence of the coughing mechanism can be harmful and even fatal in disease. On the other hand, cough may be the first overt sign of disease of the airways or lungs, when it represents more than a defence mechanism, and by its persistence becomes a helpful pointer for both patient and physician of potential disease. Nearly all conditions affecting the respiratory system and some extrapulmonary conditions may cause cough, but to the physician it is most important to exclude the most serious conditions that need prompt treatment. Cough may be persistent in incurable diseases such as in terminal lung cancer, when other chronic symptoms are also present such as dyspnoea and pain. Cough may be the most prominent symptom complained of by patients with chronic respiratory disease such as asthma [1]. Excessive persistent cough may also be present in association with chronic non-malignant disease with or without excessive mucus production. The effect of persistent cough itself may be harmful and deleterious to the patient by interfering with breathing, social activities and sleep, and by causing deterioration in the quality of life and social embarrassment, not to mention syncopal episodes, urinary incontinence, muscle ache, insomnia and fatigue. Thus, cough is a symptom with many facets: a protec-

tive mechanism for the lungs, a warning sign of disease, and a detrimental symptom when persistent.

With these several aspects of the problem of cough, the challenge to understand and adequately treat cough has been and remains daunting, from both the investigational and clinical angles. Our pathophysiological understanding of the genesis of cough is incomplete, particularly with reference to disease. This volume will focus on all the clinical, pathogenetic and treatment aspects of cough. To approach the challenge presented by cough, this first chapter will discuss the following themes: (i) the normal cough; (ii) the significance of cough in the community; (iii) the spectrum of cough presenting to the clinician; (iv) the mechanisms of increased cough sensitivity; and (v) the treatment of cough.

## The normal cough

What is a normal cough pattern? How often do healthy people cough? There are no clear data. Cough is not necessarily an 'abnormal' symptom with clinical significance. But when does a normal pattern of cough becomes an abnormal one? One presumes that a cough is necessary to clear the airways of the mucus and fluid secretion from the airways (estimated to be 20–30 mL over 24 h), and the amount of airway secretion may be related to the amount of exposure to daily irritants. City dwellers exposed to increasing pollution such as particulate materials may cough more. The fact that healthy people need to cough may be judged from the occurrence of cough during large gatherings for a lecture or concert or during intervals of concerts, and a rate of 2.5 coughs/min has been quoted for a gathering of 100 people in a lecture room [2]. In a small group of healthy people in whom cough was monitored using a portable cough counter, the frequency of cough over a 24-h period was found to be less than 16 coughs [3] and 11 bursts of cough per 24 h (range 1–34) in children [4], or a range of 0–141 (median of 10) coughs per day if children with respiratory infections are included [5]. We do not know whether the normal protective cough reflex occurs during sleep, particularly during rapid eye movement sleep; presumably it does, since there is no other obvious protective mechanism that can be invoked. The smoker with a chronic morning cough usually considers his or her cough to be normal, necessary to clear the airways of the excessive secretions induced by cigarette smoke. However, to study the normality of cough, it is important to exclude the possibility of an enhanced cough reflex response which may be induced by cigarette smoking or even perhaps daily exposure to pollutants. A cough may be provoked by a tussive stimulus, and the likelihood of this cough occurring is increased by the presence of an enhanced cough reflex. The definition of normality of cough experience needs to be studied from the point of view of the event, the type of cough and the cough sensitivity reflex, so that the significance of cough prevalence studies can be determined.

## Prevalence of cough in the community

In several epidemiological surveys, persistent cough is reported as a symptom that affects a large proportion of the general population, being prevalent for example in 18% of the US population, in up to 16% of a southeast English population and in 11% of the Swedish population [6–8]. In these surveys, there has been no estimate of how many of these reported symptoms have received medical attention, and whether the person considers the cough to be a 'normal' symptom. In investigations of the Swedish part of the European Community Respiratory Health Survey (ECRHS) [9,10], a higher prevalence of nocturnal and non-productive cough was reported in females than in males. In a more recent *trans*-European survey of ECRHS, about one-third of subjects reported that they had been woken up by an attack of cough in the last 12 months, and about 20% reported a non-productive or productive cough during the winter months [11]. There was again a pre-

ponderance of females with nocturnal and non-productive cough, and nocturnal cough was related to asthma, tobacco smoking, exposure to environmental tobacco smoke and obesity. However, there has been no detailed community survey of the potential diseases underlying the cough reported.

Exposure to pollutants or environmental irritants appears to be important, judging from the epidemiological information linking dry or productive cough with outdoor air pollution, particularly in children. In adults and schoolchildren, productive cough or chronic nocturnal dry cough has been associated with levels of the $PM_{10}$ particulates [12,13]. Increases in levels of $PM_{10}$ are also related with reductions in peak expiratory flows and with increased reporting of cough, sputum production and sore throat in children with or without asthma [14]. Living close to heavy traffic may be associated with increased asthma symptoms and longstanding cough compared to not living close to heavy traffic [15]. In the Italian Po Valley district, the increase in air pollution has been associated with an increase in cough incidence amongst females but not males [16]. Nocturnal cough in relation to indoor exposure to cat allergens was observed not only in sensitized but also in non-sensitized subjects [17]. It is possible that population surveys are picking up more cough in the community from subjects being exposed to environmental pollutants and allergens, but we do not know whether these factors induce or sensitize cough. It would seem most important to determine the prevalence of sensitivity of the cough reflex in the community and relate this to the presence of cough, and thus determine levels of normal vs. abnormal cough in the community. For example, exposure of workers to capsaicin in a chilli processing factory was associated with an increase in self-reporting of cough but no increase in capsaicin cough responsiveness in these workers, indicating a 'normal' response to exposure to capsaicin [18].

When evaluating any community surveys, it is worth remembering that up to 25–30% of the population are usually cigarette smokers. In a survey in southeast England, up to 16% of 9077 responders had cough every day or half of the days of the year, and up to 13.2% had sputum every day or on half the days of the year; in this cohort, 54% were current cigarette smokers [7]. The chronic cough of cigarette smokers is a well-known feature, and is accompanied by hypersecretion of mucus and possibly by slowing of mucociliary clearance. Chronic bronchitis has been defined as the expectoration of sputum on most days during at least three consecutive months per year over two successive years. Apart from mucus stimulation of cough, chronic smoking may increase airway sensitivity to capsaicin [19], and patients with chronic obstructive airways disease caused by cigarette smoking show an increased tussive response to capsaicin [20]. Cigarette smokers with chronic cough do not usually seek medical help unless the pattern of their cough changes.

More detailed analysis of the factors that may cause cough, its severity and an assessment of the distribution of cough responsiveness is needed in epidemiological surveys. This indicates the need to have better methods of recording the severity of cough, objective measurements and a rapid easy and safe method of measuring the cough sensitivity reflex. There are no epidemiological data on the distribution of cough responsiveness in the population, and this is important to know.

## Cough presenting to the clinician

Cough is one of the most frequent reasons for seeking a consultation with a doctor. In the US, a national medical case survey reported that in 1991 cough was the most common complaint for which patients sought medical attention, and the second most common reason for a general medical consultation [21]. Much of this is likely to be due to cough occurring with the common cold, which is a self-limiting disease. In the US, for a chest specialist practice, patients with persistent chronic cough probably account for 10–38% of outpatient practice [22,23]. In addition, treatment of cough is a substantial proportion of health care expenditure. In the UK, about 3 million prescriptions for cough preparations are given annually by general practitioners, representing a cost of £1.9 million [24]. This is, however, an underestimate of the use of cough preparations since cough mixtures can be obtained over the counter.

Faced with a patient with a chronic cough, utilization of an anatomical diagnostic protocol has been advocated [25], and application of such a protocol often leads to a cause identified in 88–100% of cases, with treatment success rates of between 84 and 98% [22,23]. Such figures are perhaps overoptimistic, dependent on the referral practice of the clinic. Other cough clinics report that in 12–31% of their patients no underlying cause of the cough can be found

despite investigation and empirical treatment for gastro-oesophageal reflux, postnasal drip and asthma [26–28]. In patients referred with a chronic cough in whom the diagnosis of cancer has been excluded, a proportion will respond to the institution of inhaled corticosteroid therapy, on the basis of which one could be confident of the diagnosis of asthma, cough-variant asthma or eosinophilic bronchitis as underlying the cough [29]. Whether the eosinophil is the pathogenic factor in the induction of the cough remains unclear. Other prevalent diagnoses that are reported to 'cause' cough are chronic rhinosinusitis often with a postnasal drip, gastro-oesophageal reflux, chronic bronchitis, bronchiectasis or taking an angiotensin-converting enzyme inhibitor medication [30]. There appears to be little value in separating chronic dry cough from chronic cough with excessive sputum production in terms of the diagnostic yield since the frequency of the causes of both symptoms appear to be similar [31]. Postnasal drip, asthma, gastro-oesophageal reflux and bronchitis were the most frequent cause of a chronic productive cough. When a 'cause' is established, one assumes that the specific treatment of that cause should relieve the cough, and it sometimes does not. This raises the issue as to whether the 'cause' is really involved in the genesis of cough, or whether the treatment is really effective for the 'cause'.

The role of postnasal drip in causing cough merits some discussion [32]. Postnasal drip is defined as the presence of secretions at the back of the throat associated with frequent throat-clearing. How could it trigger cough when there is no vagal afferent innervation of the throat and there is no evidence for aspiration of secretions from the sinuses into the lungs in patients with sinusitis [33]? Patients with gastro-oesophageal reflux and cough may not respond to treatment with proton pump inhibitors that suppress acid production, perhaps because other factors in the refluxate such as the content of pepsin may be important in the pathogenesis of cough. In spite of these uncertainties, there is a group of chronic coughers in whom there appears to be no associated cause. There are other causes that remain unidentified. For example, a condition of eosinophilic bronchitis without bronchial hyperresponsiveness has recently been established as a cause of chronic cough [34]. *Bordetella pertussis* infection has been flagged as a potential cause, when nasopharyngeal aspirates were examined for the presence of *Bordetella pertussis* by polymerase chain reaction [35].

## The increased tussive response

Many patients with a chronic cough have a sensitized cough reflex response, and patients whose cough disappears or is controlled with appropriate treatments normalize their cough reflex response [36,37]. A sensitized cough reflex is also described in many other conditions such as asthma, pulmonary fibrosis and chronic obstructive pulmonary disease (COPD) [20,38,39]. However, the prevalence of sensitized cough reflex in the population and its association with different types of cough are still to be determined. It is not necessary for the cough to be 'dry' in order for the cough to be sensitized since patients with COPD with sputum production can demonstrate sensitization.

The sensitized cough reflex has various clinical connotations. Often, there is a history that the cough was first triggered following an upper respiratory virus infection or by a cold, and that the cough persisted, despite the clearing of the infective period, which indicates the notion of a central cough sensitization process. Such patients usually present with a history of persistent cough which may have lasted for many years. The cough is described as an irritation in the throat or upper chest, ranging from a feeling of wanting to cough to severe episodes of violent coughing that cannot be stopped. The severity of the cough may be variable over periods of months with mild or asymptomatic periods interspersed with periods of severe symptoms. Typically, the cough may be triggered by stimuli such as changes in temperature of inhaled air, taking a deep breath, talking over the telephone, laughing, eating crumbly food, certain smells or perfumes and lying in a supine posture. Often, any suspected associated cause has been treated with no success in controlling the cough.

## Pathophysiology of cough

Understanding of the cough response and of how cough may become persistent is of the utmost importance. The anatomy of the cough reflex has been dissected extensively, with the airway afferents and receptors, a central pathway and efferent pathways defined. The cough reflex is subserved mainly by vagal primary afferent nerves such as bronchopulmonary rapidly adapting receptors (RARs) which can be evoked by mechanical stimulation and deformation of

the airway epithelium such as particulate matter or mucus, and by airway smooth muscle contraction induced by constrictor agents [40,41]. These are predominantly present in the larynx, trachea and carina. Activation of bronchopulmonary C fibres by chemicals such as bradykinin and capsaicin can evoke cough in conscious animals and humans [42], although these may also activate RARs. C fibres and RARs project to different subnuclei in the nucleus tractus solitarius in the brainstem, considered to be a cough centre, although these are not anatomically discrete, and the concept of a cough centre is not universally accepted. Various second-order neurones project to other nuclei associated with the regulation of breathing. Integration of the various inputs occur centrally. For example, slow-adapting receptor afferent input may have a facilitatory effect on the genesis of cough [43].

This work has paved the way for an understanding of the cough response, but there is more to be understood regarding the cough reflex in the clinical situation. One could take the cough associated with gastro-oesophageal reflux as an example of how one could work out how the refluxate could induce cough [44]. Protons within the refluxate or other components of the refluxate could directly stimulate cough receptors in the upper airways; alternatively, there could be a distal oesophageal–tracheobronchial reflex mechanism which would be mediated through the usual pathway of the cough receptor. The biochemical counterparts of the cough reflex arc remain to be elucidated, and such information may provide therapeutic targets.

One defining concept of the chronic cougher is that of an enhanced cough reflex in patients with persistent cough as being the fundamental abnormality. Through understanding how this occurs, more targeted specific suppressants of the cough response, irrespective of the cause, can be devised. The process of cough 'sensitization' remains unclear, and this may invoke both 'peripheral' (i.e. in the airways) and/or 'central' (i.e. in the brain) mechanisms, according to our current understanding of the cough reflex pathways. Central sensitization may occur by integration from various sensory nerve subtypes in the central nervous system to initiate exaggerated reflexes and sensation [45]. Substance P may be involved as an important central mechanism for sensitization of the cough reflex, and its persistence. In a model of allergic inflammation, neuroplastic changes in the response of vagal primary afferent neurones were described, such that Aδ mechanosensor RARs released substance P, when under normal conditions, they do not [46]. Substance P in the nucleus tractus solitarius can increase bronchopulmonary C fibre reflex activity [47]. Peripheral mechanisms that can heighten cough reflex mechanisms have been mainly envisaged as an effect of altered environment of the cough receptor such as the release of inflammatory mediators such as prostaglandins or bradykinin that could enhance the response of the cough receptor [48,49]. Alternatively, there may be direct interactions between inflammatory cells and the cough receptor such that the threshold of the cough receptor is altered.

It has not been possible to determine whether the cough receptor itself is abnormal in terms of the transduction of the stimulatory signals. Examination of neural afferent profiles in the airways of persistent coughers has been limited. A recent study of airway biopsies reported an increase in total intraepithelial nerve density together with augmented staining for the neuropeptide calcitonin gene-related peptide (CGRP) but not for substance P [27]. However, the significance of the increase in intraepithelial nerves is unclear since we do not know whether any of these profiles are indeed cough receptors. Detailed localization of cough fibres and their ultrastucture, particularly in an airway that demonstrates augmented tussive response, is crucial to undertake.

## Approach to the treatment of cough

The treatment of cough would be more efficacious if one could understand the mechanisms of the phenomenon of cough sensitivity, since suppression of the heightened responses would control the urge to cough. The search for new antitussives has progressed along several lines, from studies of airway afferent nerve activity *in vitro* (with the disadvantage that the activity observed is not necessarily that of a 'cough' receptor) to studies in whole organisms using tussive challenges, and more rarely using patients with enhanced cough reflex or with chronic cough. The predictive value of antitussives tested in animals to their effectiveness in humans is not known. Some investigators study rodents such as mice that cannot cough, while the best model for studying cough is the guinea-pig which produces the explosive noise similar to the human cough. The use of the capsaicin or citric acid challenge in normal subjects cannot be predictive of antitussive activity since normal volunteers do not possess an enhanced cough reflex. Even if we do not currently have an understanding of the enhanced cough reflex, it is imperative that novel antitussives be tested in patients with an enhanced cough reflex. The aim would be to inhibit the enhanced component of the cough reflex to maintain the 'normal' cough reflex. This task would be easier if the enhanced cough reflex was superimposed on the normal reflex by entirely different mechanisms rather than representing an amplification of 'normal' mechanisms.

Many targets can be defined if one considers treating the 'cause' of the cough first. Treatment of the causes of cough may include anti-inflammatory approaches such as the cough associated with eosinophilic inflammation in the airways as in asthma, cough-variant asthma or eosinophil bronchitis [29]. Inhaled corticosteroids are particularly effective here, although the eosinophil as a causation of the cough is not entirely proven. Cough and enhanced cough with a neutrophilic inflammation [20] which do not respond to inhaled corticosteroids, and approaches that suppress the neutrophilic response or neutrophil activation could be helpful. The treatment of cough associated with gastro-oesophageal reflux with acid suppressants such as histamine $H_2$-receptor antagonists or proton pump inhibitors, or associated with rhinosinusitis with antihistamines or with nasal steroid drops, is not always successful. This may mean either that these conditions are not the cause of the cough or that a central mechanism of cough sensitization has occurred.

Partly because there is no apparent cause associated with a persistent cough in many patients, it is clear that the development of effective antitussives (i.e. drugs that specifically block cough whatever the cause) is needed. Currently, the most commonly used antitussives are the centrally acting opiates such as codeine, dihydrocodeine or pholcodeine. Sometimes for the intractable cough in terminal disease, morphine or diamorphine is used, with the advantage that these also possess analgesic properties. However, at their effective doses, these antitussives cause drowsiness, nausea and vomiting, and constipation, and often cause physical dependence. Development of new antitussives has occurred on a number of fronts. An improved understanding of the cough reflex pathways and of the mechanisms by which the reflex is enhanced has led to the identification of potential targets [50]. Finally, the assessment of antitussives in clinical studies has also been improved with the use of cough reflex challenge protocols such as capsaicin or citric acid, or of measuring the cough itself in ambulatory patients [51], but experience needs to be gathered.

It would be useful in clinical practice to divide the antitussive drugs into those that are acute relievers of cough such as the opiates; and those that can prevent cough ('preventors') when taken on a regular basis, such as corticosteroid therapy for eosinophil-associated cough or proton pump inhibitors for gastro-oesophageal reflux-associated cough (these preventors would be specific to the cause of cough).

## Conclusion

This chapter has provided an overview of the clinical and pathophysiological challenges of cough, and highlighted areas of unmet needs and of future investigations. Because of the high prevalence of cough, physicians commonly encounter patients presenting with a cough problem for diagnosis and management. The potentially wide diagnostic possibilities make it necessary for a systematic protocol to be used to ensure that diagnoses are not missed. New causes of chronic persistent cough will certainly be discovered. The tools to determine the severity of a chronic cough are being developed, and these can be applied to the clinic as well as to the evaluation of new antitussive therapies. In cough pathophysiology, an understanding of the pathways that enhance the cough reflex is needed, and what biochemical or structural abnormalities constitute a hypertussive cough receptor should be determined. We need to apply the knowledge obtained from studying the cough reflex to clinical practice, which includes the discovery of new treatments for suppressing cough.

## References

1 Osman LM, McKenzie L, Cairns J, Friend JA, Godden DJ, Legge JS *et al.* Patient weighting of importance of asthma symptoms. *Thorax* 2001; 56: 138–42.

2 Loudon RG. Cough in health and disease. Current research in chronic obstructive lung disease. In: *Proceedings of the 10th Emphysema Conference.* US Department of Health, Education & Welfare, 1967: 41–53.

3 Hsu J-Y, Stone RA, Logan-Sinclair R, Worsdell M, Busst C, Chung KF. Coughing frequency in patients with persistent cough using a 24-hour ambulatory recorder. *Eur Respir J* 1994; 7: 1246–53.

4 Munyard P, Bush A. How much coughing is normal? *Arch Dis Child* 1996; 74: 531–4.

5 Chang AB, Phelan PD, Robertson CF, Newman RG, Sawyer SM. Frequency and perception of cough severity. *J Paediatr Child Health* 2001; 37: 142–5.

6 Barbee RA, Halonen M, Kaltenborn WT, Burrows B. A longitudinal study of respiratory symptoms in a community population sample. Correlations with smoking, allergen skin-test reactivity, and serum IgE. *Chest* 1991; 99: 20–6.

7 Cullinan P. Persistent cough and sputum: prevalence and clinical characteristics in south east England. *Respir Med* 1992; 86: 143–9.

8 Lundback B, Nystrom L, Rosenhall L, Stjernberg N. Obstructive lung disease in northern Sweden: respiratory symptoms assessed in a postal survey. *Eur Respir J* 1991; 4: 257–66.

9 Bjornsson E, Plaschke P, Norrman E, Janson C, Lundback B, Rosenhall A *et al.* Symptoms related to asthma and chronic bronchitis in three areas of Sweden. *Eur Respir J* 1994; 7: 2146–53.

10 Ludviksdottir D, Bjornsson E, Janson C, Boman G. Habitual coughing and its associations with asthma, anxiety, and gastroesophageal reflux. *Chest* 1996; 109: 1262–8.

11 Janson C, Chinn S, Jarvis D, Burney P. Determinants of cough in young adults participating in the European Community Respiratory Health Survey. *Eur Respir J* 2001; 18: 647–54.

12 Zemp E, Elsasser S, Schindler C, Kunzli N, Perruchoud AP, Domenighetti G *et al.* Long-term ambient air pollution and respiratory symptoms in adults (SAPALDIA study). The SAPALDIA Team. *Am J Respir Crit Care Med* 1999; 159: 1257–66.

13 Braun-Fahrlander C, Wuthrich B, Gassner M, Grize L, Sennhauser FH, Varonier HS *et al.* Validation of a rhinitis symptom questionnaire (ISAAC core questions) in a population of Swiss school children visiting the school health services. SCARPOL team. Swiss study on childhood allergy and respiratory symptom with respect to air pollution and climate. International study of asthma and allergies in childhood. *Pediatr Allergy Immunol* 1997; 8: 75–82.

14 Vedal S, Petkau J, White R, Blair J. Acute effects of ambient inhalable particles in asthmatic and nonasthmatic children. *Am J Respir Crit Care Med* 1998; 157: 1034–43.

15 Montnemery P, Bengtsson P, Elliot A, Lindholm LH, Nyberg P, Lofdahl CG. Prevalence of obstructive lung diseases and respiratory symptoms in relation to living environment and socio-economic group. *Respir Med* 2001; 95: 744–52.

16 Viegi G, Pedreschi M, Baldacci S, Chiaffi L, Pistelli F, Modena P *et al*. Prevalence rates of respiratory symptoms and diseases in general population samples of North and Central Italy. *Int J Tuberc Lung Dis* 1999; 3: 1034–42.

17 Gehring U, Heinrich J, Jacob B, Richter K, Fahlbusch B, Schlenvoigt G *et al*. Respiratory symptoms in relation to indoor exposure to mite and cat allergens and endotoxins. Indoor Factors and Genetics in Asthma (INGA) Study Group. *Eur Respir J* 2001; 18: 555–63.

18 Blanc P, Liu D, Juarez C, Boushey HA. Cough in hot pepper workers. *Chest* 1991; 99: 27–32.

19 Bergren DR. Enhanced lung C-fiber responsiveness in sensitized adult guinea pigs exposed to chronic tobacco smoke. *J Appl Physiol* 2001; 91: 1645–54.

20 Doherty MJ, Mister R, Pearson MG, Calverley PM. Capsaicin responsiveness and cough in asthma and chronic obstructive pulmonary disease. *Thorax* 2000; 55: 643–9.

21 Schappert SM. National ambulatory medical care survey: 1991: Summary. In: *Vital and Health Statistics*, Publication No. 230. US Department of Health and Human Services, 1993: 1–20.

22 Irwin RS, Curley FJ, French CL. Chronic cough: the spectrum and frequency of causes, key components of the diagnostic evaluation, and outcome of specific therapy. *Am Rev Respir Dis* 1990; 141: 640–7.

23 Irwin RS, Carrao WM, Pratter MR. Chronic persistent cough in the adult: the spectrum and frequency of causes and successful outcome of specific therapy. *Am Rev Respir Dis* 1981; 123: 413–17.

24 British Thoracic Society. *The Burden of Lung Disease*. London: BMJ Publishing, 2001.

25 Irwin RS, Madison JM. The diagnosis and treatment of cough. *N Engl J Med* 2000; 343: 1715–21.

26 Poe RH, Harder RV, Israel RH, Kallay MC. Chronic persistent cough. Experience in diagnosis and outcome using an anatomic diagnostic protocol. *Chest* 1989; 95: 723–8.

27 O'Connell F, Springall DR, Moradoghli-Haftvani A, Krausz T, Price D, Fuller RW *et al*. Abnormal intraepithelial airway nerves in persistent unexplained cough? *Am J Respir Crit Care Med* 1995; 152: 2068–75.

28 McGarvey LP, Heaney LG, Lawson JT, Johnston BT, Scally CM, Ennis M *et al*. Evaluation and outcome of patients with chronic non-productive cough using a comprehensive diagnostic protocol. *Thorax* 1998; 53: 738–43.

29 Chung KF. Assessment and measurement of cough: the value of new tools. *Pulm Pharmacol Ther* 2002; 15: 267–72.

30 Chung KF, Lalloo UG. Diagnosis and management of chronic persistent dry cough. *Postgrad Med J* 1996; 72: 594–8.

31 Smyrnios NA, Irwin RS, Curley FJ. Chronic cough with a history of excessive sputum production. The spectrum and frequency of causes, key components of the diagnostic evaluation, and outcome of specific therapy. *Chest* 1995; 108: 991–7.

32 Campanella SG, Asher MI. Current controversies: sinus disease and the lower airways. *Pediatr Pulmonol* 2001; 31: 165–72.

33 Bardin PG, Van Heerden BB, Joubert JR. Absence of pulmonary aspiration of sinus contents in patients with asthma and sinusitis. *J Allergy Clin Immunol* 1990; 86: 82–8.

34 Brightling CE, Pavord ID. Eosinophilic bronchitis: an important cause of prolonged cough. *Ann Med* 2000; 32: 446–51.

35 Birkebaek NH, Kristiansen M, Seefeldt T, Degn J, Moller A, Heron I *et al*. Bordetella pertussis and chronic cough in adults. *Clin Infect Dis* 1999; 29: 1239–42.

36 Choudry NB, Fuller RW. Sensitivity of the cough reflex in patients with chronic cough. *Eur Respir J* 1992; 5: 296–300.

37 O'Connell F, Thomas VE, Pride NB, Fuller RW. Capsaicin cough sensitivity decreases with successful treatment of chronic cough. *Am J Respir Crit Care Med* 1994; 150: 374–80.

38 Lalloo UG, Lim S, DuBois R, Barnes PJ, Chung KF. Increased sensitivity of the cough reflex in progressive systemic sclerosis patients with interstitial lung disease. *Eur Respir J* 1998; 11: 702–5.

39 Doherty MJ, Mister R, Pearson MG, Calverley PM. Capsaicin induced cough in cryptogenic fibrosing alveolitis. *Thorax* 2000; 55: 1028–32.

40 Widdicombe JG. Neurophysiology of the cough reflex. *Eur Respir J* 1995; 8: 1193–202.

41 Karlsson J-A, Sant'Ambrogio G, Widdicombe J. Afferent neural pathways in cough and reflex bronchoconstriction. *J Appl Physiol* 1988; 65: 1007–23.

42 Fox AJ. Modulation of cough and airway sensory fibres. *Pulm Pharmacol* 1996; 9: 335–42.

43 Hanacek J, Davies A, Widdicombe JG. Influence of lung stretch receptors on the cough reflex in rabbits. *Respiration* 1984; 45: 161–8.

44 Ing AJ, Ngu MC. Cough and gastro-oesophageal reflux. *Lancet* 1999; 353: 944–6.

45 Canning BJ. Interactions between vagal afferent nerve subtypes mediating cough. *Pulm Pharmacol Ther* 2002; 15: 187–92.

46 Myers AC, Kajekar R, Undem BJ. Allergic inflammation-induced neuropeptide production in rapidly adapting afferent nerves in guinea pig airways. *Am J Physiol Lung Cell Mol Physiol* 2002; 282: L775–L781.

47 Mutoh T, Bonham AC, Joad JP. Substance P in the nucleus of the solitary tract augments bronchopulmonary C fiber

reflex output. *Am J Physiol Regul Integr Comp Physiol* 2000; **279**: R1215–R1223.

48  Nichol GM, Nix A, Barnes PJ, Chung KF. Enhancement of capsaicin-induced cough by inhaled prostaglandin F2α: modulation by beta-adrenergic agonist and anticholinergic agent. *Thorax* 1990.

49  Fox AJ, Lalloo UG, Bernareggi M, Belvisi MG, Chung KF, Barnes PJ. Bradykinin and captopril-induced cough in guinea-pigs. *Nature Med* 1996; **2**: 814–7.

50  Chung KF. Cough: potential pharmacological developments. *Expert Opin Investig Drugs* 2002; **11**: 955–63.

51  Chung KF. Methods of assessing cough and antitussives in man. *Pulm Pharmacol* 1996; **9**: 373–7.

# 2

# Epidemiology of cough

*Alyn H. Morice*

## Introduction

Cough is a universal experience common to us all. It is also the commonest symptom for which medical advice is sought [1]. For the purpose of classification cough may be divided into defined, acute, self-limiting episodes and chronic persistent cough. This distinction is clinically useful since the aetiology of the two syndromes is very different. An arbitrary cut-off of 8 weeks is taken to separate acute from chronic cough.

## Acute cough

The majority of consultations with acute cough are due to viral respiratory tract infections. The UK Morbidity Statistics from General Practice survey [2] suggests an average of two consultations per year for every adult and six consultations for each child under 4. Of total primary care workload Morrell [3] found cough to be the presenting complaint in 527 per 1000 consultations with new symptoms. Even this staggering statistic, that over half of new consultations are due to cough, underestimates the true socioeconomic impact of of this symptom. Many of us do not consult a physician for viral cough, and if driven to treatment self-medicate with over-the-counter products of dubious efficacy. The market in cough and cold products in the US is estimated at over 2 billion dollars.

This enormous morbidity is caused by a wide array of viral pathogens including influenza, parainfluenza, rhinovirus, adenovirus, respiratory syncytial virus and the respiratory corona virus [4]. All of these viruses share a common short incubation period of between 1 and 4 days. Because of its ability to undergo antigenic shift and genetic recombination influenza occurs in epidemics. Why these epidemics occur during the winter months is unknown but may be related to cooling of the airway epithelium decreasing host defence [5]. Parainfluenza viruses differ from influenza viruses in that they are much more antigenically stable and of the four subtypes types one and three are particularly important, causing serious lower respiratory tract infections, croup and tracheobronchitis in infants and young children. In all, parainfluenza viruses are thought to be responsible for a fifth of all non-bacterial respiratory tract disease in childhood. Since immunity to reinfection is only transient it is one of the commonest causes of the typical infective cough which plagues families with small children.

Respiratory syncytial virus (RSV) is the single most important aetiological agent in cough in infancy [6]. RSV occurs in epidemics, usually between the autumn and early spring. Each outbreak lasts between 2 and 3 months and can involve as many as half of all families with children. There is also a second peak of infectivity in the elderly. Unfortunately, immunity to RSV infection is transient so reinfection is common.

Of the over 100 serotypes of adenovirus eight are important in the production of a syndrome of severe acute cough. Immunity following infection is good but since so many serotypes are associated with cough the likelihood of repeated adenovirus-induced cough is high. The common cold or rhinovirus again represents over 100 serotypes and is the major cause of mild upper respiratory tract infection and cough in both children and adults. Unsurprisingly, rhinovirus immunity is very poor. Coronaviruses are similar in clinical presentation to rhinoviruses and may be responsible for between 5 and 10% of human coughs and colds.

At the age of 15 a gender difference appears in consultation rates reported in the morbidity statistics in general practice. During the reproductive years consultations are twice for women what they are for men. After the age of 55 consultation rates in both men and women become equal again. Whilst this could be explicable by societal differences in that women may consult more, there are intriguing clues to the fact that women may have a heightened cough reflex compared with men. Women exposed to cough challenge with protussive agents cough twice as much as men or, conversely, cough the same amount at a lower dose [7,8]. This could be an artefact of inhaling drug into a smaller lung volume but women are also over-represented in those patients who develop angiotensin-converting enzyme (ACE) inhibitor cough [9]. In the majority of cough clinics women outnumber men and when tested with cough challenge they exhibit a heightened cough response [10]. It is possible that women have an intrinsically heightened cough reflex compared with men.

## Chronic cough

Several surveys have attempted to quantify the incidence of chronic cough within populations [11–14]. The objective of most of these surveys is to assess the symptomatology associated with cigarette smoking and so questions are directed towards discovering the prevalence of chronic bronchitis. This leads to confusion in the data analysis between cough and chronic sputum production. Despite these methodological shortcomings it is clear that chronic cough is a common problem with reported prevalence varying between 40 and 6%. In the UK four general practices undertook a postal and telephone survey of over 11 000 patients. Cough was reported every day or on over half of the days of the year by 14% of males and 10% of females. A worldwide study from 16 countries surveyed 18 277 subjects aged between 20 and 48. Nocturnal cough was present in 30%, productive cough in 10%, and non-productive cough in 10%. There was a clear dose-related effect of cigarette smoking on cough. The very high prevalence of nocturnal cough arose because a positive response to the question 'Have you been woken by an attack of coughing at any time in the last 12 months?' was taken as indicating the symptom. However, since acute cough could also lead to a positive response, significant nocturnal cough was probably overestimated in this study. Another problem is in the choice of age group in which to study cough. Chronic cough is present in older subjects as may be seen from the average age of patients seen in cough clinics (Table 2.1). Whatever the failings of individual surveys chronic cough is clearly a very common symptom which although associated with considerable morbidity goes largely unheeded.

Those patients presenting to specialist cough clinics, however, represent a subgroup of this population. Most smokers assume that their morning cough reflects their smoking habit and do not consult. Conditions such as chronic bronchitis are therefore grossly under-represented, even though they cause considerable morbidity within the population. Similarly, such tertiary referral clinics are unlikely to represent the true prevalence of conditions such as asthma as a cause of chronic cough, since at least in European practice, a therapeutic trial of antiasthma medication is usually performed by the primary physician. If such therapy is successful the patient remains in primary care and the prevalence of the condition is hidden from the tertiary referral centre.

### The three common causes of chronic cough

All of the reported series from tertiary referral centres identify the same three common causes of cough. This diagnostic triad underlies the vast majority of chronic cough seen within the population. The problem of the high morbidity from chronic cough is the failure of doctors, both generalists and specialists, to recognize that cough as an isolated symptom may be generated from any of three anatomical areas. The relative incidence of asthma or asthma-like syndrome, gastro-oesophageal reflux and rhinitis is illustrated in Table 2.1 which lists the reported prevalence.

The individual reports from cough clinics illustrate a wide variety in the prevalence of each syndrome. This variation may represent different patient populations, or the different prevalence of the underlying diseases such as asthma in each individual population and different diagnostic methods. A further source of error is the criteria for diagnosis. Some clinics only accept diagnosis when a therapeutic trial of appropriate treatment has been successful [15]. Other clinics report a positive

**Table 2.1** Commonest causes of chronic cough in patients investigated in specialist clinics.

| Author | Mean age in years (range) | Diagnosis (% of total) | | | |
|---|---|---|---|---|---|
| | | Asthma syndrome | GOR | Rhinitis | Most common other causes (%) |
| Irwin *et al.* 1981 [18] | 50.3 (17–88) | 25 | 10 | 29 | Chronic bronchitis (12) |
| Poe *et al.* 1982 [20] | ? (15–89) | 36 | 0 | 8 | Postinfectious (27) |
| Poe *et al.* 1989 [21] | 44.8 (19–79) | 35 | 5 | 26 | Idiopathic (12) |
| Irwin *et al.* 1990 [19] | 51 (6–83) | 24 | 21 | 41 | Chronic bronchitis (5) |
| Hoffstein 1994 [22] | 47 | 25 | 24 | 26 | Postinfectious (21) |
| O'Connell *et al.* 1994 [23] | 49 (19–83) | 6 | 10 | 13 | Idiopathic (22) |
| Smyrnios *et al.* 1995 [24] | 58 (18–86) | 24 | 15 | 40 | Chronic bronchitis (11) |
| Mello *et al.* 1996 [17] | 53.1 (15–83) | 14 | 40 | 38 | Bronchiectasis (4) |
| Marchesani *et al.* 1998 [25] | 51 | 14 | 5 | 56 | Chronic bronchitis (16) |
| McGarvey *et al.* 1998 [15] | 47.5 (18–77) | 23 | 19 | 21 | Idiopathic (18) |
| Palombini *et al.* 1999 [16] | 57 (15–81) | 59 | 41 | 58 | Bronchiectasis (18) |
| Brightling *et al.* 1999 [26] | * | 31 | 8 | 24 | Postviral (13) |

GOR, gastro-oesophageal reflux.
* No figures given for the total sample but mean age of 12/91 patients with eosinophilic bronchitis given as 52 (28–76) years.

diagnosis as a positive result during investigation, leading to apparent multiple diagnoses [16].

There is no doubt that a positive result in terms of diagnosis and therapy can suggest multiple causes of cough in individual patients. I believe, however, that this illustrates the plasticity of the cough reflex. Low-grade, subclinical, cough may be present in an individual but only become apparent when an additional provoking feature occurs. A good example of this phenomenon is ACE inhibitor cough, where ACE inhibitors alter the cough reflex sensitivity as shown by shift in the capsaicin dose–response curve [27] and may reveal previous low-grade cough due to gastro-oesophageal reflux or rhinitis [28].

### Cough-predominant asthma

The term cough-predominant asthma has been introduced to illustrate that cough may be one facet of an asthma syndrome which is variously represented in individual patients. In classic asthma where bronchoconstriction, and conversely bronchodilator response, can be demonstrated cough may be an additional and important feature. However, cough as an isolated symptom without bronchoconstriction or breathlessness, but with the characteristic pathological features of asthmatic airway inflammation, is the other end of the spectrum [29,30]. This so-called cough variant asthma is merely one end of a continuum. The term cough-predominant asthma may be preferred since this terminology includes patients in whom the major problem is cough but who also illustrate some or all of the other features of classic asthma [31]. Why individuals should vary so much in the expression of cough as a symptom of asthma is at present unclear. An elegant series of papers by Brightling has explored the extreme end of this spectrum, eosinophilic bronchitis. Here airways inflammation is present but there are no features of classic asthma, including bronchial hyper-responsiveness. However there are subtle differences in the cellular composition and location of the inflammation, particularly concerning mast cells and their mediators [26,32].

Between a quarter and a third of patients presenting to a tertiary referral centre with chronic cough will be suffering from cough-predominant asthma (Table 2.1). This rate of detection probably does not reflect the prevalence of cough-predominant asthma since many patients, particularly those who have features of classic asthma, are diagnosed and treated in the community. Indeed it is unusual for patients with chronic cough to be seen in tertiary clinics who have not had an unsuccessful trial of inhaled medication. The reasons for failure of therapy, even when the underlying diagnosis is of cough-predominant asthma, are all those usually associated with poor asthma control: compliance, poor inhaler technique, inappropriate choice of device, etc. In addition there are other features of cough-predominant asthma, which unless recognized, lead to failure of therapy. Clearly the usual diagnostic measures of reversibility testing or home peak flow monitoring are frequently unhelpful. Even methacholine challenge may not identify patients who respond adequately to corticosteroid therapy since those with eosinophilic bronchitis are not hypersensitive [33]. Whilst sputum examination in expert hands clearly has a role the methodological difficulties obviate its routine use. Ultimately, the diagnosis and therefore prevalence of cough-predominant asthma rests on the use of a therapeutic trial of antiasthma medication. Here again the differences between cough-predominant asthma and classic asthma may lead to confusion. Since bronchospasm may only be a minor feature or even absent, add-on therapy with long-acting β-agonists rarely proves successful and leukotriene antagonists may be the preferred add-on therapy [34]. The response to leukotriene antagonists may illustrate the hypothesized role of lipoxygenase products in the direct modulation of the putative VR1 cough receptor [35]. Ultimately, diagnosis of cough-predominant asthma may rely on the demonstration of a response to parenteral steroids.

### The oesophagus and cough

A considerable portion of patients presenting with chronic cough have a disorder of the oesophagus. It is clearly poorly recognized by many physicians, yet cough as the sole presentation of gastro-oesophageal reflux has been well described [36,37]. In addition to reflux it is becoming increasingly clear that a number of oesophageal disorders, broadly classified as dysmotility and including abnormal peristalsis and abnormal lower oesophageal sphincter tone, may give rise to cough [38]. That acid reflux alone is not the cause of cough in oesophageal disease explains the partial response seen in many patients with even high doses of proton pump inhibitors.

As with other causes of cough, diagnosis may be difficult because there can be few clues from the history. However, whilst there is some disagreement [17], in individual patients there may be a strong association with other symptoms, particularly heartburn. More unusual characteristics such as an association with hoarseness, choking sensation and postnasal symptoms are increasingly recognized as being part of a reflux phenomenon by ENT specialists. Indeed, a striking reduction of cough during sleep, which initially may be thought to count against a diagnosis of oesophageal cough, may indicate an oesophageal origin. Lower oesophageal sphincter pressure increases physiologically in recumbency preventing reflux in the early stages of the disease [39]. The clues to the diagnosis of cough of oesophageal origin may be obtained by looking for associations between food, eating and cough.

### Rhinitis and postnasal drip

There is marked geographical variation in the incidence of rhinitis and postnasal drip in the reported series of patients presenting to cough clinics. Patients in the Americas present with symptoms of postnasal drip in up to 50% of cases, whereas rhinitis is reported in approximately 10% in most European experience. The difference for this may be in part societal in that patients from North America are far more likely to describe upper respiratory tract symptoms as postnasal drip [18,19]. In addition, the diagnosis of postnasal drip or rhinitis is frequently accepted because of a response to 'specific therapy' with broad-spectrum, centrally acting antihistamines and systemic decongestants [40]. Of course, such treatment is anything but specific. Such therapy may act in upper airway disease and in asthma. Centrally acting antihistamines may work either on the central pathways of the cough or simply through a sedating mechanism unrelated to the anatomical site of cough generation.

Until such problems in the definition of postnasal drip and its subsequent specific diagnosis are resolved, rhinitis or rhinosinusitis is probably the preferred term describing this syndrome. One further problem is the numerous observations from animal species, which point to the absence of afferent cough sensory neurones within the territory of the glossopharyngeal and trigeminal nerves [41]. It is possible that the symptoms of rhinitis and postnasal drip are epiphenomena associated with inflammation in the territory of the vagus.

## Other rare causes of cough

Whilst the rarer causes of cough may not matter in the overall epidemiology of cough, they are extremely important to the individual patient since prolonged suffering may result because of a lack of firm diagnosis. The whole panoply of disorders within the territory of the vagus nerve must be considered in patients with obscure cough. The ear (from the nerve of Arnold), the oesophagus, and even the heart may be the seat of the generation of cough.

Some of the more important causes of chronic cough, which lead to considerable diagnostic and social consequences are:

• Inhaled foreign body. Whilst this can occur in any age group, typically it affects boys aged 3 [42]. There may be little or no clue from the history or chest radiography. Foreign bodies can be radiolucent and those with a lumen can produce wheezing without distal atelectasis and may be frequently misdiagnosed as asthma.

• Habit cough, a syndrome almost exclusively restricted to children and young people. The physical characteristics of the cough are unlike those of an 'organic' cough and the sound produced has been described as a 'honk'. The cough characteristically disappears when the patient is asleep. Whilst most paediatricians treat habit cough with simple measures such as reassurance and breathing exercises there remains a hard core of patients who are resistant to therapy. In these habit cough has many of the characteristics of a tic and may on close observation be associated with other mannerisms. Cough is a feature of Gilles de la Tourette syndrome in approximately 10% of cases and therapy with haloperidol or pimozide may be highly effective.

• Postviral cough. Whilst most cough associated with upper respiratory tract viral infection abates within 1 week, in some patients coughing is prolonged and may take several months to settle. Such patients have a heightened cough reflex and may have some subclinical cause of cough which is exacerbated by virus-induced vagal hypersensitivity. There is no specific therapy [43].

• ACE inhibitor cough. Similar to postviral cough, ACE inhibitor cough causes a shift in the cough sensitivity to tussigenic agents [44]. This alteration in the cough reflex may take several months to settle. Thus, although patients usually improve within a week of cessation of ACE inhibitors, a number of individuals continue coughing weeks and months after the cessation of treatment. As with postviral cough such individuals frequently have a low-grade or subclinical cough caused by other aetiologies.

## References

1 Schappert KT. National Ambulatory Medical Care Survey: 1991, Summary. Advance Data 93 A.D., Number 230. US Department of Health and Human Services, National Center for Health Statistics, 1993.

2 Office of Population Censuses and Surveys. *Morbidity Statistics from General Practice: 4th National Study 1991–1992*. London: HMSO, 1995: Series MB5, 3.

3 Morrell DC. Symptom interpretation in general practice. *J R Coll General Pract* 1972; **22**: 297–309.

4 Ison MG, Mills J, Openshaw P, Zambon M, Osterhaus A, Hayden F. Current research on respiratory viral infections: Fourth International Symposium. *Antiviral Res* 2002; **55** (2): 227–78.

5 Eccles R. An explanation for the seasonality of acute upper respiratory tract viral infections. *Acta Otolaryngol* 2002; **122** (2): 183–91.

6 Law BJ, Carbonell-Estrany X, Simoes EA. An update on respiratory syncytial virus epidemiology: a developed country perspective. *Respir Med* 2002; **96** (Suppl. B): S1–S7.

7 Fujimura M, Kasahara K, Kamio Y, Naruse M, Hashimoto T, Matsuda T. Female gender as a determinant of cough threshold to inhaled capsaicin. *Eur Respir J* 1996; **9**: 1624–6.

8 Dicpinigaitis PV, Allusson VRC, Baldanti A, Nalamati JR. Ethnic and gender differences in cough reflex sensitivity. *Respiration* 1901; **68** (5): 480–2.

9 Yeo WW, Maclean D, Richardson PJ, Ramsay LE. Cough and enalapril: assessment by spontaneous reporting and visual analogue scale under double-blind conditions. *Br J Clin Pharmacol* 1991; **31** (3): 356–9.

10 Kastelik JA, Thompson RH, Aziz I, Ojoo JC, Redington AE, Morice AH. Sex-related differences in cough reflex sensitivity in patients with chronic cough. *Am J Respir Crit Care Med* 2002; **166**: 961–4.

11 Cullinan P. Persistent cough and sputum: prevalence and clinical characteristics in south east England. *Respir Med* 1992; **86** (2): 143–9.

12 Janson C, Chinn S, Jarvis D, Burney P. Determinants of cough in young adults participating in the European Community Respiratory Health Survey. *Eur Respir J* 1991; **18** (4): 647–54.

13 Littlejohns P, Ebrahim S, Anderson R. Prevalence and diagnosis of chronic respiratory symptoms in adults. *Br Med J* 1989; **298**: 1556–60.

14 Boezen HM, Schouten JP, Postma DS, Rijcken B. Relation between respiratory symptoms, pulmonary function and peak flow variability in adults. *Thorax* 1995; **50**: 121–6.

15 McGarvey LP, Heaney LG, Lawson JT, Johnston BT, Scally CM, Ennis M, Shepherd DR, MacMahon J. Evalua-

tion and outcome of patients with chronic non-productive cough using a comprehensive diagnostic protocol. *Thorax* 1998; **53** (9): 738–43.

16 Palombini BC, Villanova CA, Araujo E, Gastal OL, Alt DC, Stolz DP, Palombini CO. A pathogenic triad in chronic cough: asthma, postnasal drip syndrome, and gastroesophageal reflux disease. *Chest* 1999; **116** (2): 279–84.

17 Mello CJ, Irwin RS, Curley FJ. Predictive values of the character, timing, and complications of chronic cough in diagnosing its cause. *Arch Intern Med* 1996; **156** (9): 997–1003.

18 Irwin RS, Corrao WM, Pratter MR. Chronic persistent cough in the adult: the spectrum and frequency of causes and successful outcome of specific therapy. *Am Rev Respir Dis* 1981; **123** (4 Part 1): 413–17.

19 Irwin RS, Curley FJ, French CL. Chronic cough. The spectrum and frequency of causes, key components of the diagnostic evaluation, and outcome of specific therapy. *Am Rev Respir Dis* 1990; **141** (3): 640–7.

20 Poe RH, Israel RH, Utell MJ, Hall WJ. Chronic cough: bronchoscopy or pulmonary function testing? *Am Rev Respir Dis* 1982; **126** (1): 160–2.

21 Poe RH, Harder RV, Israel RH, Kallay MC. Chronic persistent cough. Experience in diagnosis and outcome using an anatomic diagnostic protocol. *Chest* 1989; **95** (4): 723–8.

22 Hoffstein V. Persistent cough in nonsmoker. *Can Respir J* 1994; **1**: 40–7.

23 O'Connell F, Thomas VE, Pride NB, Fuller RW. Capsaicin cough sensitivity decreases with successful treatment of chronic cough. *Am J Respir Crit Care Med* 1994; **150**: 374–80.

24 Smyrnios NA, Irwin RS, Curley FJ. Chronic cough with a history of excessive sputum production. The spectrum and frequency of causes, key components of the diagnostic evaluation, and outcome of specific therapy. *Chest* 1995; **108** (4): 991–7.

25 Marchesani F, Cecarini L, Pela R, Sanguinetti CM. Causes of chronic persistent cough in adult patients: the results of a systematic management protocol. *Monaldi Arch Chest Dis* 1998; **53** (5): 510–14.

26 Brightling CE, Ward R, Goh KL, Wardlaw AJ, Pavord ID. Eosinophilic bronchitis is an important cause of chronic cough. *Am J Respir Crit Care Med* 1999; **160** (2): 406–10.

27 Morice AH, Lowry R, Brown MJ, Higenbottam T. Angiotensin converting enzyme and the cough reflex. *Lancet* 1987; **ii**: 1116–18.

28 Ojoo JC, Kastelik JA, Morice AH. Duration of angiotensin converting enzyme inhibitor (ACEI) induced cough. *Thorax* 1902; **56**: 89.

29 Glauser FL. Variant asthma. *Ann Allergy* 1972; **30** (8): 457–9.

30 Corrao WM, Braman SS, Irwin RS. Chronic cough as the sole presenting manifestation of bronchial asthma. *N Engl J Med* 1979; **300** (12): 633–7.

31 Pratter MR, Bartter T, Akers S, Dubois J. An algorithmic approach to chronic cough. *Ann Intern Med* 1993; **119** (10): 977–83.

32 Brightling CE, Ward R, Woltmann G, Bradding P, Sheller JR, Dworski R, Pavord ID. Induced sputum inflammatory mediator concentrations in eosinophilic bronchitis and asthma. *Am J Respir Crit Care Med* 2000; **162** (3 Part 1): 878–82.

33 Gibson PG, Dolovich J, Denburg J, Ramsdale EH, Hargreave FE. Chronic cough: eosinophilic bronchitis without asthma. *Lancet* 1989; **1**: 1346–8.

34 Dicpinigaitis PV, Dobkin JB. Effect of zafirlukast on cough reflex sensitivity in asthmatics. *J Asthma* 1999; **36** (3): 265–70.

35 Hwang SW, Cho H, Kwak J, Lee SY, Kang CJ, Jung J, Cho S, Min KH, Suh YG *et al.* Direct activation of capsaicin receptors by products of lipoxygenases: endogenous capsaicin-like substances. *Proc Natl Acad Sci USA* 2000; **97** (11): 6155–60.

36 Irwin RS, Zawacki JK, Curley FJ, French CL, Hoffman PJ. Chronic cough as the sole presenting manifestation of gastroesophageal reflux. *Am Rev Respir Dis* 1989; **140** (5): 1294–300.

37 Ing AJ, Ngu MC. Cough and gastro-oesophageal reflux. *Lancet* 1999; **353**: 944–6.

38 Kastelik JA, Aziz I, Thompson R *et al.* Gastroesophageal dysmotility as a cause of chronic persistent cough. *Thorax* 2003 (in press).

39 Mittal RK, Balaban DH. The esophagogastric junction. *N Engl J Med* 1997; **336** (13): 924–32.

40 Irwin RS, Madison JM. Anatomical diagnostic protocol in evaluating chronic cough with specific reference to gastroesophageal reflux disease. *Am J Med* 2000; **108** (Suppl. 4a): 126S–30S.

41 Widdicombe JG. Afferent receptors in the airways and cough. *Respir Physiol* 1998; **114** (1): 5–15.

42 Hoeve LJ, Rombout J, Pot DJ. Foreign body aspiration in children. The diagnostic value of signs, symptoms and preoperative examination. *Clin Otolaryngol* 1993; **18** (1): 55–7.

43 Ojoo JC, Kastelik JA, Morice AH. A boy with a disabling cough. *Lancet* 2003; **361**: 674.

44 Morice AH, Brown MJ, Higenbottam T. Cough associated with angiotensin converting enzyme inhibition. *J Cardiovasc Pharmacol* 1989; **13** (Suppl. 3): S59–S62.

# 3

# A brief overview of the mechanisms of cough

*John G. Widdicombe*

## Introduction

The aim of this chapter is to review briefly the patho-physiological mechanisms of cough so that the clinical reader can see their relevance to the understanding of the conditions being studied. It is an introduction to, but not a substitute for, the detailed description of the pathophysiology of cough given in Section 4 of this book; the latter will provide the detailed basis of the mechanisms of cough, and point to future developments in the understanding and treatment of cough.

Of all the specialized and forceful acts of breathing (ignoring vocalization)—e.g. cough, sneeze, sigh/gasp, yawn, hiccup—cough has special distinctive features: it usually signals disease; it is not stereotyped but can take many forms; it has a voiceprint that identifies the subject; it can be produced and mimicked voluntarily and accurately; and it is used as a form of communication. Possibly the last two features apply in part also to yawns and sighs.

## Definition and description

Cough has three defining features: an initial deep breath, a brief powerful expiratory effort against a closed glottis, and opening of the glottis with closure of the nasopharynx and vigorous expiration through the mouth. Within this definition there are several variants. The act may be a single deep inspiration followed by a single glottic closure interrupting an almost complete expiration near to residual volume; the same but with multiple glottic closures during the single expiration; or a 'bout' of coughing with each expiratory effort either completed or partial. Other acts, such as the 'huff' of clearing the throat and the expiratory effort with glottic closure due to touching the vocal folds or trachea (the 'expiration reflex'), are by definition not cough but may be fragments of a cough.

The problem is that we know virtually nothing about the *differences* in activation of neural mechanisms that determine the patterns of cough. Nor do we understand the secondary mechanisms whereby a cough, once initiated, may itself strongly influence its own pattern by feedback from the airway receptors stimulated by the cough. Just as we do not understand the physiological basis for different patterns of cough, the clinician can seldom define the underlying causes of cough by observing and measuring it, apart from the broad distinction between 'wet' and 'dry' cough.

Cough is the most vigorous respiratory act to involve the body. The commonest cause is probably cigarette smoking, which has been very little studied because subjects do not usually go to the physician. Acute cough due to upper respiratory tract infection inflicts virtually everyone in developed countries at least once a year, but again has been little studied because patients prefer the pharmacist to the physician. Chronic cough, the commonest symptom of respiratory disease, can have over 100 underlying causes, but the complexity of its mechanisms has baffled both the clinician and the basic scientist.

## Physiological mechanisms of cough

Cough is said to be exclusively mediated via the vagus nerves [1]. If so, this may explain cough due to irritation of the external ear, which is innervated by a small branch of the vagus. It should follow that pharyngeal irritation due, for example, to postnasal drip cannot itself cause cough, since the pharynx has no vagal innervation; the mucus and its inflammatory mediators must first reach the larynx. In experimental animals no-one has shown that stimulation restricted to the pharynx induces cough.

Cough can be initiated from the larynx, including its supraglottal part, from the trachea and from the larger bronchi. Irritation of the smaller bronchi, the bronchioles and the alveoli does not cause cough; cough initiated from such sites would not be very effective because the luminal airflows and velocities would be too low to have shear forces adequate to clear airway mucus and debris [2,3].

## Sensory mechanisms of cough

The airway zones that can initiate cough, from larynx to bronchi, all contain rapidly adapting pulmonary stretch receptors (RARs), and there is abundant evidence that these mediate cough [4–6]. They have small-diameter myelinated nerve fibres, the block of which prevents cough, and all the mechanical, chemical and pathological conditions that stimulate them also induce cough. As their name implies, they adapt rapidly to a maintained stimulus, which might limit a continuous bout of coughing that could be harm-

ful; however, they do not accommodate to repeated stimulation [7].

The morphology of RARs has not been clearly delineated [4,8–10]. However, they are almost certainly the branching terminals of non-myelinated nerve fibres under, and possibly in, the epithelium [10] (Fig. 3.1). This gives them an ideal site for sensing inhaled irritants and locally released inflammatory mediators. These terminals link to vagal thin myelinated fibres, with cell bodies mainly in the nodose ganglia.

The RARs are exquisitely mechanosensitive, and also respond to acid and to non-isosmolar solutions [7,11,12]. Their membranes have receptors and channels for these stimuli, all of which can cause cough. However, in vitro the RARs are insensitive to a wide range of chemicals and mediators that can produce cough: histamine, bradykinin, prostaglandins, 5-hydroxytryptamine, capsaicin, tachykinins, etc. The explanation of this paradox is that RARs can be sensitized or stimulated by mechanical events in the airway wall, including smooth muscle contraction, vasodilatation and oedema, mucus secretion and decrease in lung compliance. All these changes occur in inflammatory conditions such as asthma, either by the direct action of inflammatory mediators released in the tissues, or by the local actions of tachykinins released from C-fibre receptors in the epithelium and mucosa (mediating the local reflex effects known as neurogenic inflammation) [13].

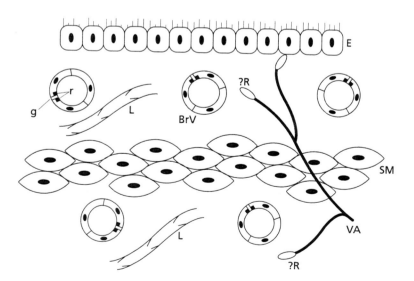

Fig. 3.1 Hypothetical location and structure of a rapidly adapting pulmonary stretch receptor that causes cough. It is proposed that the receptor is localized in the extracellular space in close proximity to bronchial venules. An increase in interstitial pressure in the venules, or vasoactive substances such as histamine or substance P, will increase extravascular fluid volume and stimulate the receptors. Irritant gases in the airways will also stimulate the endings. VA, vagal afferent fibre; BrV, bronchial venule; L, lymphatic; g, gaps between endothelial cells; r, pharmacological receptors; SM, smooth muscle, E, epithelial cells. From [9].

There has been some advocacy for the view that these C-fibre receptors can directly cause cough [14], based on the relative insensitivity of RARs *in vitro* to tussigenic chemical stimuli [15]. However, as explained above, C-fibre receptors can release tachykinins with mucosal responses that secondarily excite the RARs. There is no convincing evidence that C-fibre receptors can directly cause cough, and much evidence against this belief [3,4,6]. The issue is an important one in view of the current interest in peripherally acting antitussive drugs; we need to know how they act on the RAR–C-fibre mediator–mucosal response complex, and this complex must first be mapped out.

Other airway receptors are unlikely to play an important role in cough, although slowly adapting receptors (SARs), responsible for the Hering–Breuer reflex and for controlling breathing pattern, can have a facilitatory effect on the cough reflex [4].

(See also Chapter 16.)

## Central nervous mechanisms of cough

The old-fashioned concept of a 'cough centre' in the brainstem has been discarded in the light of recent understanding of the neuronal circuitry of cough and its relation to the respiratory rhythm generator [16–21]. The subject is complex and at least some conclusions are hypothetical. But since this is the site where centrally acting antitussive agents act it is a topic with important clinical implications.

The vagal fibres for cough enter the brainstem and relay in the nucleus of the solitary tract with connections to second-order neurones [4,21]. Here their pathways overlap and interact with those from other airway afferents—C-fibre receptors and SARs. The interaction of multiple inputs is such that, for example, C-fibre activity will potentiate that of RARs, i.e. augment the cough reflex. The neurotransmitters involved have been studied and include glutamate and the tachykinins substance P and neurokinin A [4,21].

If the activity of RARs increases sufficiently then coughing is produced. This involves:
1 a gating process which determines whether the 'cough input' is adequate to cause cough; the gates are in turn controlled by afferent inputs, for example from SARs, and probably from higher centres;
2 a complex interaction with the respiratory rhythm generator. Obviously we cannot cough and breathe at the same time so, if cough is induced, breathing has to

be switched off, even although the same motor outputs are involved in both activities; and
3 a coordination of motor activities to diaphragm, abdominal and intercostal muscles, and the larynx and upper airway muscles mainly via the nuclei retroambigualis and ambiguus; here further integrative processes take place and there are distinctive differences between motor controls for breathing and for cough.

Recent studies on the brainstem cough generator circuit show several important features.
1 The gating systems for cough from the tracheobronchial tree and for that from the larynx are different and with different control activities; at the same time centrally acting antitussive agents can have different actions on the cough from the two regions [18]. If humans behave like experimental animals, at least potentially physicians should give different cough remedies for laryngeal compared with lower airway inflammation.
2 Although cough and breathing have the same final common integrative pathways, they can be dissociated both physiologically and pharmacologically [18,19]; this explains why appropriate antitussive agents can block cough without inhibiting breathing, and why agents that depress breathing may not be antitussive.
3 Antitussive drugs can inhibit some components of the cough while leaving others intact [19,22]; for example, codeine can block the frequency of cough without affecting the pattern of the individual cough cycle. This fits with experience of antitussive agents on the pattern of cough in humans, where cough frequency is usually affected more than is cough pattern [23].

Increasing knowledge of the neurotransmitters involved in the central cough complex has incriminated, as well as the tachykinins and glutamate, 5-hydroxytryptamine, γ-aminobutyric acid, N-methyl-D-aspartate and dopamine; various types of opioid receptors have been described, and also nociceptin receptors [8,21]. The scope for development of novel centrally acting antitussive drugs is great.

Recently the role of the cerebral cortex in influencing cough has been studied [24,25]. Of course we can voluntarily produce cough, but voluntary *inhibition* of cough due to upper respiratory tract infection (URTI) has now been measured. Of course there are limits; it would be impossible to inhibit cough due to touching the vocal folds. These studies should be compared with recent evidence that the standard dose of over-the-counter dextromethorphan is little more effective than placebo [25] (although this view is disputed [23,26]). It is proposed that both a small dose of the antitussive and the placebo act on cortical or subcortical pathways; this opens another avenue for antitussive research. Figure 3.2 illustrates a possible neuronal system that includes the cerebral cortex [24].

This view of the importance of higher centres in cough is supported by the observation that some patients with stroke exhibit a weak or absent cough reflex [27], which may increase the likelihood of aspiration pneumonias. A similar condition is seen in Parkinson's disease, where the cough reflex may be inhibited and its pattern altered [22].

(See also Chapters 17, 22 and 25.)

## Motor actions of cough

Typical cough consists of four phases [1] (Fig. 3.3).
1 Inspiratory, when a near-maximal deep inspiration is taken.
2 Compressive, when the glottis closes and forced expiration takes place. The closure is for about 200 ms, and intrapleural and intra-alveolar pressures as high as 300 mmHg can be achieved.
3 Expulsive, when the glottis opens and forced expiration takes place. Velocities as great as 28 000 cm/s (85% of the speed of sound) have been reported, but it is impossible to determine the gas velocity at points of airway constriction, where the greatest shearing forces will be developed. During this phase there is dynamic collapse in the bronchial tree, with large pressure gradients across the collapsed segment. Maximum expirato-

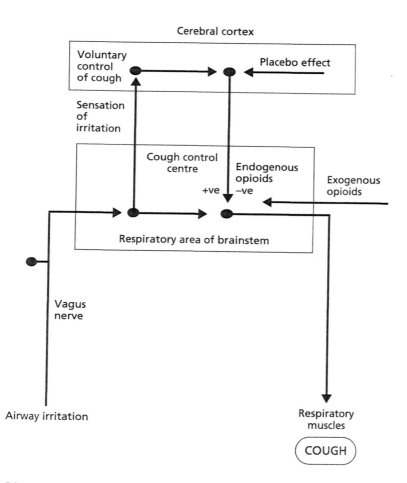

Fig. 3.2 Cough model to illustrate reflex and voluntary control mechanisms. Irritation of airway receptors may cause reflex cough via a brainstem control area. A sensation of irritation may cause cough via higher centres such as the cerebral cortex. Cough can be voluntarily initiated and inhibited via the cerebral cortex that influences cough by two pathways: via the brainstem and via a descending pathway to the spinal cord. Cough can also be inhibited by endogenous or exogenous opioids. Cough associated with common cold may be a mixture of both voluntary and reflex cough. From [24].

# Cough in the Clinic

# 4 Clinical assessment of cough

*Lorcan P.A. McGarvey*

## Introduction

Cough frequently accompanies the common cold and is usually self-limiting, causing little more than a nuisance [1]. In this circumstance, many individuals self-medicate, as is implied by the considerable annual expenditure on 'over-the-counter' antitussive preparations [2,3]. Although there is a close association between smoking and cough, smokers may become so accustomed to their cough that it becomes less apparent to them on a daily basis [4].

Despite these two well-recognized scenarios, cough remains one of the most common symptoms for which patients seek medical attention [5]. Patients requesting medical help for a chronic cough are often concerned that 'something is wrong', a number report exhaustion from sleep deprivation and many become socially self-conscious [6]. Coughing can be so severe as to induce vomiting, incontinence and syncope, and is known to significantly impair quality of life [7].

In the last 30 years there has been expanding clinical and research interest in the whole area of cough. Recommendations on the management of cough have been published, but the cost-effectiveness of the suggested strategies needs to be evaluated [8]. Acceptable guidelines must consider the availability of laboratory tests to the general and specialist physician in both hospital and general practice and address the role of empirical therapy.

To date, no completely satisfactory agreement on the clinical assessment and treatment of cough exists. The aim of this chapter is to review the current diagnostic approach to the adult presenting with a cough, provide some additional suggestions for effective clinical as-sessment and consider the areas of contention that remain to be resolved.

## An overview of current diagnostic protocols

An effective cough involves a complex reflex arc initiated by stimulation of afferent structures, innervated by the vagus nerve and its branches [9] (see Fig. 4.1). The neurophysiological mechanisms underlying cough have already been extensively covered elsewhere in this book. In 1981, a protocol to evaluate patients with chronic cough was devised [10]. This approach was based on the systematic evaluation, using history, examination and laboratory investigations directed at the anatomical sites of cough receptors which comprise the afferent limb of the cough reflex. Suspected aetiologies were confirmed if the cough resolved or significantly improved after a trial of diagnosis-specific therapy. It was termed the 'anatomic diagnostic protocol' and encouraged physicians to consider both pulmonary and extrapulmonary conditions as potential causes for cough. The findings have contributed significantly to what are now accepted as the main disease processes which underpin chronic cough. The main observations have been supported by a repeat study almost 10 years later [11] and by a number of prospective studies in both community and hospital settings, using modifications of the protocol [12–16]. The consistent findings from all these studies are summarized as follows.

1 A cause for chronic cough could be determined in most cases (82–100%).

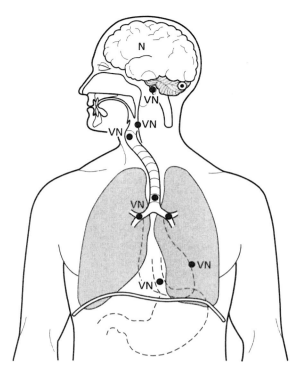

**Fig. 4.1** The anatomy of the afferent limb of the cough reflex. Solid dots represent receptors, circled dot represents the cough centre. N, cortical input; VN, vagus nerve. (Reprinted from Gibson *et al.* (2003), *Respiratory Medicine*, 3rd Edn. © (2003), with permission from Elsevier.)

2 In nearly every case, postnasal drip syndrome (PNDS), asthma, and gastro-oesophageal reflux disease (GORD) either alone or in combination accounted for the cough.

3 Multiple causes for cough were frequently identified (approximately one-quarter of cases).

4 Despite extensive investigation and treatment a subgroup of patients with idiopathic or unexplained cough remained (up to 30%).

Despite the consistencies between studies, a wide variation in the frequencies of the three most common causes of cough exists. This is most likely attributable to differences in how diagnoses are established and some variation in the study populations. In one prospective study, patients were treated empirically for PNDS as first line with cough improvement in 87% of cases [17]. This extremely high prevalence of upper airway disease contrasts with other studies reporting fre-

quencies of between 13% and 21% [13,15]. The failure to use optimal diagnostic methods may also explain differences in diagnostic frequencies reported. One group suggested that their use of barium swallow rather than a more sensitive and specific test, namely ambulatory oesophageal pH monitoring, contributed to a lower frequency of GORD-associated cough [13]. Cough symptom duration may differ between study populations and consequently modify the diagnostic outcomes. One study group with relatively short average cough duration reported postviral cough in 27% of patients evaluated [12]. It is widely appreciated that asthma, gastro-oesophageal reflux (GOR) and post nasal drip coexist and may simultaneously contribute to the cough, and failure to appreciate this leads to treatment failure. However, a complex protocol, which serially investigated these aetiologies in all patients, reported all three causes concurrently causing cough in 15% of patients [16].

Alternative management strategies include trials of empirical therapy alone or in combination with laboratory investigations. There is some evidence that empirical treatment of GORD is more cost-effective than investigation followed by treatment in chronic cough [18]. There is at least general agreement as to the importance of a protocol, which considers the most common causes of cough. In general clinics and hospitals where no such approach exists, extrapulmonary causes are often overlooked and consequently treatment success is poor [19,20].

What follows is a commentary on the current approach to clinical assessment of patients with cough including a suggested management pathway incorporating courses of empirical therapy.

## The clinical assessment of an adult with cough

### History

It is unlikely for the history alone to provide sufficient information to support a diagnosis for the cough. Nonetheless, a careful history should include questioning of the duration, characteristics, associated symptoms and timing of the cough.

*Cough duration*
Classification of cough based on symptom duration is somewhat arbitrary. A cough lasting less than 3 weeks

is termed *acute* and one lasting longer defined as *chronic*. Acute cough is usually a result of a viral upper respiratory tract infection as almost all such coughs resolve within this time period [1]. A postinfective cough may, however, persist for considerable periods of time It may be more satisfactory to define chronic cough as one lasting greater than 8 weeks and to recognize an overlap period of between 3 and 8 weeks.

### Sputum production

Attempts to accurately measure sputum volume may be difficult, as the amount swallowed is variable. The cough may be dry or productive of only scanty amounts of phlegm. A productive cough has been defined as one productive of more than 30 mL of sputum per day [14]. In practical terms what is more relevant is the finding of expectoration of large volumes of purulent phlegm on a daily basis or the presence of haemoptysis. Furthermore, the diagnostic approach and outcome is almost identical, whether the cough is productive or not [14].

### Cough characteristics

Experience from specialist cough clinics suggests that the character and timing of a cough are not diagnostically helpful [21]. The history may establish that the cough is associated with frequent throat clearing or the sensation of postnasal drip, occurs mainly at night or after meals, or is made worse with exercise or cold air. Reliance solely on the characteristics may be misleading: the symptoms of postnasal drip in a patient may reflect only coexistent rhinitis and the absence of dyspepsia does not rule out reflux as the cause of cough. In one study, the predictive values for cough characteristics and associated symptoms were calculated and the findings have been outlined in Table 4.1 [15].

A cough with a 'honking' or 'barking' quality and which disappears with sleep has been suggested as typical of a psychogenic or habit cough. Such characteristics have been frequently reported in the paediatric literature. Such features obtained at history in adults with cough are not helpful [21]. Furthermore, sleep is known to suppress the cough reflex. In a series of patients with lung disease and nocturnal cough, spontaneous cough was almost abolished during stage 3 and 4 sleep [22].

### Smoking history

There is a threefold greater prevalence of cough among smokers compared to never smokers. The causes of cough identified in current or ex-smokers are quite different from never smokers and usually due to chronic bronchitis. A cough which is productive of phlegm on most days for 3 months for 2 consecutive years, satisfies the diagnosis of chronic bronchitis [23]. However, smokers account for only about 5% of those seeking specialist help for their cough [11]. Over time, presumably they attribute their symptom to the direct effects of tobacco exposure. In one study, half of the smokers with an initial cough complaint denied it as a problem 8 years later [4]. In a smoker, the onset of a new cough, a change in cough character, or presence of haemoptysis should raise the suspicion of a bronchogenic carcinoma. Smoking cessation is associated with resolution or improvement of the cough in over 90% of individuals, with over 50% reporting disappearance of cough within 1 month [24].

### Occupational history

A thorough occupational history may identify a possible aetiological factor. Cough has been reported as consequence of working with tussive irritants [25,26].

**Table 4.1** Predictive value of symptom characteristics obtained from history. Reproduced from [15] with permission.

| | Number with positive history | Number correctly identified | Positive predictive value (%) |
|---|---|---|---|
| Asthma (nocturnal cough, precipitated by cold air, exercise, aerosols) | 27 | 15 | 56 |
| PNDS (throat clearing, sensation of postnasal drip, nasal discharge, previous sinusitis) | 27 | 14 | 52 |
| GORD (dyspepsia, cough worse after meals) | 20 | 8 | 40 |

PNDS, postnasal drip syndrome; GORD, gastro-oesophageal reflux disease.

Sensitization to a growing list of agents in the work place may explain the increasing prevalence of occupational asthma and asthma-like symptoms including cough [27].

*Drug history*

Angiotensin-converting enzyme (ACE) inhibitors are increasingly used in the treatment of hypertension and heart failure and although usually well tolerated, a persistent cough has been reported as the most common side-effect, occurring in around 10% patients treated [28]. Typically the cough is dry and tickly and more common among women. It can develop within a week or not for some months after starting therapy. The drug should be withdrawn or substituted with another family of antihypertensive or heart failure medication. When this is necessary, the cough usually subsides within a few days but may take a few months in some cases. Any drug that induces parenchymal lung damage may be associated with cough.

## Physical examination

The physical examination of the patient with cough may demonstrate clinical signs of obstructive lung disease, lung cancer, bronchiectasis, pulmonary fibrosis or cardiac failure. More often though, the examination reveals less specific findings.

*Acute cough*

At the outset of the common cold there may be clinical evidence of a rhinitis and pharyngitis with inflamed nasal mucosa and posterior pharynx with adherent or draining secretions. Inspection of the ears may reveal a serous otitis. A computed tomographic (CT) study of the nasal passages and sinuses in the common cold has demonstrated that a widespread rhinosinusitis, which clears on resolution of the infection, is most typical [29]. The findings on high-resolution CT of the lung have been reported in a group of 76 young adults with the common cold [30]. No important pulmonary changes were reported which is consistent with the normal findings usually reported on examination of the lower respiratory tract.

Acute cough is common in any patient who has a pneumonia. Physical findings on examination of the chest are often very helpful and include dullness on percussion, bronchial breathing and crackles on auscultation.

Rarely, on examination of a patient with an acute cough there may be distinguishing features suggesting specific infective aetiologies. These include bullous myringitis in patients with a *Mycoplasma pneumoniae* infection and subconjunctival haemorrhages described in acute pertussis infection.

*Chronic cough*

Physical examination should concentrate on the afferent sites identified as most commonly associated with chronic cough.

An ear, nose and throat (ENT) examination may reveal evidence of nasal obstruction due to inflamed turbinates or the presence of polyps. The appearance of secretions draining in the posterior pharynx may be apparent. A 'cobblestone' appearance of the oropharyngeal mucosa has been suggested but is an uncommon finding in the routine examination of patients with chronic cough [15]. A more comprehensive discussion on the physical findings in rhinitis, sinusitis and postnasal drip can be found elsewhere in the text. Evidence of irritation of the larynx and pharynx on indirect laryngoscopy could suggest proximal GOR [31].

Examination of the chest is not useful in differentiating reversible airflow obstruction from fixed or partially reversible airflow limitation. Likewise, there are no features that easily distinguish cough-variant asthma. Asking the patient to inhale may trigger paroxysms of coughing. Chest auscultation may reveal rhonchi and a prolonged expiratory phase on auscultation. Coarse crackles may be a prominent finding on examination of a patient with bronchiectasis while widespread fine late inspiratory crackles are typical of diffuse parenchymal lung disease.

The presence of finger clubbing in a smoker together with evidence of a pleural effusion or lobar collapse on examination almost certainly points to a diagnosis of bronchogenic carcinoma.

## Assessing frequency and severity of cough

Clinical assessment involves an appreciation of the severity of cough in terms of its frequency and intensity and any impact on psychological well-being. A cough-specific quality of life questionnaire has recently been validated and may prove a useful tool in routine clinical assessment of both acute and chronic cough [32]. Subjective assessment including cough diaries and symptom scores have been used but are often inaccurate. In relation to nocturnal cough, for example, scoring of cough severity by children and their parents correlated poorly with objective monitoring [33]. Ambulatory cough monitoring is more objective but not widely available and limited by cost and size of the device together with insufficient computer memory. Current advances in technology should resolve these problems and widen the opportunity to accurately record cough frequency.

A wide range of tussigenic agents may be delivered by inhalation challenge to assess cough severity and treatment efficacy [34]. A full discussion of these is outside the scope of this chapter and has been covered elsewhere within the book.

## Clinical investigations

The routine clinical assessment of cough should include a number of baseline investigations. These, together with any additional tests, should reflect the pulmonary and extrapulmonary diseases known to commonly cause chronic cough. Investigations should be requested until a cause is identified but given that cough may have a multiplicity of aetiologies, the diagnostic strategy may become unwieldy and expensive.

The sequence in which investigations are ordered and the degree to which they are pursued will depend on the clinician's impression of each case. However, the dominant factor in many scenarios will be what tests are available to the physician either in hospital or in general practice. The investigations relevant to the most common causes of chronic cough, namely asthma, PNDS and GOR, will be dealt with in detail in the pertinent chapters of this book.

However, the following section aims to provide an overview of the diagnostic tests that may be available to the physician. An outline of the most common investigations is provided in Table 4.2.

### Chest radiograph

A chest radiograph is mandatory at an early stage as a significant abnormality will alter the diagnostic algorithm and avoid unnecessary investigation. In the selected population assessed at specialist clinics, the chest radiograph is almost always normal. In a series of studies the chest radiograph was abnormal less than 10% of the time [10,11]. The frequency of abnormal chest radiographs among unselected cases presenting with chronic cough to a general respiratory clinics has been reported to be 30% [19].

### Spirometry and peak expiratory flow measurements

When available, spirometry both before and after an inhaled bronchodilator should be performed at an early stage in the routine diagnostic testing of all patients with cough. Testing may demonstrate significant reversibility, establishing the diagnosis of asthma. Spirometry is not readily available in primary care and it has been advocated that peak flow meters should be used as an alternative [35]. It is unclear if daily peak expiratory flow (PEF) monitoring at home or the use of a

Table 4.2 Investigations used in the evaluation of patients with chronic cough.

| Investigation | Comment |
| --- | --- |
| Chest radiograph | Essential investigation in all patients |
| Spirometry and reversibility testing | A baseline investigation; not readily available in primary care |
| Peak flow recording | May reliably demonstrate diurnal variability |
| Bronchial challenge | A negative study effectively rules out asthma but not steroid responsive cough |
| 24-h ambulatory pH monitoring | If available; helpful in patients with no reflux symptoms to assess duration and frequency of reflux episodes and any temporal association with cough |
| Paranasal sinus radiograph (or CT scan) | May reveal sinus opacity, mucosal thickening and air–fluid levels |
| Fibreoptic bronchoscopy | Diagnostic utility is low if chest radiograph is normal |
| Non-invasive assessment of airway inflammation | Induced sputum useful in identifying an eosinophilic bronchitis; best reserved for patients with negative bronchoprovocation test |

peak flow meter to assess bronchodilator reversibility are diagnostically reliable for patients with persistent cough. An analysis of the value of measuring diurnal peak flow variability in patients with cough concluded that this method provided accurate diagnostic information [36]. However, peak expiratory flow measurements are not reliable for use in assessing bronchodilator response in primary care patients with persistent cough [37].

*Bronchoprovocation testing*

If doubt remains about the diagnosis of asthma, bronchoprovocation testing should be considered. As bronchial hyperresponsiveness is invariably present in symptomatic asthma, a positive test is persuasive evidence to begin treatment with inhaled steroids and a favourable response confirms the diagnosis of asthma. A negative test reliably rules out asthma [15] but does not exclude a steroid-responsive cough [38]. Eosinophilic bronchitis has none of the airway dysfunction typically associated with asthma. Critically, the diagnosis relies in part on the demonstration of normal airway hyperresponsiveness (provocative concentration of methacholine producing a 20% decrease in $FEV_1$ ($PC_{20}$) $> 16 mg/mL$) [38]. Therefore, a negative bronchial challenge may trigger additional tests aimed at assessing the cellular characteristics of the airway. The nature of such investigations will be discussed below.

*Upper airway provocation studies*

It has been suggested that asthma-like symptoms in particular cough are associated with extrathoracic airway dysfunction. Using flow–volume loops, variable extrathoracic upper airway obstruction has been observed in a series of patients with cough due to PNDS, which improved with treatment [39]. Extrathoracic airway responsiveness can be assessed by recording the maximal inspiratory flow/volume curve during conventional bronchial challenge testing [40]. Extrathoracic airway hyperresponsiveness in the absence of bronchial hyperresponsiveness may be an indicator of upper airway disease as a cause for cough [41].

*Sinus imaging*

Empirical trials of therapy for postnasal drip have been advocated but the place of sinus imaging in cough evaluation has yet to be established [17]. A plain radiograph of the sinuses may reveal evidence of opacity,

mucosal thickening and air–fluid levels in individuals with sinusitis but is rather less helpful when rhinitis is the prominent element. Plain sinus radiography alone has low specificity but improves when combined with history and findings at ENT inspection [42]. When the cough is productive, sinusitis accounts for postnasal drip in 60% of cases [14] and in this circumstance ordering sinus radiograph has been recommended [8].

CT imaging of the sinuses and nasal passages has superior specificity to plain radiography [43]. Screening coronal CT studies have reduced both cost and radiation exposure without compromising accuracy [44]. In a prospective evaluation of a diagnostic protocol for cough which included routine CT sinus imaging, the predictive value of the scan was no better than ENT examination in accurately identifying upper airway disease [15]. Sinus CT scanning should be reserved for refractory cases, which may require surgical referral.

*Gastrointestinal investigations*

If symptoms of GOR seem prominent from the history then an empirical trial of an antireflux regimen should precede investigation of the upper gastrointestinal tract. In a double blind randomized study of patients with chronic cough, empirical treatment with a high-dose proton pump inhibitor proved cost-effective when compared with routine gastrointestinal investigation [18]. However, typical symptoms of GOR are frequently absent and investigations may be necessary.

Barium swallow has been extensively used in the diagnosis of GOR. However, free reflux of barium is not uncommonly observed in healthy individuals and often not at all in those with known GOR [45]. The low sensitivity and specificity exclude barium swallow as a routine diagnostic tool for cough. Endoscopy accurately identifies oesophagitis but does not establish that the cough is due to oesophageal reflux. Twenty-four-hour oesophageal pH monitoring is regarded as the most sensitive and specific test for diagnosing GOR. Hypothetically it has the additional advantage of identifying any temporal association between an acid reflux event and a cough episode. A series of prospective studies of diagnostic cough protocols have reported positive predictive values for the investigation in the range of 68–100% [11,15,16]. All studies agreed, however, that a negative test effectively excluded GOR as the cause for the cough. Nevertheless, as the oesophageal pH profile may not predict response to antireflux therapy, and factors other than acid may be contributing to oesophageal cough, caution is needed in particular when interpreting a negative study [46]. The role of ambulatory 24-h oesophageal pH monitoring in the evaluation of chronic cough needs further scrutiny.

*Fibreoptic bronchoscopy*

Fibreoptic bronchoscopy together with a chest radiograph are the first tests to consider in evaluating a smoker with cough. However, the diagnostic yield from bronchoscopy in the routine evaluation of chronic cough is low, about 5% [8]. This reflects the low frequency of smokers and radiograph abnormalities among patients seeking medical attention for their cough. In spite of this, bronchoscopy has significant diagnostic potential in selected patients where the more common causes have been rigorously excluded [47]. In this study diagnoses were found in 7 of 25 patients undergoing bronchoscopy for unexplained cough. They included broncholithiasis, tracheobronchopathia and laryngeal dyskinesia. Aspirated foreign bodies may go unrecognized for prolonged periods of time although bronchoscopy is probably only indicated when there is a clue in the medical history.

Fibreoptic bronchoscopy provides the opportunity for airway sampling by either mucosal biopsy or bronchial lavage. There has been expanding interest in the role of non-invasive methods to assess airway inflammation and this will be discussed below.

*Thoracic CT scanning*

Diagnoses including diffuse parenchymal lung disease or bronchiectasis not appreciated on history or chest radiograph may be identified on high-resolution CT scanning of the thorax. Only one study has employed thoracic CT scanning routinely in the evaluation of patients referred to a specialist cough clinic [16]. In this report, an abnormality was identified in over a quarter of tests performed with a positive predictive value of 83%. The diagnosis in each case was bronchiectasis but it was not clear if this could have been made on history, examination and/or chest radiograph alone. The addition of thoracic CT scanning to baseline investigations is unlikely to be cost-effective.

*Assessing airway inflammation*

Eosinophilic bronchitis has now been added to the spectrum of diseases that commonly cause chronic cough [48]. It may account for between 10 and 15% of cases referred for specialist attention [38,41]. It has

therefore been suggested that the assessment of airway inflammation should be an important addition to the clinical evaluation of cough [38]. The development of non-invasive techniques such as induced sputum provides a means by which this may be achieved. The methodology involved has been well documented [49] but is not widely employed outside of specialist cough clinics. A greater than 3% sputum eosinophil count has been taken as indicative of eosinophilic bronchitis and warranting a trial of corticosteroid therapy [38].

Exhaled nitric oxide (NO) represents an alternative non-invasive technique for assessing airway inflammation. Exhaled NO levels appear to be lower in non-asthmatic coughers allowing some differentiation from asthmatic cough [50]. Conversely, elevated levels of exhaled NO have been reported in eosinophilic bronchitis [51]. The technique and interpretation of measurements has yet to be fully evaluated. For the near future, in the evaluation of cough at least, the role of exhaled NO outside of a research capacity is likely to remain limited.

*Psychological assessment*

A psychogenic or 'habit' cough has been most frequently reported in children and adolescents [52]. In a very few case reports detailing adults with refractory cough, psychotherapy was the only successful intervention [53,54]. Criteria to help identify patients with unexplained cough, or even those in whom a cause has been established, who may benefit from psychological intervention, have not been established.

## Suggestions for the effective clinical assessment of cough

A revised protocol for evaluating patients with chronic cough should continue to appreciate the three most common aetiologies, which may operate singly or simultaneously. It should ensure both correct interpretation of diagnostic tests and the timely inclusion of empirical therapeutic trials which must be of adequate dose and duration. One such protocol has been outlined in Fig. 4.2.

The objective of the history, physical examination and baseline investigations (which at a minimum should include chest radiograph and spirometry) is to identify any primary pulmonary pathology. ACE inhibitor therapy should be stopped or replaced with an

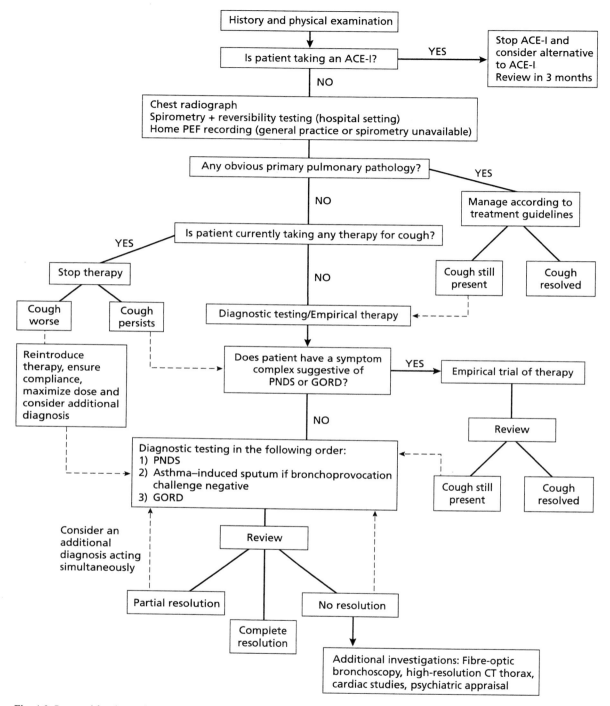

**Fig. 4.2** Protocol for the evaluation of chronic cough in an adult. Adapted with permission from [8]. ACE-I, angiotensin-converting enzyme inhibitor; PEF, peak expiratory flow; PNDS, postnasal drip syndrome; GORD, gastro-oesophageal reflux disease; CT, computed tomography.

alternative. As patients attending specialist cough clinics are rarely treatment naïve, stopping any existing cough treatment can be a useful next step. If as a consequence, symptoms worsen, treatment should be reintroduced, compliance checked, dose maximized and if necessary a coexistent aetiology sought.

The next stage involves a combination of diagnostic testing and trials of empirical therapy. Patients reporting symptoms suggestive of GORD or PNDS should be first offered a trial of empirical therapy. In a placebo-controlled trial in patients with GORD-associated cough, omeprazole 40 mg o.d. for 8 weeks produced an effective and sustained resolution of symptoms [55]. Older (first-generation) antihistamines in combination with decongestants have been recommended as empirical therapy for PNDS [8,17].

In the absence of symptoms, diagnostic testing should be arranged systematically in an order which reflects the three most likely possibilities, i.e. PNDS, asthma and GORD. A further advance in current protocols is the place of induced sputum in the diagnosis of eosinophilic bronchitis. Where available, induced sputum should be reserved for patients with a negative bronchoprovocation test.

In the event of any positive investigation, an appropriate trial of therapy should be commenced, ensuring that both patient compliance and effective doses are prescribed. If the outcome of treatment effects only a partial response, then another cause acting simultaneously should be considered. Each case should be considered on its own merits but testing should be continued until a cause is determined. In general, once the most common causes for cough have been reliably excluded, additional tests may prove valuable. These may comprise fibreoptic bronchoscopy, high-resolution thoracic CT scanning and psychiatric appraisal.

## Cost-effectiveness of clinical assessment of cough

Current management strategies for cough have undergone cost-effectiveness analysis [56]. The approach to 'test all then treat' similar to that advocated by Palombini and colleagues [16] was the most expensive approach but had the shortest treatment duration. In contrast, treating sequentially starting with PNDS as recommended by Pratter and coworkers [17], was the cheapest option but had the longest treatment dura-

tion. The challenge therefore appears to be balance of cost against time to treatment success.

## Conclusions

Although the clinical approach to cough has been well defined it needs to be continually refined. Based on current experience, a large proportion of patients with cough can be successfully managed using existing strategies. However, important questions remain as to the complexity and cost-effectiveness of cough algorithms. Identifying more precise and reliable diagnostic tests, determining the specific role of empirical therapeutic trials and understanding more completely pathogenic mechanisms of cough remain the challenges for future research.

## References

1 Curley FJ, Irwin RS, Pratter MR. Cough and the common cold. *Am Rev Respir Dis* 1988; **138**: 305–11.
2 Couch RB. The common cold: control? *J Infect Dis* 1984; **150**: 167–73.
3 Higgenbottom T. Cough induced by changes of ionic composition of airway surface liquid. *Bull Eur Physiopathol Respir* 1984; **20**: 553–62.
4 Barbee RA, Halonen M, Kaltenborn WT, Burrows B. A longitudinal study of respiratory symptoms in a community population sample. Correlations with smoking allergen skin-test reactivity and serum IgE. *Chest* 1991; **99**: 20–6.
5 Schappert SM. National ambulatory medical care survey 1991; Summary. In: *Adv Data Stat No. 230*. US Department of Health and Human Services. March 29, 1993: 1–20.
6 Irwin RS, Curley FJ. The treatment of cough: a comprehensive review. *Chest* 1991; **99**: 1477–84.
7 French CL, Irwin RS, Curley FJ, Krikorian CJ. Impact of chronic cough on quality of life. *Arch Intern Med* 1998; **158**: 1657–61.
8 Irwin RS, Boulet LP, Cloutier MM *et al.* Managing cough as a defence mechanism and as a symptom. A consensus panel report of the American College of Chest Physicians. *Chest* 1998; **114**: 133S–181S.
9 Korpas J, Tomori Z. *Cough and Other Respiratory Reflexes*, 12th edn. Basel: S. Karger, 1979.
10 Irwin RS, Corrao WM, Pratter MR. Chronic persistent cough in the adult: the spectrum and frequency of cases and successful outcome of specific therapy. *Am Rev Respir Dis* 1981; **123**: 414–7.

11 Irwin RS, Curley FJ, French CL. Chronic cough: the spectrum and frequency of causes, key components of the diagnostic evaluation and outcome of specific therapy. *Am Rev Resp Dis* 1990; **141**: 640–7.

12 Poe HR, Harder RV, Israel RH. Chronic persistent cough: experience in diagnosis and outcome using an anatomic diagnostic protocol. *Chest* 1989; **95**: 723–7.

13 O'Connell F, Thomas VE, Fuller RW *et al*. Cough sensitivity to inhaled capsaicin decreases with successful treatment of chronic cough. *Am J Respir Crit Care Med* 1993; **150**: 374–80.

14 Smyrnios NA, Irwin RS, Curley FJ. Chronic cough with a history of excessive sputum production: The spectrum and frequency of causes, key components of the diagnostic evaluation, and outcome of specific therapy. *Chest* 1995; **108**: 991–7.

15 McGarvey LPA, Heaney LG, Lawson JT *et al*. Evaluation and outcome of patients with chronic non-productive cough using a comprehensive diagnostic protocol. *Thorax* 1998; **53**: 738–43.

16 Palombini BC, Villanova CA, Araujo E *et al*. A pathogenic triad in chronic cough: asthma, postnasal drip syndrome and gastrooesophageal reflux disease. *Chest* 1999; **116**: 279–84.

17 Pratter MR, Bartter T, Akers S, Dubois J. An algorithmic approach to chronic cough. *Ann Intern Med* 1993; **119**: 977–83.

18 Ours TM, Kavuru MS, Schilz RJ, Richter JE. A prospective evaluation of esophageal testing and a double blind, randomized study of omeprazole in a diagnostic and therapeutic algorithm for chronic cough. *Am J Gastroenterol* 1999; **94**: 3131–8.

19 McGarvey LPA, Heaney LG, MacMahon J. A retrospective survey of diagnosis and management of patients presenting with chronic cough to a general chest clinic. *Int J Clin Pract* 1997; **52**: 158–61.

20 Al-Mobeireek AF, Al-Sarhani A, Al-Amri S, Bamgboye E, Ahmed S. Chronic cough at a non-teaching hospital: Are extrapulmonary causes overlooked? *Respirology* 2002; **7**: 141–6.

21 Mello CJ, Irwin RS, Curley FJ. The predictive values of the character, timing and complications of chronic cough in diagnosing its cause. *Arch Intern Med* 1993; **119**: 997–1003.

22 Power JT, Stewart IC, Connaughton JJ *et al*. Nocturnal cough in patients with chronic bronchitis and emphysema. *Am Rev Respir Dis* 1984; **130**: 999–1001.

23 Medical Research Council. Committee report on the aetiology of chronic bronchitis: Definition and classification of chronic bronchitis for clinical and epidemiological purposes. *Lancet* 1965: 775–8.

24 Wynder EL, Kaufman PL, Lesser RL. A short term follow up study on ex-cigarette smokers: With special emphasis on persistent cough and weight gain. *Am Rev Respir Dis* 1967; **96**: 645–55.

25 Blanc P, Liu D, Juarez C, Boushey HA. Cough in hot pepper workers. *Chest* 1991; **99**: 27–32.

26 Gordon SB, Curran AD, Turley A, Wong C, Rahman S, Wiley K, Morice AH. Glass bottle workers exposed to low dose irritant fumes cough but do not wheeze. *Am J Respir Crit Care Med* 1997; **156**: 206–10.

27 Chan-Yeung M, Malo J. Aetiological agents in occupational asthma. *Eur Respir J* 1994; **7**: 346–71.

28 Israili ZH, Hall WD. Cough and angioneurotic oedema associated with angiotensin-converting enzyme inhibitor therapy: a review of the literature and pathophysiology. *Ann Intern Med* 1992; **117**: 234–42.

29 Gwaltney JM Jr, Phillips CD, Miller RD, Riker DK. Computed tomographic study of the common cold. *N Engl J Med* 1994; **330**: 25–30.

30 Puhakka T, Lavonius M, Varpula M *et al*. Pulmonary imaging and function in the common cold. *Scand J Infect Dis* 2001; **33**: 211–4.

31 Koufman JA. The otolaryngologic manifestations of gastroesophageal reflux disease (GERD): a clinical investigation of 225 patients using ambulatory 24-hour pH monitoring and an experimental investigation of the role of acid and pepsin in the development of laryngeal injury. *Laryngoscope* 1991; **101**: 1–78.

32 French CT, Irwin RS, Fletcher KE, Adams TM. Evaluation of a cough specific quality of life questionnaire. *Chest* 2002; **121**: 1123–31.

33 Chang AB, Newman RG, Carlin JB, Phelan PD, Robertson CF. Subjective scoring of cough in children: parent-completed vs child-completed cards vs an objective method. *Eur Respir J* 1998; **11**: 462–6.

34 Morice AH, Kastelik JA, Thompson R. Cough challenge in the assessment of cough reflex. *Br J Clin Pharmacol* 2001; **52**: 365–75.

35 Global Initiative for Asthma. *Global Strategy for Asthma Management and Prevention*, Publ. 95-3659. Washington, DC: National Heart, Lung and Blood Institute, National Institutes of Health, 1995: 1–176.

36 Thiadens HA, De Bock GH, Dekker FW *et al*. Value of measuring diurnal peak flow variability in the recognition of asthma: a study in general practice. *Eur Respir J* 1998; **12**: 842–7.

37 Thiadens HA, De Bock GH, Van Houwelingen JC *et al*. Can peak expiratory flow measurements reliably identify the presence of obstruction and bronchodilator response as assessed by FEV(1) in primary care patients presenting with a persistent cough? *Thorax* 1999; **54**: 1055–60.

38 Brightling C, Ward R, Goh KL, Wardlaw AJ, Pavord ID. Eosinophilic bronchitis is an important cause of chronic cough. *Am J Respir Crit Care Med* 1999; **160**: 406–10.

39 Irwin RS, Pratter MR, Holland PS, Corwin RW, Hughes JP. Postnasal drip causes cough and is associated with reversible upper airway obstruction. *Chest* 1984; **85**: 346–52.

40 Bucca C, Rolla G, Brussino L, De Rose V, Bugiani M. Are asthma-like symptoms due to bronchial or extrathoracic airway dysfunction? *Lancet* 1995; **346**: 791–5.

41 Carney IK, Gibson PG, Murree-Allen K, Saltos N, Olson LG, Hensley MJ. A systematic evaluation of mechanisms in chronic cough. *Am J Respir Crit Care Med* 1997; **156**: 211–6.

42 Pratter M, Bartter T, Lotano R. The role of sinus imaging in the treatment of chronic cough in adults. *Chest* 1999; **116**: 1287–91.

43 Davidson TM, Brahme FJ, Gallagher ME. Radiographic evaluation for nasal dysfunction: computed tomography versus plain films. *Head Neck* 1989; **11**: 405–9.

44 Goodman GM, Martin DS, Klein J, Awwad E, Druce HM, Sharafuddin M. Comparison of a screening coronal CT versus contiguous coronal CT for the evaluation of patients with presumptive sinusitis. *Ann Allergy Asthma Immunol* 1995; **74**: 178–82.

45 Richter J, Castell DO. Gastroesophageal reflux. Pathogenesis, diagnosis and therapy. *Ann Intern Med* 1982; **97**: 93–103.

46 Irwin RS, Zawacki JK, Wilson MM, French CT, Callery MP. Chronic cough due to gastroesophageal reflux disease: failure to resolve despite total/near-total elimination of esophageal acid. *Chest* 2002; **121**: 1132–40.

47 Sen RP, Walsh TE. Fibreoptic bronchoscopy for refractory cough. *Chest* 1991; **99**: 33–5.

48 Gibson PG, Dolovich J, Denberg JA, Ramsdale EH, Hargreave FE. Chronic cough: eosinophilic bronchitis without asthma. *Lancet* 1989, 1346–8.

49 Pavord I, Pizzichini MM, Pizzichini E, Hargreave FE. The use of induced sputum to investigate airway inflammation. *Thorax* 1997; **52**: 498–501.

50 Chatkin JM, Ansarin K, Silkoff PE *et al.* Exhaled nitric oxide as a noninvasive assessment of chronic cough. *Am J Respir Crit Care Med* 1999; **159**: 1810–3.

51 Berlyne GS, Parmeswaran K, Kamada D, Efthimiadis A, Hargreave FE. A comparison of exhaled nitric oxide and induced sputum as markers of airway inflammation. *J Allergy Clin Immunol* 2000; **106**: 638–44.

52 Lokshin B, Lindgren S, Weinberger M, Koviach J. Outcome of habit cough in children with a brief session of suggestion therapy. *Ann Allergy* 1991; **67**: 579–82.

53 Riegal B, Warmoth JE, Middaugh SJ *et al.* Psychogenic cough treated with biofeedback and psychotherapy. A review and case report. *Am J Phys Med Rehabil* 1995; **74**: 155–8.

54 Mastrovich JD, Greenberger PA. Psychogenic cough in adults: a report of two cases and review of the literature. *Allergy Asthma Proc* 2002; **23**: 27–33.

55 Kiljander T, Salomaa ERM, Hietanen EK, Terho EO. Chronic cough and gastro-oesophageal reflux: a double-blind placebo-controlled study with omeprazole. *Eur Respir J* 2000; **16**: 633–8.

56 Lin L, Poh KL, Lim TK. Empirical treatment of chronic cough: A cost-effective analysis. *Proc AMIA Symp* 2001, 383–7.

# 5 Measurement and assessment of cough

*Kian Fan Chung*

## Introduction

The assessment of cough by the clinician should include both tools that measure the amount and severity of the cough, and also investigations that may lead to unravelling the cause of the cough, in terms of both disease and disease processes. An anatomical approach to the investigation of the patient with chronic cough has been successfully advocated [1], and many investigations that are part of the work-up of the patient with persistent cough (Table 5.1) contribute to this approach. However, not only anatomical evaluation but assessing disease processes must be part of the investigation. In this chapter, I will focus on the measurement of the cough itself, and on the assessment of airway inflammation in chronic cough. Other aspects of measurement and assessment of patients with cough are covered elsewhere.

## Measuring cough

The measurement of cough is important in order to determine its severity, following which an approach to treating the cough can be planned. A reliable measure is needed so that the evolution of a persistent cough in a particular patient can be measured and the effectiveness of treatments can be determined.

Cough severity can be measured in several ways (Table 5.2) but the clinician can simply ask the patient how the cough affects his or her daily living and activities, the frequency and intensity of episodes of cough, and his or her own appreciation of the overall severity, and thus obtain a subjective evaluation of the patient's perception of this symptom. Perception of severity on a linear cough symptom score scale ranging from mild to severe has been widely used, but there has been few comparative studies performed with other measures of cough. The notation of the patient, scaling of cough intensity and frequency, and patients' diaries have been used to assess severity [2–4]. Table 5.3 shows a scale that rests on the frequency and intensity of the cough, although the intensity component is not included at the lower scores. The table also uses a scoring system for the daytime as well as the night-time although the reliability of such a measure at night-time is not known.

Although this is the most convenient tool that the clinician has to assess severity of cough, it remains a relatively unvalidated measure. For example, one does not know whether this scale is linear and whether this represents the physical or mental effects of the persistent cough. The sensitivity of the scale is not known and the basis for any changes reported on the score is unclear (for example, psychological factors or the intensity or the frequency of the cough itself).

The impact of cough on patients has been evaluated using a cough-specific health-related quality of life questionnaire [5]. Such a tool provides a more quantitative reflection, but what do changes in the score reflect? In a study of chronic persistent coughers of unknown cause, we found that according to a general health questionnare (the SF-36) the mental but not the physical scores were impaired (R.G. Stirling & K.F. Chung, unpublished data), which is not surprising since chronic coughing itself is unlikely to be associated with any physical impairment, except in the very severe cougher. It also indicated the potential mental effects of

**Table 5.1** Tests used to investigate cough.

Chest radiograph
Lung function tests
Bronchodilator reversibility
Methacholine or histamine bronchial responsiveness
Exercise-induced bronchoconstriction
Exhaled nitric oxide
Induced sputum eosinophilia
Fibreoptic bronchoscopy
High-resolution computed tomography of thorax
High-resolution computed tomography of the nose and
   sinuses
Barium swallow studies
Gastro-oesophagoscopy
24-h monitoring of acid in oesophagus
Oesophageal manometry
Total serum immunoglobulin E
Skin prick tests to common allergens

**Table 5.2** Analysis of cough severity.

1 Clinical history
2 Cough symptom score
3 Cough-specific quality of life
4 Ambulatory cough counts
5 Ambulatory cough intensity
6 Spectral analysis of cough sound
7 Cough sensitivity (to capsaicin or citric acid)

**Table 5.3** Cough symptom score.

*Daytime*
0 No cough
1 Cough for one short period
2 Cough for more than two short periods
3 Frequent cough not interfering with usual activities
4 Frequent cough interfering with usual activities
5 Distressing cough most of the day

*Night-time*
0 No cough
1 Cough on waking only/cough on going to sleep only
2 Awoken once or woken early due to coughing
3 Frequent waking due to coughing
4 Frequent coughs most of the night
5 Distressing cough

chronic cough. For this reason, it is important to examine objective measures of cough so as to determine what components of the cough response contribute to the 'integrated' severity profiles measured either from the cough symptom score or from a cough-specific quality of life assessment. One has to hypothesize that the severity of the cough symptom may depend on its frequency of occurrence and on its intensity. The cough reflex measurement may be considered as similar to the relationship of methacholine or histamine bronchial hyperresponsiveness to asthma severity but there is much less investigation of the cough reflex. Other potential contributions to the severity of cough may include bronchial hyperresponsiveness and submucosal inflammatory changes.

## Monitoring cough counts

The quantitative recording of cough over a representative period of time is necessary for the objective evaluation of cough associated with different diseases and for the assessment of the efficacy of different treatments for chronic cough. Early methods recorded cough in non-ambulatory patients, usually limited to short periods of time [6–11]. Pneumographic recording of thoracic pressure change during cough and measurement of airflow have been used to count cough numbers and the use of the cassette recorder using a free-air microphone was described in the 1960s [12,13]. A variety of methods have been developed initially recording cough in the non-ambulatory subject while sitting in a room and usually limited to short periods of time by having an observer count cough sounds as they occur. Such recordings are limited because the patients are not exposed to the presumed tussive stimuli that they encounter in their daily activities. Monitoring of patients with a cold while sitting in a room shows that cough counts fall significantly over the first 60 min [14].

The intensity and duration of cough have been examined by recording of the pneumogram on a kymograph [15], but the most common method has been to record the coughs onto a tape recorder either fixed on the wall of the patient's room or placed in close contact to the patient's throat [16,17]. Cough sounds have also been recorded with a dynamic microphone placed in the acoustic focus of a paraboloid mirror [18]. Cough intensity has also been measured using an integrated surface abdominal electromyogram [19].

Recent developments have given rise to ambulatory methods of monitoring cough over a period of days [20,21]. A 24-h ambulatory system using a solid-state, multiple channel recorder to measure the number of coughs has been devised. Coughs were measured as the simultaneous occurrence of the digitized cough sound recorded by a microphone and the electromyographic signals from the lower respiratory muscles. The signals were analysed visually, and it was possible in this way to distinguish a cough from sneezing, Valsalva manoeuvre, laughing and speaking loudly. What probably remains most difficult to distinguish from cough is throat-clearing but the intensity of the noise induced by throat-clearing is less. The data could be analysed either as single cough events or as episodes of successive burst of coughs, termed epochs, and there was an excellent correlation between the cough epochs and the total number of coughs.

Another system that has been described is the acquisition of only the cough sound from a computerized audiotimed portable recorder connected to a transmitter using telemetry to send the collected sound signals to a computer in the home that digitizes and stores the signals [22]. The volunteer is free to move within 100 m of the computer. The parameters that were measured included the cough count, the cough latency (periods between coughs), the cough effort (integral of the cough acoustic power spectrum), cough intensity (cough effort divided by cough count) and the 'wetness' of the cough. It is interesting that there is no system commercially available for ambulatory cough monitoring for clinical use. The automatic computerized analysis of cough events is still an issue. The ability to record high-fidelity cough sounds acquired on a sound card with subsequent computerized analysis is likely to be the way forward. Cough frequency, in addition to other parameters from the cough sound such as the range of frequencies of the cough, spectral bursts and duration of cough, can be measured [23].

## Analysis of cough counts and intensity

Most of the coughs of patients with chronic persistent cough occurred during the awake hours, with reduced or little activity during the sleeping hours [20]. This is in agreement with studies showing a depression of the cough reflex during rapid eye movement sleep [24]. In chronic coughers, there was a good correlation between daytime coughs and the self-assessment cough scores (Fig. 5.1). In both adults and children, a correlation has been demonstrated between a cough scoring system and the cough counts, particularly during the day [20,25]. However, the correlation is not perfect, indicating that the cough scoring system may also reflect other parameters than just the cough numbers, such as the intensity of the cough or the physical effects of cough.

## Pharmacological assessment

In children with recurrent cough, the effects of salbutamol or beclomethasone (beclometasone) were examined on the cough counts. Overall, these drugs did not inhibit cough. However, a 70% reduction in cough counts was taken as representing success of treatment and, on individual assessment, 4 out of 21 and 12 out of

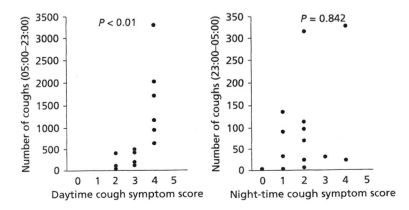

Fig. 5.1 Relationship of cough counts with cough symptom scores during the day or night. From [20].

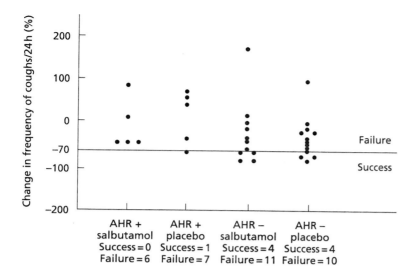

Fig. 5.2 Effect of salbutamol treatment on cough counts in children with a chronic cough. AHR, airway hyper-responsive. From [26].

22 children had a therapeutic response following salbu-tamol and beclomethasone, respectively [26] (Fig. 5.2). The telemetric method of acquisition of cough sounds has been used mainly to test the effects of antitussives during acute cough associated with an upper respirat-ory tract virus infection. The effects of a reliever anti-tussive, dextromethorphan, were examined by compar-ing recordings over a 1-h baseline period with a 3-h postdose period. In a meta-analysis of six studies in-volving 710 subjects, dextromethorphan was signifi-cantly effective in reducing cough counts (by 13%), cough intensity (by 6%) and cough effort (by 17%), and increasing cough latency period (by 17%) [27]. In a similar study of 43 subjects who were observed in a non-ambulatory study, dextromethorphan had no sig-nificant effect on the cough counts [28]. The study with the ambulatory monitoring indicates that large cohorts are needed to show an effect of dextromethorphan. The remaining question is how significant are the changes in the objective measurements observed?

The use of ambulatory monitoring of chronic persis-tent cough is still surprisingly limited. What are the is-sues raised and the potential advantages that the 24-h ambulatory cough monitoring system will provide? First, it is necessary to determine the variability of the cough count and intensity: patients with chronic cough often mention a variable course of chronic cough. This could be related to various environmental factors, and triggers may be identified. Secondly, it would be pos-sible to relate temporally specific triggers with the cough event, such as an episode of gastro-oesophageal reflux, timed with a decrease in oesophageal pH. In one study where cough was noted by the patient as it oc-curred, about 46% of coughs were temporally associat-ed with acid reflux as measured by oesophageal pH monitoring [29]. Thirdly, it would be possible to relate the measures of count and intensity to the cough re-sponsiveness to capsaicin, to the cough symptom score and to cough-associated quality of life score. Finally, we may obtain useful ways of determining the effects of therapy in particular patients and also for trials of drug or other therapies as illustrated above.

## Can quantitative analysis of the cough sound help in the diagnosis?

An interest in quantitative analysis of the cough sound has been generated with the hope that such analysis may be used for diagnostic purposes, as well as for as-sessing the severity of the disease process [30]. Analysis of the cough sound (the tussiphonogram) can often dis-cern two components, with the first sound originating at the level of the tracheal bifurcation or below, while the second sound probably from the vocal cords. The second cough sound is often absent in voluntary cough-ing, in patients following laryngectomy or chordec-tomy, during laryngeal paralysis and in patients with a cough due to psychological reasons [31]. Abnormali-ties of the first cough sound such as a prolongation is due to tracheobronchial collapse. The presence of mucus in the airways could lead to doubling or tripling of the first cough sound. Changes in airway calibre resulting from pharmacological drugs do not appear to change the quality of the cough sound. Various characteristics have been described in terms of the cough sounds associated with tracheitis, bronchitis and laryngitis, but these have not been put to test in clinical practice. A barking cough is typical of subglottic stenosis with the deep hollow cough sounds also coming from the trachea. Whoops are typical of pertussis infections. A brassy sound is characteristic of bronchial compression.

The intensity of the sound at a wide range of frequency levels can be analysed using a fast Fourier transformation (spectral analysis). Using this analysis, the spontaneous cough of an asthmatic has been characterized by relatively long duration with a prolonged wheezing sound and by a lower frequency than those patients with chronic bronchitis or with tracheobronchial collapse [32,33]. Differences in the cough spectrogram have also been reported between asthmatic and non-asthmatic children [34] and exercise changed cough sound of the asthmatic child but not that of the non-asthmatic child [35]. Spectrographic differences in children with cystic fibrosis, acute bronchiolitis and whooping cough have been described. Different patterns of cough spectra may provide possible discrimination between normal and abnormal cough sounds [36]. Higher frequencies of voluntary cough spectrograms were reported in patients with asthma, chronic bronchitis, bronchial carcinoma and laryngeal nerve paralysis compared with healthy volunteers [37]. However, there are inherent difficulties in the use of this analysis in diagnostic work, and these have limited the usefulness of such an approach. The frequency distribution of the cough sound is variable between subjects and also within the same subject under different conditions. One disappointing feature of spectral analysis of cough is that it does not appear to be different within the same subject when challenged with different tussive stimuli such as with capsaicin or prostaglandin $F_{2\alpha}$ or chloride-deficient solutions.

## Assessment of airway inflammation in chronic cough

Many of the tests in the assessment of airway inflam-

mation relate to the diagnosis of asthma or cough-variant asthma, because these conditions are associated typically with airway eosinophilia. Sputum can be induced by inhalation of hypertonic solutions of salt, and the resulting expectorate can be examined for inflammatory cells such as eosinophils [38]. The value of performing fibreoptic bronchoscopy in patients with persistent cough of indeterminate cause remains unclear [39], mainly because the significance of inflammatory cells in the submucosa apart from eosinophils remains uncertain. Other non-invasive measures that may help in the diagnostic process of confirming asthma or asthma-associated cough include exhaled nitric oxide.

## Assessment of airway inflammation by induced sputum

In asthma, one expects to see high levels of eosinophil counts, often related to the severity of the disease [40]; in addition, raised levels of neutrophils can also be seen in patients with more severe asthma needing oral corticosteroid therapy [41]. There are three conditions of persistent cough associated with eosinophilic inflammation as assessed by induced sputum (Table 5.4).

Cough-variant asthma, first described in six patients with chronic persistent cough without wheezing or dyspnoea or airflow obstruction, but with bronchial hyperresponsiveness [42], responds well to bronchodilator therapy and inhaled corticosteroids. In a comparative study, serum eosinophil cationic protein levels and the percentage of eosinophils in bronchoalveolar lavage fluid and in bronchial biopsy specimens were elevated in patients with cough-variant asthma and comparable to those levels found in patients with classic asthma associated with wheeze [43]. Increased thickness of the bronchial basement membrane has also been described in patients with cough-variant asthma, indicating that a similar process of 'airway remodelling' as observed in asthma may be present in cough-variant asthma [44]. The relationship of bronchial hyperrresponsiveness to the cough reflex to capsaicin in this group of patients is interesting. These patients have been divided into those hyperresponsive to methacholine whose coughs were responsive to bronchodilators, and into those who were normoresponsive and whose cough did not respond to

Table 5.4 Common causes of cough with eosinophilia.

| | Peak flow variability | BHR | Sputum | Sputum eosinophils | Steroid responsiveness |
|---|---|---|---|---|---|
| Asthma | + | + | ± | + | + |
| Cough-variant asthma | ± | + | − | + | + |
| Eosinophilic bronchitis | − | − | + | + | + |

Eosinophil-associated cough: +, present; ±, variable; −, absent.
BHR, bronchial hyperresponsiveness.

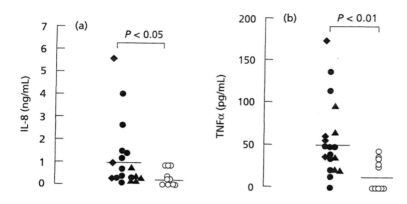

Fig. 5.3 Levels of interleukin-8 (IL-8) and tumour necrosis factor-α (TNFα) in supernatants of induced sputum from non-asthmatic chronic coughers (closed symbols) and from control non-coughing volunteers (open symbols). From [52].

bronchodilators [45]. The former group had a normal capsaicin cough threshold, while the latter had a hypertussive response to capsaicin, which reverted to normal when treated with steroids or anti-H$_1$ histamine drugs. In this group, eosinophilia was not present in bronchoalveolar lavage fluid, but there was a small number of eosinophils in the subepithelium of the trachea and bronchi [46].

Eosinophilic bronchitis is a condition presenting with chronic cough, and characterized by sputum eosinophilia but without any evidence of variable airflow obstruction or airway hyperresponsiveness [47,48]. It is found in 10–20% of patients presenting with a persistent cough to a hospital cough clinic [49]. Sputum eosinophilia ranging between 3 and 95% has been reported with normal bronchial responsiveness to histamine but with a hypertussive response to capsaicin. With inhaled corticosteroid treatment, the cough improves with a reduction in capsaicin tussive response and with a significant reduction (not suppression) of the sputum eosinophilia [50].

In patients with eosinophilic bronchitis, similar to

asthmatics, gene expression of the cytokines interleukin-5 (IL-5) and granulocyte–macrophage colony-stimulating factor (GM-CSF), measured by in situ hybridization were expressed in bronchoalveolar lavage cells from most of these patients [51]. By contrast, in cells obtained from patients whose cough did not respond to inhaled corticosteroids, these cytokines were not expressed. Similar to patients with asthma, patients with steroid-responsive cough demonstrate expression of IL-5 and GM-CSF. On the other hand, in a study of patients with chronic cough without asthma or asthma-related conditions, examination of sputum revealed no eosinophils but an excess of neutrophils [52]. These included patients with 'idiopathic' cough or cough associated with postnasal drip or gastro-oesophageal reflux. There were also increased levels of interleukin-8 and tumour necrosis factor-α which are neutrophil-associated cytokines (Fig. 5.3). Interestingly, patients with chronic obstructive pulmonary disease of moderate severity, a condition associated with neutrophilic inflammation, have an enhanced capsaicin tussive response [53].

Wark *et al.* have looked at the measurement of induced eosinophil count in the assessment of asthma and chronic cough, and concluded that this may be a useful guide to therapy, especially in the assessment of persistent symptoms in asthmatics on corticosteroids, and in the assessment of non-asthmatic subjects with cough [54]. Of interest, in cough patients without sputum eosinophilia, inhaled corticosteroids had no effect on the cough [55].

Overall, one could define a group of chronic cough associated with eosinophilic inflammation ('eosinophilic cough'), an enhanced cough reflex to capsaicin, and a suppression of the cough to inhaled corticosteroids. These patients reflect the spectrum of conditions ranging from asthma to eosinophilic bronchitis. Clinically, these conditions can be grouped together because of their good therapeutic response to inhaled steroids. We do not know whether cough due to gastro-oesophageal reflux is an eosinophil-associated condition: in a small study that included two patients with gastro-oesophageal reflux and in another larger study there was no sputum eosinophilia [52,56] but, in a bronchoalveolar lavage study, eosinophilia was reported [57].

## Exhaled nitric oxide

Nitric oxide is an intracellular messenger with actions as an inflammatory mediator, vasodilator and a non-adrenergic non-cholinergic neurotransmitter. Increased levels of exhaled nitric oxide are observed in patients with asthma, after upper airway viral infections and in bronchiectasis [58]. Raised levels of exhaled nitric oxide have been used as a non-invasive marker of airway inflammation. Exhaled nitric oxide levels are raised in patients presenting with chronic cough in whom asthma has been documented with an increased methacholine hyperresponsiveness [59], while in chronic cough not attributable to asthma, levels are within normal. The sensitivity and specificity of exhaled nitric oxide for detecting asthma in patients with chronic cough were 75% and 87%, respectively. Exhaled nitric oxide is not elevated in patients with cough associated with gastro-oesophageal reflux [56], nor in non-asthmatic coughing children [60,61]. Therefore, a normal level of exhaled nitric oxide may confidently exclude the diagnosis of asthma-associated cough, although these measurements should be made

with patients not taking inhaled corticosteroids since this inhibits exhaled nitric oxide levels [62]. The levels of exhaled nitric oxide in eosinophilic bronchitis are not known. The relationship between exhaled nitric oxide levels and induced sputum eosinophils or submucosal eosinophils in chronic asthmatic coughers is not known. In mild asthma, exhaled nitric oxide correlates with bronchial hyperresponsiveness but not with sputum eosinophilia [63,64].

## Bronchial mucosal biopsies

There are limited data regarding the inflammation observed in bronchial biopsies from patients with chronic cough, and therefore the interpretation of the presence of inflammatory cells in these biopsies remains unclear. In addition, it is possible that coughing itself could perpetuate a chronic inflammatory airway response. This issue remains unresolved. Bronchial biopsies from 25 patients with a chronic dry cough as an isolated symptom over a 3-week period revealed in 21 patients an infiltrate with eosinophils, of whom five were hyperresponsive to methacholine; in the other four, a lymphocytic infiltrate was found [65]. The significance of airway lymphocytic inflammation in chronic cough is not known but this has also been observed by other groups [66]. In a group of non-asthmatic patients with chronic cough associated with postnasal discharge, chronic sinusitis, gastro-oesophageal reflux, or without any associated cause, endobronchial biopsies showed increased epithelial desquamation and the presence of inflammatory cells, particularly mononuclear cells [66]. In addition, submucosal fibrosis, squamous cell metaplasia and loss of cilia are also described. The significance of these changes are unclear and more detailed analysis is necessary.

## Conclusion

This chapter has reviewed the measurement and assessment of airway inflammation in chronic persistent cough. Measurement of cough severity needs more validated tools, which are also required for the proper evaluation of antitussive drugs. Assessment of airway inflammation by invasive and non-invasive techniques is required for investigating the cause of cough, but may also provide clues to the pathogenesis of cough.

## References

1 Irwin RS, Curley FJ, French CL. Chronic cough: the spectrum and frequency of causes, key components of the diagnostic evaluation, and outcome of specific therapy. *Am Rev Respir Dis* 1990; **141**: 640–7.
2 Aylward M, Maddock J, Davies DE, Protheroe DA, Leideman T. Dextromethorphan and codeine: comparison of plasma kinetics and antitussive effects. *Eur J Respir Dis* 1984; **65**: 283–91.
3 Gulsvik A, Refvem OK. A scoring system on respiratory symptoms. *Eur Respir J* 1988; **1**: 428–32.
4 Ellul-Micallef R. Effect of terbutaline sulphate in chronic 'allergic' cough. *Br Med (Clin Res Ed)* 1983; **287**: 940–3.
5 French CL, Irwin RS, Curley FJ, Krikorian CJ. Impact of chronic cough on quality of life. *Arch Intern Med* 1998; **158**: 1657–61.
6 Barach AL, Bickerman HA, Beck GJ. Clinical and physiological studies on the use of metacortandracin in respiratory disease. 1. Bronchial asthma. *DC* 1955; **27**: 515–22.
7 Bickerman HA, Borach AL. The experimental production of cough in human subjects induced by citric acid aerosols. Preliminary studies on the evaluation of antitussive agents. *Am J Med Sci* 1954; **228**: 156–63.
8 Morris DJ, Shane SJ. Human bioassay of a new antitussive agent. *Can Med Assoc J* 1960; **83**: 1093–5.
9 Prime FJ. The assessment of antitussive drugs in man. *Br Med J* 1961; **1**: 1149–51.
10 Calesnik B, Christensen JA, Munch JC. Antitussive action of 1-propoxyphene in citric acid-induced cough response. *Am J Med Sci* 1961; **242**: 560–4.
11 Chernish SM, Lewis G, Kraft B, Howe J. Clinical evaluation of a new antitussive preparation. *Ann Allergy* 1963; **21**: 677–82.
12 Loudon RG, Brown LC. Cough frequency in patients with respiratory disease. *Am Rev Respir Dis* 1967; **96**: 1137–43.
13 Reece CA, Cherry AC, Reece AT, Hatcher AT, Diehl AM. Tape recorder for evaluation of cough in children. *Am J Dis Child* 1966; **112**: 124–8.
14 Eccles R, Morris S, Jawad M. Lack of effect of codeine in the treatment of cough associated with acute upper respiratory tract infection. *J Clin Pharm Ther* 1992; **17**: 175–80.
15 Gravenstein JS, Devloo RA, Beecher HK. Effect of antitussive agents on experimental and pathological cough in man. *J Appl Physiol* 1954; **7**: 119–39.
16 Woolf CR, Rosenberg A. The cough suppressant effect of heroin and codeine: a controlled clinical study. *Can Med Assoc J* 1962; **87**: 810–4.
17 Sevelius H, Colmore JP. Objective assessment of antitussive agents in patients with chronic cough. *J New Drugs* 1966; **6**: 216–33.
18 Salmi T, Sovijarvi ARA, Brander P, Piirila P. Long-term recording and automatic analysis of cough using filtered acoustic sign movements on static charge sensitive bed. *Chest* 1988; **94**: 970–5.
19 Cox ID, Wallis PJW, Apps MCP, Hughes DTD, Empey DW, Osman RCA et al. An electromyographic method of objectively assessing cough intensity and use of the method to assess effects of codeine on the dose–response curve to citric acid. *Br J Clin Pharmacol* 1984; **18**: 377–82.
20 Hsu J-Y, Stone RA, Logan-Sinclair R, Worsdell M, Busst C, Chung KF. Coughing frequency in patients with persistent cough using a 24-hour ambulatory recorder. *Eur Resp J* 1994; **7**: 1246–53.
21 Chang AB, Phelan PD, Robertson CF, Newman RG, Sawyer SM. Frequency and perception of cough severity. *J Paediatr Child Health* 2001; **37**: 142–5.
22 Subburaj S, Parvez L, Rajagopalan TG. Methods of recording and analysing cough sounds. *Pulm Pharmacol* 1996; **9**: 269–79.
23 Dalmasso F, Isnardi E, Sudaro L, Bellantoni R. Bioacoustics of cough during bronchial inhalation challenge (BIC) with methacholine. *Eur Resp J* 2001; **18** (33): 135s.
24 Power JT, Stewart IC, Connaughton JJ, Brash HM, Shapiro CM, Flenley DC et al. Nocturnal cough in patients with chronic bronchitis and emphysema. *Am Rev Respir Dis* 1984; **130**: 999–1001.
25 Chang AB, Newman RG, Carlin JB, Phelan PD, Robertson CF. Subjective scoring of cough in children: parent-completed vs child-completed diary cards vs an objective method. *Eur Respir J* 1998; **11**: 462–6.
26 Chang AB, Phelan PD, Carlin JB, Sawyer SM, Robertson CF. A randomised, placebo controlled trial of inhaled salbutamol and beclomethasone for recurrent cough. *Arch Dis Child* 1998; **79**: 6–11.
27 Pavesi L, Subburaj S, Porter-Shaw K. Application and validation of a computerized cough acquisition system for objective monitoring of acute cough: a meta-analysis. *Chest* 2001; **120**: 1121–8.
28 Lee PCL, Jawad MS, Eccles R. Antitussive efficacy of dextromethorphan in cough associated with acute upper respiratory tract infection. *J Pharm Pharmacol* 2000; **52**: 1137–42.
29 Avidan B, Sonnenberg A, Schnell TG, Sontag SJ. Temporal associations between coughing or wheezing and acid reflux in asthmatics. *Gut* 2001; **49**: 767–72.

30  Korpas J, Sadlonova J, Vrabec M. Analysis of the cough sound: an overview. *Pulm Pharmacol* 1996; **9**: 261–8.

31  Korpas J, Sadlonova J, Salat D, Masarova E. The origin of cough sounds. *Bull Eur Physiopathol Respir* 1987; **23** (Suppl. 10): 47s–50s.

32  Piirila P, Sovijarvi AR. Differences in acoustic and dynamic characteristics of spontaneous cough in pulmonary diseases. *Chest* 1989; **96**: 46–53.

33  Salat D, Korpas J, Salatova V, Korpasova Sadlonova J, Palecek D. The tussiphonogram during asthmatic attack. *Acta Physiol Hung* 1987; **70**: 223–5.

34  Thorpe CW, Toop LJ, Dawson KP. Towards a quantitative description of asthmatic cough sounds. *Eur Respir J* 1992; **5**: 685–92.

35  Toop LJ, Dawson KP, Thorpe CW. A portable system for the spectral analysis of cough sounds in asthma. *J Asthma* 1990; **27**: 393–7.

36  Debreczeni LA, Korpas J, Salat D. Spectral analysis of cough sounds recorded with and without a nose clip. *Bull Eur Physiopathol Respir* 1987; **23** (Suppl. 10): 57s–61s.

37  Debreczeni LA, Korpas J, Salat D, Sadlonova Korpasova J, Vertes C, Masarova E *et al.* Spectra of the voluntary first cough sounds. *Acta Physiol Hung* 1990; **75**: 117–31.

38  Jayaram L, Parameswaran K, Sears MR, Hargreave FE. Induced sputum cell counts: their usefulness in clinical practice. *Eur Respir J* 2000; **16**: 150–8.

39  Markovitz DH, Irwin RS. Is bronchoscopy overused in the evaluation of chronic cough? Bronchoscopy is overused. *J Bronchol* 1997; **4**: 332–6.

40  Peleman RA, Rytila PH, Kips JC, Joos GF, Pauwels RA. The cellular composition of induced sputum in chronic obstructive pulmonary disease. *Eur Respir J* 1999; **13**: 839–43.

41  Jatakanon A, Uasuf C, Maziak W, Lim S, Chung KF, Barnes PJ. Neutrophilic inflammation in severe persistent asthma. *Am J Respir Crit Care Med* 1999; **160**: 1532–9.

42  Carrao WM, Braman SS, Irwin RS. Chronic cough as the sole presenting manifestation of bronchial asthma. *N Engl J Med* 1979; **300**: 633–7.

43  Niimi A, Amitani R, Suzuki K, Tanaka E, Murayama T, Kuze F. Eosinophilic inflammation in cough variant asthma. *Eur Respir J* 1998; **11**: 1064–9.

44  Niimi A, Matsumoto H, Minakuchi M, Kitaichi M, Amitani R. Airway remodelling in cough-variant asthma. *Lancet* 2000; **356**: 564–5.

45  Fujimura M, Kamio Y, Hashimoto T, Matsuda T. Cough receptor sensitivity and bronchial responsiveness in patients with only chronic non-productive cough: in view of effect of bronchodilator therapy. *J Asthma* 1994; **31**: 463–72.

46  Fujimura M, Ogawa H, Yasui M, Matsuda T. Eosinophilic tracheobronchitis and airway cough hypersensitivity in chronic non-productive cough. *Clin Exp Allergy* 2000; **30**: 41–7.

47  Gibson PG, Dolovich J, Denburgh J, Ramsdale EH, Hargreave FE. Chronic cough: Eosinophilic bronchitis without asthma. *Lancet* 1989; **1**: 1246–7.

48  Brightling CE, Pavord ID. Eosinophilic bronchitis: an important cause of prolonged cough. *Ann Med* 2000; **32**: 446–51.

49  Brightling CE, Ward R, Goh KL, Wardlaw AJ, Pavord ID. Eosinophilic bronchitis is an important cause of chronic cough. *Am J Respir Crit Care Med* 1999; **160**: 406–10.

50  Brightling CE, Ward R, Wardlaw AJ, Pavord ID. Airway inflammation, airway responsiveness and cough before and after inhaled budesonide in patients with eosinophilic bronchitis. *Eur Respir J* 2000; **15**: 682–6.

51  Gibson PG, Zlatic K, Scott J, Sewell W, Woolley K, Saltos N. Chronic cough resembles asthma with IL-5 and granulocyte-macrophage colony-stimulating factor gene expression in bronchoalveolar cells. *J Allergy Clin Immunol* 1998; **101**: 320–6.

52  Jatakanon A, Lalloo UG, Lim S, Chung KF, Barnes PJ. Increased neutrophils and cytokines, TNF-alpha and IL-8, in induced sputum of non-asthmatic patients with chronic dry cough. *Thorax* 1999; **54**: 234–7.

53  Doherty MJ, Mister R, Pearson MG, Calverley PM. Capsaicin responsiveness and cough in asthma and chronic obstructive pulmonary disease. *Thorax* 2000; **55**: 643–9.

54  Wark PA, Gibson PG, Fakes K. Induced sputum eosinophils in the assessment of asthma and chronic cough. *Respirology* 2000; **5**: 51–7.

55  Pizzichini MM, Pizzichini E, Parameswaran K, Clelland L, Efthimiadis A, Dolovich J *et al.* Nonasthmatic chronic cough: no effect of treatment with an inhaled corticosteroid in patients without sputum eosinophilia. *Can Respir J* 1999; **6**: 323–30.

56  Parameswaran K, Allen CJ, Kamada D, Efthimiadis A, Anvari M, Hargreave FE. Sputum cell counts and exhaled nitric oxide in patients with gastroesophageal reflux, and cough or asthma. *Can Respir J* 2001; **8**: 239–44.

57  McGarvey LP, Forsythe P, Heaney LG, MacMahon J, Ennis M. Bronchoalveolar lavage findings in patients with chronic nonproductive cough. *Eur Respir J* 1999; **13**: 59–65.

58  Kharitonov SA, Barnes PJ. Clinical aspects of exhaled nitric oxide. *Eur Respir J* 2000; **16**: 781–92.

59  Chatkin JM, Ansarin K, Silkoff PE, McClean P, Gutierrez C, Zamel N *et al.* Exhaled nitric oxide as a noninvasive assessment of chronic cough. *Am J Respir Crit Care Med* 1999; **159**: 1810–3.

60  Avital A, Uwyyed K, Berkman N, Godfrey S, Bar-Yishay E, Springer C. Exhaled nitric oxide and asthma in young children. *Pediatr Pulmonol* 2001; **32**: 308–13.

61  Formanek W, Inci D, Lauener RP, Wildhaber JH, Frey U,

Hall GL. Elevated nitrite in breath condensates of children with respiratory disease. *Eur Respir J* 2002; **19**: 487–91.

62 Kharitonov SA, Yates DH, Barnes PJ. Inhaled glucocorticoids decrease nitric oxide in exhaled air of asthmatic patients. *Am J Respir Crit Care Med* 1996; **153**: 454–7.

63 Jatakanon A, Lim S, Kharitonov SA, Chung KF, Barnes PJ. Correlation between exhaled nitric oxide, sputum eosinophils, and methacholine responsiveness in patients with mild asthma. *Thorax* 1998; **53**: 91–5.

64 Dupont LJ, Rochette F, Demedts MG, Verleden GM. Ex-haled nitric oxide correlates with airway hyperresponsiveness in steroid-naive patients with mild asthma. *Am J Respir Crit Care Med* 1998; **157**: 894–8.

65 Lee SY, Cho JY, Shim JJ, Kim HK, Kang KH, Yoo SH *et al.* Airway inflammation as an assessment of chronic nonproductive cough. *Chest* 2001; **120**: 1114–20.

66 Boulet LP, Milot J, Boutet M, St Georges F, Laviolette M. Airway inflammation in non-asthmatic subjects with chronic cough. *Am J Respir Crit Care Med* 1994; **149**: 482–9.

# Cough sensitivity: the use of provocation tests

*Rick W. Fuller*

## Introduction

Cough has been identified as a significant symptom in the population. Everybody will experience cough at some time, either during a respiratory infection or as one of a significant number of people who will have chronic cough from other causes [1]. Almost any disease of the respiratory tract, as well as some non-respiratory conditions, such as gastro-oesophageal reflux, can cause cough. Traditionally the study of cough has relied on patient reports via questionnaires or by mechanical recording of cough events. Provocation tests provide another mechanism to study cough [2]. Despite the demonstration in 1957 [3] that cough provocation could be safely and reliably performed, such methodology has not been as well developed as those for provoking bronchoconstriction. Nevertheless, there are data on cough provocation studies in three areas, which I will discuss in this chapter. They are the epidemiology of cough, the clinical management of cough and the clinical research of cough.

## Epidemiology

Cough is a symptom which is found commonly in all communities with an incidence varying from 5 to 40% [1]. Environmental and lifestyle factors, e.g. smoking, appear to have the greatest influence on the frequency with which cough is reported. A recent study in Europe [4] has shown that three distinct types of cough can be identified in the population: productive cough, non-productive cough and nocturnal cough. These different cough types have different associations with the data

gained in the survey, i.e. increased body mass and cigarette exposure contributed to all three whereas rhinitis and gender did not. The question is whether cough provocation testing, as an index of the sensitivity of the cough reflex in those populations, would have enriched the information. Unfortunately no true epidemiology study has used cough reflex testing as a variable; there are, however, data from small studies, which point to its possible value.

Data in patient groups have been gathered using challenges such as low $Cl^-$ solutions [5], which is a timed tidal breathing challenge, and single breath challenges with citric acid [6] and capsaicin [7], although the methods used tend to vary from group to group. Broadly speaking, the studies show that in the non-coughing population there is little variability in the cough reflex sensitivity, i.e. very few people do not cough or have very sensitive reflexes (Fig. 6.1). There is some evidence that children are more sensitive than adults [8], which may well be an artifact of dosing due to their smaller airways. In addition, a clear difference can be defined between males and females (the females being more sensitive) with low $Cl^-$ challenge [9] and in some studies with the single breath challenges [10] but not others [7]. The explanation is likely to be anatomical differences in airway size and therefore a dose issue until proven otherwise.

The cough reflex has been studied in a number of different patient groups with respiratory diseases with and without cough. Patients with stable disease without cough, chiefly asthma, have a normal reflex (Table 6.1); however, if the disease is associated with dry cough then an increased sensitivity of the reflex has been observed [7] (Table 6.1). The exception in the study in Table 6.1 was a patient group with postnasal drip who complained of a dry cough but had on average a normal reflex; however, the variability was large and the sample small so the conclusion may not stand the test of time. On the other hand the patients who had productive cough were likely to have a normal cough

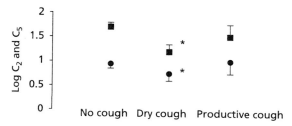

**Fig. 6.1** The log concentration (µmol/L) of capsaicin that caused at least 2 ($C_2$, ●) or at least 5 ($C_5$, ■) coughs. In patients with no cough, dry cough and productive cough, the data are significantly (*$P<0.05$) different in the no cough compared to the other patients. Data from [7].

reflex (Fig. 6.1). In this series (Table 6.1) the exception was a group of patients with bronchiectasis with active infection who as a group had an increased reflex sensitivity likely to be due to the acute inflammation associated with the infection. There is some variability in the data on chronic obstructive pulmonary disease (COPD) who as a group were normal in our study whereas others [11] have seen increases in the sensitivity of the reflex. Our group was stable and screened to rule out acute disease while in the other series the disease activity status was less clear and any active inflammation would change the picture.

In summary, an abnormal reflex is observed in some patient groups with cough and it does relate to the presence of non-productive cough. I would submit that this is sufficiently similar to the early information on bronchial hyperreactivity in asthma to support the use of cough reflex testing to enhance the data of epidemiology studies in respiratory diseases.

**Table 6.1** The various disease groups in the population covered in Fig. 6.1.

| Patient group | $n$ | $C_2 \pm 95\%$ CI | $C_5 \pm 95\%$ CI |
|---|---|---|---|
| (a) *No cough* | | | |
| Normal | 90 | $1.04 \pm 0.02$ | $1.81 \pm 0.14$ |
| ACE-I | 35 | $0.94 \pm 0.18$ | $1.8 \pm 0.1$ |
| Hypertension | 15 | $0.91 \pm 0.27$ | $1.77 \pm 0.36$ |
| Asthma | 18 | $0.87 \pm 0.22$ | $1.49 \pm 0.37$ |
| (b) *Dry cough* | | | |
| Idiopathic | 65 | $0.6 \pm 0.12$ | $1.08 \pm 0.37$ |
| Postnasal drip | 13 | $1.3 \pm 0.49$ | $1.93 \pm 0.39$ |
| Post viral | 5 | $0.59 \pm 0.35$ | $1.14 \pm 0.62$ |
| Asthma | 23 | $0.65 \pm 0.25$ | $1.06 \pm 0.41$ |
| GOR | 14 | $0.54 \pm 0.07$ | $0.8 \pm 0.12$ |
| (c) *Productive cough* | | | |
| Bronchiectasis | 12 | $1.25 \pm 0.41$ | $1.94 \pm 0.38$ |
| Bronchiectasis with infection | 7 | $0.5 \pm 0.22$ | $1.11 \pm 0.58$ |
| COPD | 11 | $0.92 \pm 0.43$ | $1.44 \pm 0.52$ |
| Inflammatory lung disease | 12 | $1.29 \pm 0.53$ | $1.5 \pm 0.51$ |

$C_2$ = log concentration (µmol/L) of capsaicin causing 2 or more coughs.
$C_5$ = log concentration (µmol/L) of capsaicin causing 5 or more coughs.
ACE-I, angiotensin-converting enzyme inhibitor; COPD, chronic obstructive pulmonary disease; GOR, gastro-oesophageal reflux.
Data from [7].

## Clinical management

Cough provocation testing has a potential role in three areas of clinical management: first, as an aid in diagnosis; second, as a guide to prognosis; and finally, as a tool for monitoring the course of treatment.

### Diagnosis

The symptom of cough as noted in the previous section can have several attributes attached to it, i.e. dry (no sputum), productive (sputum), temporal (night, etc.) or provoking (cold air, etc.) events. Unfortunately, none of these attributes narrow down the cause of the cough. Standard history-taking and routine investigations may help identify the cause, which can then be investigated by more specific tests and eventually therapeutic trials. A cough-specific test, which could pinpoint the diagnosis, would therefore be of great clinical value. Does cough provocation testing meet this need? Unfortunately, as the data in Table 6.1 and Fig. 6.1 show, provocation testing can differentiate between productive and dry coughing but not for various causes within those subsets. It can therefore be used only to confirm that aspect of the history which may have some limited value. In addition, it can be used to rule out psychogenic or fictitious cough if the test is performed blind to the subject and yet is still abnormal. These findings appear to be true of all the provocation tests studied sufficiently to date. It is unlikely that provocation testing will be used as a routine in clinical diagnosis but will be reserved as a research tool.

### Prognosis

Like diagnosis, the prognosis of a patient with cough once chronic cannot be easily judged until the success or failure of a therapeutic trial is known. This is not to say that it is not a safe bet to reassure the sufferer of an acute cough during a respiratory infection that their suffering will be relatively short-lived! Theoretically the relative abnormality of a cough provocation test could inform on prognosis. However, there is insufficient information in the studies such as those in Fig. 6.2 to know whether this is a possibility. This question is clearly an area that would benefit from systematic evaluation.

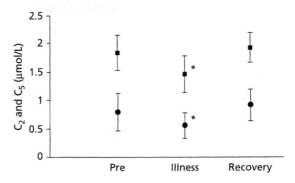

**Fig. 6.2** The log concentration (μmol/L) of capsaicin that caused at least 2 ($C_2$, ●) or at least 5 ($C_5$, ■) coughs. In 31 patients before (Pre), during (Illness) and after (Recovery) upper respiratory infection, the data are significantly different (*$P < 0.05$) in the illness compared to the 'Pre' and 'Recovery' data. Data from [15].

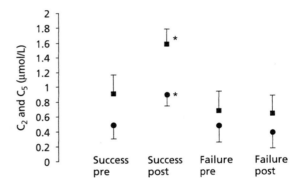

**Fig. 6.3** The log concentration (μmol/L) of capsaicin that caused at least 2 ($C_2$, ●) or at least 5 ($C_5$, ■) coughs. In patients before (pre) and after (post) successful (success $n = 48$) or unsuccessful (failure $n = 39$) treatment of the underlying cause for their cough, the data for the successfully treated patients are significantly (*$P < 0.05$) different from the 'pre' data. Data from [42].

### Monitoring

The monitoring of the clinical course of cough and the response to therapy is a more fruitful area than cough provocation tests. The data exemplified in Figs 6.2 and 6.3 show that an abnormal cough provocation test, if identified, will be present while the disease is active and resolve with the disease. The use of provocation testing can clearly help in this aspect of management especially in a patient with no clear diagnosis that may require a number of therapeutic interventions before the diagnosis is finally made.

A clear case for use of cough provocation comes in the management of neurological diseases where respiratory infection is a common sequela [12]. The loss of a functioning cough reflex is thought to be behind the mechanism for these respiratory infections in patients with a loss of neurological functions.

Efferent testing of cough reflex by asking the patient to cough will usually inform on the capacity of that limb of the reflex. However, it does not inform on the function of the sensory input. Cough provocation will so inform, as a negative provocation test in a patient who can cough voluntarily identifies the perturbation of the sensory limb of the reflex. Data to support such an abnormality are limited to date [13]; however, what data there are support the hypothesis and in view of its importance to the mobility of the patient it does require comprehensive assessment.

## Cough provocation in clinical research

### Pathophysiology

Cough provocation is able to provide an objective measure of the sensitivity of the cough reflex so that its function can be assessed in respiratory disease. It is therefore possible to use it to understand the pathophysiology of cough. Cough is a response either to the need to clear the airway of unwanted material or to an alteration in the sensitivity of the cough reflex as in dry cough. It is therefore of value to understand what may change the sensitivity of the reflex. Cross-sectional studies have shown that in some diseases the reflex can be normal or abnormal, with a suggestion that this is related to the level of activity of the diseased state. Prospective studies have confirmed that in angiotensin-converting enzyme inhibitor-associated cough [14] and common cold-associated cough [15], patients with cough start with a normal reflex which becomes exaggerated with the cough and returns to normal with the resolution of the condition.

What causes this change in the response of the reflex is not fully elucidated. Airway biopsy in a small series of dry cough patients [16] with an abnormal reflex has shown an increase in airway nerve and neuropeptide associated with those nerves. However, prospective studies have yet to be performed. Additional data has been obtained that inhaled $PGE_2$ [17] but not bradykinin or substance P can invoke a temporary change in the sensitivity of the reflex. This would suggest that hyperalgesic mediators could increase the sensory limb of the reflex, probably not by altering the number of fibres in view of the rapidity of the response. The unravelling of the mechanisms behind the change in sensitivity of the cough reflex would give a new basket of targets for developing antitussive drugs.

### Pharmacology

Most of the investigations of the pharmacology of the cough reflex have been made using cough provocation either by citric acid, low $Cl^-$ solution or capsaicin in normal volunteers. In addition there has been some limited investigation of the pharmacology of the exaggerated reflex in patients with dry cough.

Table 6.2 summarizes the results of studies using cough challenge in normal volunteers. This list may well not contain all data, as it is likely that a number of negative investigations are not in the public domain. There is consistent and predictable evidence that local anaesthesia [18] and centrally acting opiates [19] reduce the sensitivity of the reflex, however tested. Other results are either conflicting, e.g. bronchodilatation and inhaled diuretics which have shown positive results in some, but by no means all studies, or are based on the unconfirmed results of one study. If the results are confirmed, then humans [20] like cats [21] may have a 5-HT-dependent cough-suppressing mechanism, which could be exploited for antitussive therapies. Other than that there is little of encouragement from the extensive studies to date.

Equally disappointing is the data in patients with dry cough. A 4-week study with nedocromil sodium was negative [22] and despite anecdotal evidence of non-steroidal anti-inflammatory drugs working in angiotensin-converting enzyme inhibitor cough, controlled trials failed to show an effect on dry cough [23] overall.

## Conclusion

Cough challenge is a safe and easy method for assessing the sensitivity of the cough reflex. However, there are not yet any standards agreed for the methodology,

**Table 6.2** Results of pharmacological studies on cough provocation tests.

| Pharmacological tool (Reference) | Capsaicin | Low Cl⁻ | Citric acid | Other |
|---|---|---|---|---|
| Local anaesthesia [18,24] | ↓ | | ↓ | ↓ |
| Opiates [19,25] | ↓ | | ↓ | ↓ |
| $\beta_2$-Agonists [5,6,26,27] | 0 | ↓ | ± | ↓ |
| Antimuscarinics [6,26,41] | 0 | ↓ | | |
| Antihistamines [28] | 0 | | | |
| 5-HT$_3$ antagonists [29] | 0 | | | |
| 5-HT$_1$ agonists [20] | 0 | | | |
| NSAID [30,31] | 0 | | | |
| Sodium cromoglycate [32] | 0 | | | |
| Nedocromil sodium [33] | 0 | | | |
| Baclofen [34] | ↓ | | | |
| $\alpha_2$-Agonists [35] | 0 | | | |
| Diuretics [36] | 0 | | | |
| MAO-I [37] | 0 | | | |
| Demulcents [38,39] | ↓ | | ↓ | |
| Antileukotriene [40] | 0 | | | |

MAO-I, monoamine oxidase inhibitor; NSAID, non-steroidal anti-inflammatory drug.
↓, Reduced; ±, equivocal or conflicting data; 0, no effect.

which tend to be laboratory specific making comparisons between studies difficult. As well as data compatibility issues, the different methodologies occasionally lead to results that need explaining, such as differences between males and females, adults and children and in COPD. These differences could be true physiological variability or artefacts of methodology and this needs to be resolved through a consensus on methodology.

Despite the methodological issues there is sufficient evidence that the provocation tests can detect differences in the sensitivity of the reflex in disease. These differences make the cough challenge of likely value in epidemiology studies, some aspects of clinical management and in particular in hypothesis testing. In hypothesis testing it is difficult to imagine a strategy to unravel the pathophysiology and pharmacology of the reflex without using cough challenge even if the results require validation in large studies using more clinical end-points.

# References

1 Fuller RW, Jackson DM. Physiology and treatment of cough. *Thorax* 1990; **45**: 425–30.

2 Prime FJ. The assessment of antitussive drugs in man. *Br Med J* 1961; April 22: 1149–51.

3 Tiffeneau R. The acetylcholine cough test. *Dis Chest* 1957; **31**: 404–22.

4 Janson C, Chinn S, Jarvis D, Burney P. Determinants of cough in young adults participating in the European Community Respiratory Health Survey. *Eur Respir J* 2001; **18**: 647–54.

5 Lowry R, Wood A, Johnson T, Higenbottam T. Antitussive properties of inhaled bronchodilators on induced cough. *Chest* 1988; **93/6**: 1186–9.

6 Pounsford JC, Birch MJ, Saunders KB. Effect of bronchodilators on the cough response to inhaled citric acid in normal and asthmatic subjects. *Thorax* 1985; **40**: 662–7.

7 Choudry NB, Fuller RW. Sensitivity of the cough reflex in patients with chronic cough. *Eur Respir J* 1992; **5**: 296–300.

8 Chang AB, Phelan PD, Roberts RGD, Robertson CF. Capsaicin cough receptor sensitivity test in children. *Eur Respir J* 1996; **9**: 2220–3.

9 Stone RA. *Investigations into the neural control of the cough reflex*. PhD thesis, Department of Thoracic Medicine, Royal Brompton National Heart and Lung Institute, University of London, December 1992.

10 Dicpinigaitis PV, Rauf K. The influence of gender on cough reflex sensitivity. *Chest* 1998; **113**: 1319–21.

11 Doherty MJ, Mister R, Pearson MG, Calverley PMA. Capsaicin responsiveness and cough in asthma and chronic obstructive pulmonary disease. *Thorax* 2000; **55**: 643–9.

12 Smith Hammond CA, Goldstein LB, Zajac DJ, Gray L, Davenport PW, Bolser DC. Assessment of aspiration risk in stroke patients with quantification of voluntary cough. *Neurology* 2001; **56**: 502–6.

13 Addington WR, Stephens RE, Gilliland KA. Assessing the laryngeal cough reflex and the risk of developing pneumonia after stroke—an interhospital comparison. *Stroke* 1999; **30**: 1203–7.

14 McEwan JR, Choudry N, Street R, Fuller RW. Change in cough reflex after treatment with enalapril and ramipril. *Br Med J* 1989; **299**: 13–6.

15 O'Connell F, Thomas VE, Studham JM, Pride NB, Fuller RW. Capsaicin cough sensitivity increases during upper respiratory infection. *Respir Med* 1996; **90**: 279–86.

16 O'Connell F, Springall DR, Moradoghli-Haftvani A, Krausz T, Price D, Fuller RW, Polak JM, Pride NB. Abnormal intraepithelial airway nerves in persistent unexplained cough? *Am J Respir Crit Care Med* 1995; **152**: 2068–75.

17 Choudry NB, Fuller RW, Pride NB. Sensitivity of the human cough reflex: effect of inflammatory mediators prostaglandin E2, bradykinin and histamine. *Am Rev Rep Dis* 1989; **140**: 137–41.

18 Choudry NB, Fuller RW, Anderson N, Karlsson J-A. Separation of cough and reflex bronchoconstriction by inhaled local anaesthetics. *Eur Respir J* 1990; **3**: 579–83.

19 Fuller RW, Karlsson J-A, Choudry NB, Pride NB. Effect of inhaled and systemic opiates on responses to inhaled capsaicin in humans. *Am Physiol Soc* 1988; **88**: 1125–30.

20 Stone RA, Worsdell YM, Fuller RW, Barnes PJ. Effect of 5-hydroxytryptamine and 5-hydroxytryptophan on sensitivity of the human cough reflex. *J Appl Physiol* 1993; **74**: 396–401.

21 Karlsson J-A, Fuller RW. Pharmacological regulation of the cough reflex—from experimental models to antitussive effects in man. *Pulm Pharmacol Ther* 1999; **12**: 215–28.

22 Choudry NB. *Investigation of the sensitivity of the cough reflex in humans*. MD thesis, Faculty of Medicine, University of London, December 1990.

23 McEwan JR, Choudry NB, Fuller RW. The effect of sulindac on the abnormal cough reflex associated with dry cough. *J Pharmacol Exp Ther* 1990; **255**: 161–4.

24 Addington WR, Stephens RE, Goulding RE. Anesthesia of the superior laryngeal nerves and tartaric acid-induced cough. *Arch Phys Med Rehabil* 1999; **80**: 1584–6.

25 Empey DW, Laitinen LA, Young GA, Bye CE, Hughes DTD. Comparison of the antitussive effects of codeine phosphate 20 mg, dextromethorphan 30 mg and noscapine 30 mg using citric acid-induced cough in normal subjects. *Eur J Clin Pharmacol* 1979; **16**: 393–7.

26 Choudry NB, Fuller RW. Effect of airway calibre on the sensitivity of the human cough reflex. *Thorax* 1990; **45**: 311P–12P.

27 Katsumata U, Sekizawa K, Inoue H, Sasaki H, Takishima T. Inhibitory actions of procaterol, a beta-2 stimulant, on substance P-induced cough in normal subjects during upper respiratory tract infection. *Tohoku J Exp Med* 1989; **158**: 105–6.

28 Studham J, Fuller RW. The effect of oral terfenadine on the sensitivity of the cough reflex in normal volunteers. *Pulm Pharmacol*, 1992; **5** (1): 51–2.

29 Choudry NB, McEwan JR, Lavender EA, Williams AJ, Fuller RW. Human responses to inhaled capsaicin are not inhibited by granisetron. *Br J Clin Pharmacol* 1991; **31** (3): 337–9.

30 Stone RA, Barnes PJ, Fuller RW. The low-chloride cough response is not inhibited by a single, high dose of aspirin. *Br J Clin Pharmacol* 1992; **34**: 370–2.

31 Dicpinigaitis PV. Effect of the cyclooxygenase-2 inhibitor celecoxib on bronchial responsiveness and cough reflex sensitivity in asthmatics. *Pulm Pharmacol Ther* 2001; **14**: 93–7.

32 Collier JG, Fuller RW. The effect of inhaled capsaicin in man and the action of SCG on this response. *Br J Pharmacol* 1984; **81**: 113–7.

33 Hansson L, Choudry NB, Fuller RW, Pride NB. Effect of nedocromil sodium on the airway response to inhaled capsaicin in normal subjects. *Thorax* 1988; **43**: 935–6.

34 Dicpinigaitis PV, Dobkin JB. Antitussive effect of the GABA-agonist baclofen. *Chest* 1997; **111**: 996–9.

35 O'Connell F, Thomas VE, Fuller RW, Pride NB, Karlsson J-A. Effect of clonidine on induced cough and bronchoconstriction in guinea pigs and humans. *J Appl Physiol* 1994; **76**: 1082–7.

36 Karlsson JA, Choudry NB, Zackrisson C, Fuller RW. A comparison of the effect of inhaled diuretics on airway reflexes in humans and guinea pigs. *J Appl Physiol* 1992; **1**: 72 (2), 434–8.

37 Choudry NB, Studham J, Harland D, Fuller RW. Modulation of capsaicin induced airway reflexes in humans: effect of monoamine oxidase inhibition. *Br J Clin Pharmacol* 1993; **35**: 184–7.

38 Packman EW, London SJ. The utility of artificially induced cough as a clinical model for evaluating the antitussive effects of aromatics delivered by inunction. *Eur J Respir Dis* 1980; **110** (Suppl.): 101–9.

39 Fuller RW, Haase G, Choudry NB. The effect of dextromethophan cough syrup on capsaicin-induced cough in normal volunteers. *Am Rev Respir Dis* 1989; **139**: A11.

40  Dicpinigaitis PV, Dobkin JB. Effect of zafirlukast on cough reflex sensitivity in asthmatics. *J Asthma* 1999; **36** (3): 265–70.

41  Fuller RW. Pharmacology of inhaled capsaicin in humans. *Respir Med* 1991; **85** (Suppl. A): 31–4.

42  O'Connell F, Thomas VE, Pride NB, Fuller RW. Capsaicin cough sensitivity decreases with successful treatment of chronic cough. *Am J Respir Crit Care Med* 1994; **150**: 374–80.

# 7 Causes, assessment and measurement of cough in children

*Anne B. Chang*

## Introduction

The prevalence of childhood cough without wheeze is high, 12.8–15.5% [1] in community studies based on parent-completed questionnaires, and that of nocturnal cough varies from 4.9 to 28.1% [2,3]. This high prevalence raises the question as to when childhood cough should be considered 'normal' or pathological. In childhood, cough may be 'normal' [4] or a symptom of any respiratory illness and rarely of a non-respiratory illness. The management of childhood cough [4,5] differs from that of adults [6]; and paediatricians worldwide have long been passionate about managing childhood illness differently from that of adults, and about the dangers of extrapolating adult data to young children. The pattern of respiratory illness in children can be clearly different from that in adults. For example, viruses associated with the common cold in adults can cause life-threatening illness in children, such as bronchiolitis and croup; the natural history of asthma in children is dominated by decreasing severity with age and, in some, complete resolution [7] whereas asthma acquired in adulthood usually persists. The aetiology and management of childhood cough should also be clearly distinguished from adult cough. Extrapolation of adult cough literature to children can be harmful, for example the suggestion of fundoplication for gastro-oesophageal reflux as the sole symptom of cough without evidence of secondary aspiration [8] is inappropriate for children. Indeed current evidence suggests that it is erroneous to extrapolate the three commonest causes of cough in adults (cough-variant asthma, postnasal drip, gastro-oesophageal reflux) to children [9,10]. This chapter discusses the issues of cough unique to children.

## Causes of cough in children

The aetiology of cough can be broadly divided into groups of primary pathophysiology, although there is undoubtedly an overlap in the pathophysiology of some diseases (Table 7.1). The first clinical challenge that faces the physician is deciphering whether the cough is 'normal' or 'expected', non-specific or specific. Non-specific overlaps with both 'normal/expected' and specific cough, but 'expected' cough is distinctly separate from specific cough (Fig. 7.1). The relative frequency of each category will depend on the setting, and general practitioners would more likely encounter 'expected/normal' cough whereas in a tertiary setting specific cough would dominate. These descriptions and the common and/or controversial aetiologies of childhood cough are briefly discussed below. A complete clinical review of each specific aetiology is beyond the scope of this chapter and can be found in standard paediatric respiratory textbooks.

## Cough categories

### 'Normal' or 'expected' cough

Diagnosing this category of cough requires the most skill and experience [4]. All cough is arguably representative of some process. However, as the cough reflex is subjected to cortical modulation [9] and can be

**Table 7.1** Causes of cough in children.

---

*Infectious*
Acute, subacute
  Viral infections, mycoplasma, chlamydia, pneumocystis, etc.
Chronic
  Tuberculosis, non-TB mycobacteria, fungal
Suppurative lung disease
  Cystic fibrosis, ciliary dyskinesia, postpneumonia, immunodeficiency (primary or
    secondary)

*Allergy/inflammatory*
Asthma
Postviral
Nasal space disease (see text)
? Eosinophilic bronchitis

*Airway clearance*
1 Aspiration
  (a) Primary: bulbar lesions, laryngopalatal discoordination, cerebral palsy,
      Moebius syndrome, vocal cord palsy
  (b) Secondary: gastro-oesophageal reflux
  (c) Anatomical: laryngeal cleft, tracheo-oesophageal fistula, tonsil–adenoid
      hypertrophy
2 Airway lesions
  (a) Primary: laryngomalacia, bronchomalacia, tracheomalacia
  (b) Secondary: external compression (vascular slings, tumours, etc.), intraluminal
      lesions, foreign body

*Pulmonary toxicants*
Tobacco
Particulate matter
Gaseous
Biomass combustion

*Primary lung disease*
Interstitial lung disease
Pulmonary hypertension
Congenital bronchiolitis of infancy
Tumours
Follicular bronchiolitis
Bronchiolitis obliterans
Pulmonary vascular congestion

*Non-pulmonary disease*
Drugs
  Angiotensin-converting enzyme inhibitors
Cardiac disease
  Arrhythmias
Psychological
  Psychogenic cough
  Habit, tic
Gastro-oesophageal reflux without aspiration

---

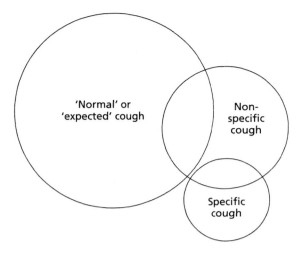

**Fig. 7.1** Broad categories of childhood cough. The diagram depicts the overlap between the categories of childhood cough. Non-specific cough overlaps with both specific cough and 'normal or expected cough', whereas specific cough is distinct from 'normal or expected cough'.

**Table 7.2** Specific cough pointers.

*Presence of*:
Haemoptysis
Recurrent pneumonia
Exertional dyspnoea
Chronic sputum production
Wheeze
Stridor
Immune deficiency
Cardiac abnormality
Swallowing difficulties
Dyspnoea
Chest deformity
Clubbing
Ausculatory abnormality
Poor growth

voluntarily initiated, it is not surprising that cough (1–34 per 24 h) can be found in 'normal' children free of a respiratory infection in the previous 4 weeks [11]. In another study, age-, sex- and season-matched 'normal controls' have 0–141 coughs per day (median 10) [12]. In this study, children with recent viral infections were not excluded but were considered well by their parents. Children can have 6–8 viral acute respiratory infections (ARIs) per year, especially when they are in daycare centres, and arguably childhood cough within this spectrum can be considered 'normal' or 'expected'. Children with recurrent cough who present to a tertiary centre do have a higher cough frequency than controls, and have a higher cough frequency during the day than the night [12].

## Specific cough

Specific refers to cough to which a definable cause (or causes) can be attributed. In specific cough, pointers of respiratory impairment are usually present. The aetiology and necessity of further investigations is usually evident from the presence of these pointers (Table 7.2).

## Non-specific cough

In non-specific cough, the cough is dry and pointers of respiratory impairment are absent. The aetiology may be ill-defined and we suspect that the majority is related to postviral cough and/or increased cough receptor sensitivity [13,14]. In non-specific cough, there is no serious underlying condition and the child is otherwise well.

## Brief overview of common causes and controversies

### Cough and respiratory infections

The spectrum of respiratory infections causing cough varies from benign (e.g. common cold) to life-threatening infections (e.g. lung abscess, pneumocystis pnuemonia). The manifestation of the infection depends on various pathogens, 'host or patient' factors (asthma, immunodeficiency, established cardiopulmonary impairment, malnutrition, genetics, etc.) and environmental factors (smoke, biomass combustion exposure).

ARIs and post-ARI-associated cough are the most common causes of childhood cough. In Australia, the reported use of medications for coughs and colds in the 2 weeks before assessment was 167 and 87 per 1000 for children under 5 years and children between 5 and 14 years, respectively, corresponding to the most frequently and third most frequently used medications in their respective age groups [15]. Approximately US $2 billion per year is spent on cough and cold remedies in the US [16]. A national US survey reported that approximately 35% of 8145 preschool-aged children had used 'over the counter' medications for cough in the past 30 days [16].

It is sometimes argued that 'the common cold', an upper respiratory infection, should not cause cough, and the presence of cough reflects the presence of a lower respiratory tract infection. However, lower airway inflammation has been demonstrated in children with colds, not only in the active phase but also in those who were asymptomatic 1–14 days before a bronchoalveolar lavage was taken [17]. Also, clinically unapparent alterations in lower airway function occur during upper ARI in infants, children and adults [18].

There are few prospective epidemiological data on the length of cough associated with a common cold in children. In one study, 80% of adults were cough free by 2 weeks [19] and cough sensitivity has been shown to be increased during upper ARIs [20]. Transient enhanced cough sensitivity has also been shown in children with influenza infection [21]. Like the clinical manifestation of ARIs, the length of cough most likely depends on patient and environmental factors.

## Cough and asthma in children

There is little doubt that children with asthma may present with cough and that wheeze may be absent during physical examination. Isolated cough has been postulated as a marker of asthma, and improper interpretation of cough as a symptom was previously thought to be a key factor in the underdiagnosis of asthma. However, more recently increasing numbers of children are misdiagnosed as having asthma on the basis of cough alone [22–24], although there is also ongoing concern that children with significant asthma symptoms are still being missed and consequently undertreated [25]. The importance of cough in the diagnosis of asthma and the frequency of cough-variant asthma is debatable [23]. Current epidemiological, inflammatory and cohort studies suggest that most cough in children is not asthma [23,26,27] and most cough in children spontaneously resolves [26,28]. A review on this is available elsewhere [9].

Recent work on airway inflammatory markers in community children with isolated persistent cough show that, unlike in the adult, most children with persistent isolated cough do not have asthma, since their airway inflammatory markers are significantly differ-ent from those in children with asthma [27,29]. How many children in the community with persistent cough do indeed have asthma is unknown. There are only two randomized controlled trials on the use of current asthma medications in children with isolated cough [30,31]. Both studies objectively measured cough, which is crucial, since cough as an outcome measure is subjective and unreliable [32]. Neither recommended prolonged or high doses of asthma-type therapy when managing these children [30,31].

Indeed, the misdiagnosis of isolated cough as asthma is not uncommon [23,24,33]. We recently showed that the overdiagnosis of asthma and the overuse of asthma treatments with significant side-effects, in children with persistent cough referred to a respiratory clinic, is common [24]. While a trial of asthma-type medications may be considered, the child must be reviewed and, if the cough does not respond to the asthma therapy, the diagnosis must be withdrawn and the medications stopped [4,5]. Failure to do so will lead to escalating doses being used with significant side-effects [24]. There is however, difficulty in defining what constitutes a response to treatment, particularly when the natural resolution of the underlying condition such as viral respiratory infection may mimic a response to treatment. Recurrence of cough on cessation and elimination of cough upon commencement of inhaled corticosteroids is sometimes necessary for confident diagnosis [4]. The original studies describing cough as a manifestation of asthma showed that the cough responded within a week to medications used for asthma during that era (theophylline and hypnotics) [34,35]. It could be argued that the currently available more potent anti-inflammatory medications for asthma would reduce the symptoms as efficaciously, if not more so. However, following an acute exacerbation of asthma, cough was present in 23% of children [36]. In this group of children whether the cough is related to concurrent viral respiratory infections, the cause of asthma exacerbations in 80% of children [37], or a marker of non-resolution of asthma is unknown. Markers of cough severity are known to correlate poorly with clinical, inflammatory and spirometry markers of asthma severity [38]. The relationship between cough and asthma is complex [39,40] and beyond the scope of this chapter.

The existence of cough-dominant asthma, where cough is a dominant feature of asthma exacerbations in patients with classical asthma, is recognized in both the paediatric [41] and the adult literature [42]. However, whether cough-dominant asthma represents a truly different phenotype is not yet confirmed at the cellular or genetic level. Increasingly asthma phenotypes are recognized and 'treatment response genes' to $\beta_2$-receptor agonists have recently been described. However, for clinicians, the aetiology of isolated cough in children with asthma can be difficult to determine, when objective markers such as spirometry are unavailable. Cough is included in asthma severity scales [43], and in children without wheeze the presence of this isolated symptom can categorize children into the moderately severe group. Isolated cough in children with asthma can be associated with any other respiratory illness, or with environmental exposure. Several studies on air pollution (environmental tobacco smoke, bioaerosols) have shown that air pollution is more likely to affect children with asthma than those without, and cough is the major symptom manifestation [44]. Many studies have shown a poor relationship between cough and other markers of asthma (day and night oxygen saturations $(S_pO_2)$, lung volumes, airway resistance $(R_{aw})$, peak expiratory flow (PEF) and variability, spirometry) in children with asthma during a non-acute phase as well in the recovery phase of an acute exacerbation, as recently summarized [40].

## Does 'allergic or atopic cough' exist in children?

This poorly defined condition is probably an overlap with asthma and eosinophilic bronchitis, a condition well recognized in adults but not well defined in children. The association between atopy and respiratory symptoms has been the subject of many epidemiological studies [45,46]. Some have described greater respiratory symptom chronicity [1] but others have not [45,46]. In the seminal prospective study of infants followed up to 11 years old, the Tuscon group showed that recurrent cough present early in life resolved in the majority of children [26]. These children with recurrent cough and without wheeze did not have airway hyperresponsiveness (AHR) or atopy and significantly differed from those with classical asthma with or without cough [26]. These important differences were: maternal allergy, wheezing, airway respiratory infection, high IgE, atopy, reduced maximal flow $(\dot{V}_{max})$ at functional residual capacity (FRC) (significant for asthma) and exposure to tobacco smoke (significant for recurrent cough). In laboratory and clinical studies, others have studied the association between

atopy, AHR, asthma and cough [14,30,47]. In these studies, AHR is an important confounder associated with atopy and is independent of other respiratory symptoms [48,49]. Studies where confounding variables were not controlled, and where standard criteria for AHR were not observed, can be misleading in their conclusions [47].

## Cough and gastro-oesophageal reflux (GOR) in children

Aspiration lung disease can result from laryngopalatal discoordination or discoordinated swallowing (primary aspiration), or severe GOR (secondary aspiration). Children with primary aspiration may present with chronic cough but usually in the context of severe developmental or neurological disturbance. The investigatory evidence for aspiration lung disease can be difficult but it is important to exclude this diagnosis in the correct setting as recurrent aspiration may lead to chronic respiratory illnesses such as bronchiectasis and bronchiolitis obliterans. Oesophageal disorders can undoubtedly trigger cough in children which may cause cough by at least three mechanisms: aspiration of gastric contents, acid reflux and volume reflux. However, while GOR can cause cough, cough can also cause GOR and causative links are hard to identify [50]. The relationship between the two is probably complex. The view that GOR is a frequent cause of cough in adults has been challenged [51,52]. Like the difference between the paediatric and adult literature for asthma and cough, there is indeed little evidence that GOR without aspiration is a specific or frequent cause of cough in children. As cough is very common in children and respiratory symptoms may exacerbate GOR, it is difficult to delineate cause and effect. Infants regularly regurgitate [53], yet few, if any, well infants cough with these episodes.

## Cough and nasal space disease

In adults, sinusitis/postnasal drip is a common cause of cough. In children, there is little supportive evidence for this condition [10]. There are no cough receptors in the pharynx or postnasal space [42]. Although sinusitis is common in childhood, it is not associated with asthma or cough once allergic rhinitis, a common association, is treated [54]. The relationship between nasal secretions and cough is more likely linked by common aetiology (infection and/or inflammation causing both) or due to throat clearing of secretions reaching the larynx. In a prospective study, 50% of 137 children aged under 13 years had CT sinus scans consistent with sinusitis but all were asymptomatic [55]. Abnormal sinus radiographs may be found in 18–82% of asymptomatic children [56]. Using a continuous infusion of 2.5 mL/min of distilled water into the pharynx of asymptomatic adults, Nishino *et al.* demonstrated that laryngeal irritation and cough only occurred in the presence of hypercapnia (45–55 mmHg) [57], suggesting that pharyngeal secretion itself does not cause cough.

## Cough and chronic suppurative lung disease

This is an essential diagnosis that should never be missed. Children with bronchiectasis have a chronic moist or productive cough and are typically but not always finger-clubbed. The cough is characteristically worse in the mornings. Physical findings are non-specific; clubbing, pectus carinatum, and coarse crepitations and localized wheeze may or may not be present. Plain chest radiography will suggest features in severe disease (dilated and thickened bronchi may appear as 'tramtracks') but is insensitive in mild disease. Confirmation is by high-resolution computed tomography (CT) scan of the chest (routine CT scan provides insufficient detail). A child with suspected bronchiectasis should be referred for investigation of a specific cause and specific treatment instituted when indicated (e.g. cystic fibrosis, primary ciliary dyskinesia, immunodeficiency).

## Cough and airway lesions in children

Cough can be due to intrinsic (tracheomalacia and bronchomalacia) [58,59] and extrinsic (foreign bodies and other endobronchial obstruction) airway lesions. An inhaled foreign body usually presents in the acute stage, with a history of acute cough following a choking event, but may be found many years later [24]. When the foreign body causes a ball-valve effect, air trapping seen in an expiratory film when compared with an inspiratory chest radiograph (CXR) may be useful. When suspected, bronchoscopy allows for the definitive diagnostic and concomitant therapeutic procedure. Airway malacia disorders (tracheomalacia, bronchomalacia) are well recognized causes of persistent and/or recurrent cough in children [24,58,59], but not

in adults [60]. In one study, 75% of children with tracheomalacia secondary to congenital vascular anomaly had persistent cough at presentation [58], whereas of 24 adults with tracheomalacia secondary to vascular rings 16 were symptomatic and none complained of cough [60]. The pathophysiology of cough in the presence of airway lesions is poorly understood but is possibly related to a localized bronchitic process.

## Environmental causes

*In utero* tobacco smoke exposure alters pulmonary development and physiology [61]. How this influences the developmental aspects of the central and peripheral cough pathways as well as the plasticity of the cough pathway is unknown. Exposure to environmental smoke and other ambient pollutants (particulate matter [62], nitrogen dioxide, etc.) is associated with increased cough in children, especially in the presence of other respiratory illness such as asthma [62]. Irrespective of the primary aetiology of cough, exposure to environmental smoke can exacerbate the frequency and severity of cough.

## Other causes of cough

Other than habitual cough, non-respiratory causes of cough are rare, but should be considered when appropriate clinical features are present.

## Habitual and psychogenic cough

Habitual cough or cough as a 'vocal tic' may be transient or chronic. While psychogenic cough is more common in adolescents, the habitual cough occurs in younger children. The mean age of diagnosis for habitual cough ranges from 4 to 15 years [63]. The typical psychogenic cough (honking cough) is recognizable and can often be heard even before the child is seen. Irrespective of the cause of cough, psychological influences on severity of cough have been documented in both children [64] and adults.

## Assessment in children

Cough is a very common symptom of respiratory disease. As cough is audible and can interfere with sleep and may represent serious underlying disorders such as cystic fibrosis, it is not surprising that parents are often anxious about their children's cough and often seek medical advice and remedy. Parental concerns may differ significantly from physicians' concerns. Physicians are usually concerned about the aetiology of cough and getting the correct diagnosis. Parental concerns, however, often relate to their perceived effects of cough on their child (sleep, choking, permanent chest damage) [65].

## Clinical assessment

When presented with a child with a cough, the key questions are aimed at clearly defining the nature and impact of the cough on the child and family:
1 Is it a symptom of an underlying problem?
2 Are there possible modifiers of exacerbation and/or contributing factors?
3 How does the cough affect the child and parents?
4 Is it necessary to investigate?
5 Are any treatment modalities available or necessary?

The clinical assessment of cough can be approached from many ways, e.g. dry vs. moist, age of the child and length of cough. Each obviously influences the others and none can be considered in isolation. A suggested pathway primarily based on the length of cough is presented (Fig. 7.2) [5]. The aetiology of cough that backdates to infancy is clearly different to that of recent onset. A history of chronicity or exertional dyspnoea may not be offered unless specifically asked for. Cough associated with pointers of respiratory impairment (Table 7.2) are immediately differentiated (pathway III in Fig. 7.2c) irrespective of the historical length of cough. These pathways are only a guide and based on clinical experience and available scientific literature. In paediatrics there are indeed insufficient data to provide a comprehensive evidence-based approach.

In a child with persistent cough, the initial clinical challenge is deciphering whether the persistent cough is specific or non-specific. The definition of persistent or chronic cough varies (> 3–6 weeks) and the aetiological factors in children vary from the benign to life-threatening causes. Specific pointers should be sought from a thorough history and examination (Table 7.2). In specific cough, the aetiology and necessity of further investigations is usually evident from the presence of coexisting symptoms and signs. The presence of any of these pointers suggests that the cough is likely to represent an underlying disorder and that further complex investigations are probably indicated, other than symmetrical polyphonic wheeze representative of asthma. The type of investigations depends on the clinical findings. Diagnoses that need to be considered include bronchiectasis, retained foreign body, aspiration lung disease, atypical respiratory infections, cardiac anomalies and interstitial lung disease, amongst other diseases. The diagnosis and management of cough associated with an underlying disorder is most appropriately undertaken by paediatric respiratory physicians and will not be discussed further in this chapter.

In deciding the aetiology of the child's cough, Bush [4] suggests that the child's cough can be placed in one of the five categories:
1 Normal.
2 A serious illness such as cystic fibrosis (rare but essential to get right).
3 An unserious but treatable cause (e.g. GOR).
4 A child with an asthma syndrome.
5 Overestimation of symptoms for psychological or other reasons by either or both child or family.

An additional category to the above would be:
6 A non-respiratory cause such as habitual cough, medications (ACE inhibitors), etc.

Exposure to tobacco smoke is the most important modifier of childhood cough and is known to increase susceptibility to respiratory infections [66], cause adverse respiratory health outcomes and increase coughing illnesses [67]. When appropriate, a non-judgmental discussion of how tobacco smoke affects children forms part of any clinical management of a child with a cough.

### Effect on parents and child

In childhood illnesses, parental expectations often drive presentations to medical personnel [68]. In adults with asthma, asthma severity determined emergency presentations whereas in paediatrics, parental anxiety was found to be the most important factor [69]. In a study on upper respiratory tract infection, the main reason for repeated consultations for the same episode occurred when parental expectations about the natural history of the illness were not fulfilled [68]. When adopting a 'wait and see' approach in a child with non-specific cough, discussing parental expectations, concerns and anxiety often proves useful, diagnostically and therapeutically.

(a)

## Pathway I: Coughing child and length of cough

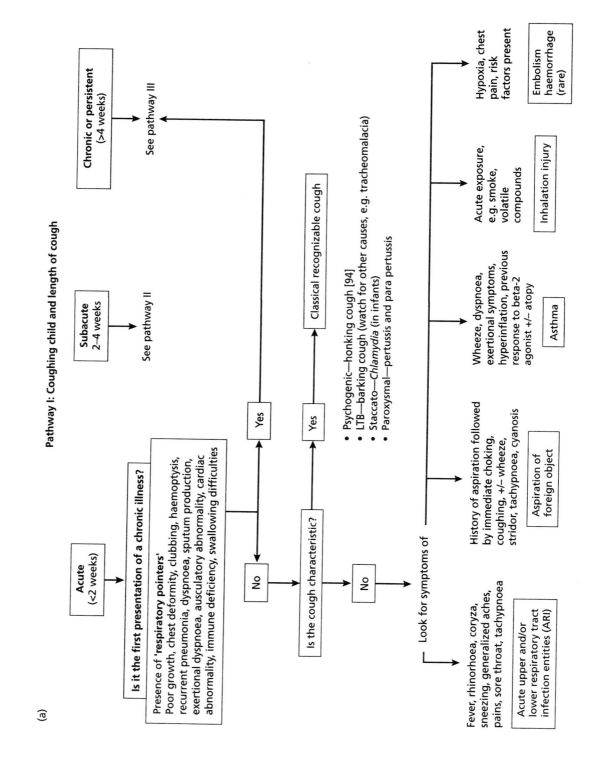

**Acute (<2 weeks)**

**Subacute 2–4 weeks**

See pathway II

**Chronic or persistent (>4 weeks)**

See pathway III

**Is it the first presentation of a chronic illness?**

Presence of 'respiratory pointers'
Poor growth, chest deformity, clubbing, haemoptysis, recurrent pneumonia, dyspnoea, sputum production, exertional dyspnoea, ausculatory abnormality, cardiac abnormality, immune deficiency, swallowing difficulties

Yes

No

**Is the cough characteristic?**

Yes

Classical recognizable cough

- Psychogenic—honking cough [94]
- LTB—barking cough (watch for other causes, e.g. tracheomalacia)
- Staccato—*Chlamydia* (in infants)
- Paroxysmal—pertussis and para pertussis

No

Look for symptoms of

Fever, rhinorrhoea, coryza, sneezing, generalized aches, pains, sore throat, tachypnoea

Acute upper and/or lower respiratory tract infection entities (ARI)

History of aspiration followed by immediate choking, coughing, +/− wheeze, stridor, tachypnoea, cyanosis

Aspiration of foreign object

Wheeze, dyspnoea, exertional symptoms, hyperinflation, previous response to beta-2 agonist +/− atopy

Asthma

Acute exposure, e.g. smoke, volatile compounds

Inhalation injury

Hypoxia, chest pain, risk factors present

Embolism haemorrhage (rare)

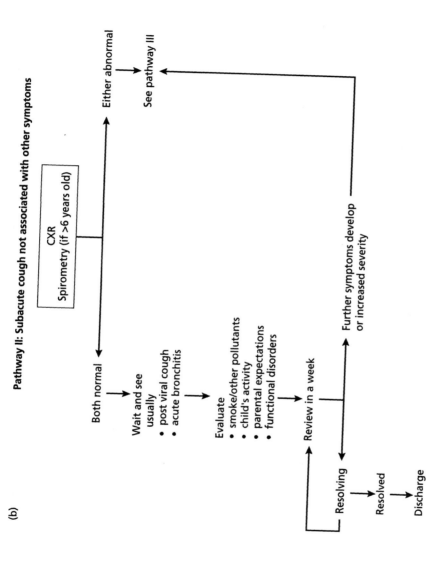

**Pathway II: Subacute cough not associated with other symptoms**

**Fig. 7.2** An approach to cough based on length of cough. These pathways are a guide to the approach to a child with a cough. However, most childhood coughs are benign and do not require drug therapy or investigations. The suggested approach depends on the length of cough (pathway I) and whether any symptoms and/or signs are present ('pointers' listed in pathway I). Symptoms and signs can be age dependent and thus the child's age and severity of illness must also be considered when approaching a child with cough. It would not be possible to factor the various possible combinations in these pathways. Note: ARI could coexist with another diagnosis. ARI, acute respiratory infection; CRS, cough receptor sensitivity; CXR, chest X-ray; FTT, failure to thrive; GOR, gastro-oesophageal reflux; HRCT, high-resolution computed tomography of the chest; LTB, laryngotracheobronchitis; TOF, tracheo-oesophageal fistula; TB, tuberculosis; UA, upper airway. Adapted with permission from [5]. (*Continued on p. 66.*)

(c)

**Pathway III: Chronic/persistent cough (>4 weeks) or acute/subacute cough associated with other symptoms**

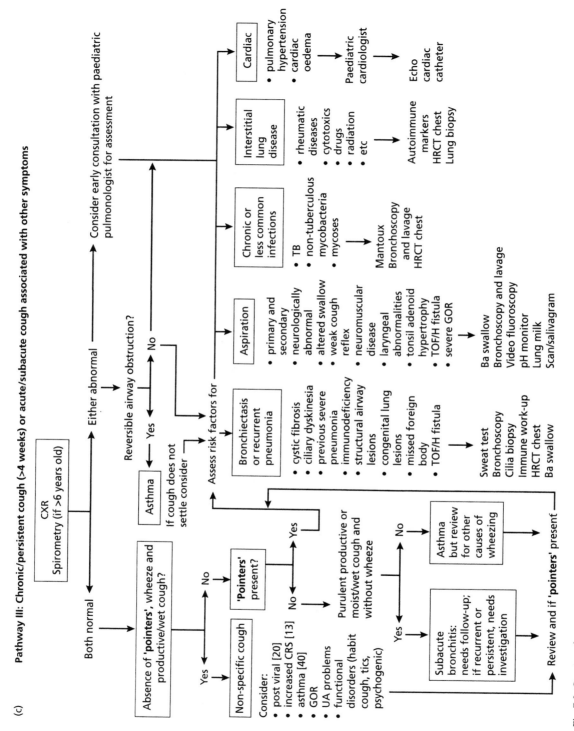

Fig. 7.2 *Continued.*

Exploring the effects of the cough on the child includes how the child deals with the cough in school, exercise and other activities. Children are sometimes requested to leave the class and prevented from participating in physical activity, and these negative elements may perpetuate or intensify cough. In our clinical experience, parents usually restrain their child's physical activities and we suspect that this can lead to 'sick child' syndrome.

## Investigative assessment

Investigation for a child with a cough may be appropriate and intensive, depending on history and examination of the clinical setting (pathway III, Fig. 7.2c). The majority of children with cough will, however, have cough of short duration and the cough is 'expected' or within the limits of normality of childhood illness [4]. In the primary care setting, the majority of children with cough do not require further investigations. The approach in a tertiary setting would clearly be different. In children with persistent cough, however, the minimum investigations are spirometry (if over 6 years old) and a chest radiograph. The more controversial and research-based investigations are described below.

### Is AHR determination useful in children?

In paediatrics, unlike work on adults, the demonstration of AHR in a child with isolated cough is unhelpful in predicting the later development of asthma [70] or the response to asthma medications [30]. However others who have stated that the presence of AHR in children with cough is representative of asthma did not use placebo-controlled studies, or confounders were not adjusted for, or an unconventional definition of AHR was used [35,71]. In a randomized placebo-controlled trial on the use of inhaled salbutamol and corticosteroids in children with recurrent cough, the presence of AHR could not predict the efficacy of these medications for cough [30]. A recent study has shown that AHR to hypertonic saline is significantly associated with wheeze and dyspnoea but not associated with dry cough or nocturnal cough once confounders were accounted for [72]. Koh et al. suggested that children with 'cough-variant asthma' (CVA) required a greater amount of methacholine to induce a wheeze which was only audible when their $FEV_1$ was lower, when compared with children with classical asthma [73]. However in their study the investigators were not blinded to

the category of the child and wheeze was determined subjectively. The concept that children with CVA require a greater fall in $FEV_1$ to induce a wheeze is interesting but questionable. Moreover, if this was so, a decrease in $FEV_1$ should still be detectable despite the absence of wheeze during a coughing episode in those with 'CVA', given that $PC_{20}$ (the concentration of methacholine that caused a 20% fall in $FEV_1$) was not different between the two groups [73].

### Airways resistance by the interrupter technique ($R_{int}$)

This measurement, not yet established in clinical practice, may prove to be useful in detecting isolated cough associated with asthma [74]. Despite its application in research, there are still problems with intersubject variability and hence validity of its measurements when undertaken by different investigators [75].

### Is cough sensitivity determination clinically useful?

The concept of 'hyperresponsiveness of cough receptors' in childhood respiratory disease was first raised by Mitsuhashi et al. [76]. Using acetic acid to assess cough reflex sensitivity (CRS), the study described a group of children with asthma who had increased CRS. However the groups were not matched for age and apart from atopy no clinical associations were made [76]. Later, using nebulized citric acid in a group of children who had been questioned 2 years before the cough challenge test, Riordan et al. studied the relationship between CRS and respiratory symptoms, and found no relationship [77]. Since then several other studies have described altered CRS in different diseases using better methods of measuring CRS and symptom ascertainment [14,21,41].

Adults with chronic cough that are subsequently well controlled demonstrate invariably a normalization of their pretreatment-enhanced capsaicin tussive response [78]. This has not been shown in children but normalization of the cough sensitivity has been shown in children with asthma [41] and recurrent cough [14] upon resolution of their cough. Although children grouped into different respiratory illnesses have significantly different cough sensitivities (Fig. 7.3) [13], this test has not been evaluated on an individual basis to identify its role in the clinic.

### Are inflammatory markers useful?

Several groups have examined airway indices in children with cough. Fitch et al. examined the

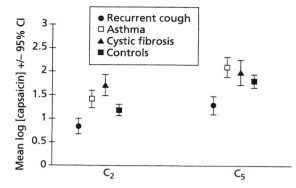

**Fig. 7.3** Cough receptor sensitivity (CRS) outcome measures in children with recurrent cough, asthma, cystic fibrosis and controls. Means and CI are adjusted for age, sex and $FEV_1$. $C_2$ and $C_5$ of children with recurrent cough were significantly lower ($P=0.00001$) when compared with all groups. CRS was similar in children with asthma and controls. Children with recurrent cough have an enhanced cough sensitivity (thus lower threshold to cough in the capsaicin cough sensitivity test) when compared with those with asthma, cystic fibrosis and controls [13]. While differences in cough sensitivity can be found in cohorts of children grouped according to disease process [13,14], their relevance for an individual child is not yet defined. Reproduced from *Arch Dis Child* 1997; 77: 331–4, with permission from the BMJ Publishing Group.

bronchoalveolar lavage in children with untreated unexplained persistent cough and showed that only a minority of children had asthma-type airway inflammation [29]. Zimmerman *et al.* [79] studied children with postinfectious cough and treated and untreated children with asthma, and concluded that postinfectious cough in children has different pathophysiological features than allergic asthma and represents a different disease. Although 6 of the 11 children with postinfectious cough had AHR, airway eosinophils and eosinophil cationic protein were normal [79]. In a community-based survey of children with chronic respiratory symptoms, Gibson *et al.* examined airway markers of four groups of children (wheeze, cough, recurrent chest colds and controls), and found elevated eosinophils (>2.5%) in all children with wheeze and AHR, but only in half of the children with wheeze alone. Other airway cell differentials were similar in all three symptom groups and sputum eosinophil cationic protein (ECP) levels were non-discriminatory between the groups [27].

In a longitudinal prospective study, children with

asthma and chronic cough were found to have elevated serum ECP and urinary eosinophil protein X (EPX) when compared with controls [80]. However, the authors failed to control for atopy, an important confounder. Also ECP may be elevated in neutrophilic inflammation, a known association in children with chronic cough [29,79].

When comparing data between groups in a cohort, differences may be found but application in the clinical setting for individual patients has not yet been shown in paediatrics. As single markers are context- and time-dependent, inflammatory markers are unlikely to be useful clinically if used in isolation [81]. This is in contrast to adults where examination of airway cells has a role in the clinical setting for evaluation of eosinophilic bronchitis.

## Measurement of cough in children

In the clinic, the severity and progress of cough is determined historically. Cough, however, can be measured and defined in other ways, most of which are used in research but not yet clinically. Cough measurements can be broadly divided into objective and subjective methods, but only some methods have been used in children. Of the objective methods that evaluate physical aspects of the cough (frequency, flow, amplitude), only cough frequency (static cough devices such as tape recorders and ambulatory cough meters) [82,83] have been used in children. Cough sensitivities or cough thresholds to a variety of stimuli (capsaicin, citric acid, osmotic agents, tartaric acid, etc.) are the only other objective measurements used in children. The many other objective measurements of cough in adults (e.g. airflow, cough sounds and spectrographs) have not yet been tested in children, which is necessary given the difference between adults and children in frequency of sound and airflow generation. Subjective measurements include measurement of 'cough tendency' (recording a number expressing a need or wish to cough but not actually coughing) [84] and diary cards using a variety of scales (Likert, visual analogue) and can be completed by parent or child. Which of these objective and/or subjective measurements are most clinically relevant is, however, yet to be defined. It is possible that the most relevant outcome measure may depend, at least in part, on the reason for performing the measurement, like determinants of asthma severity and types of airway hyperresponsiveness. Unlike the adult literature, a cough-specific quality of life measurement is unavailable in children.

There are also few data on how these measurements relate to one another. Daytime cough severity subjectively reported correlates to objectively measured cough, but the confidence intervals for the correlation coefficients were wide (0.11–0.74). Thus the severity of cough defined on diary cards does not necessarily represent cough frequency [85]. Such data are unavailable in adults. Thus the different outcomes of cough would most likely reflect different aspects of cough. Various methods of measuring cough are described in more detail below.

The need to objectively measure cough in clinical research is reflected in the several documented limitations when cough is used as an outcome measure. Firstly, questions on isolated cough are largely poorly reproducible [86]. The $\kappa$-value relating the chance-corrected agreement between answers to questions on cough ranges from 0.14 to 0.57 [86,87]. In contrast, questions on wheeze and asthma attacks are highly reproducible with $\kappa$-values of 0.7–1.0 [86]. Secondly, nocturnal cough is unreliably reported when compared to objective measurements [32,85]. Thirdly, cough is subjected to the period effect (spontaneous resolution of cough when studied) [88]. Thus non-placebo-controlled intervention studies have to be interpreted with caution. Fourthly, cough is also subjected to psychological influences [64]. In adults with cough, subjective scoring of cough does not correlate with cough frequency over a 20-min period but correlates with mood scores [89]. Rietveld et al. showed that children were more likely to cough under certain psychological settings [64]. Furthermore, subjective perception of cough severity depends on the population studied [12]. Finally, 'normal' children do cough as described in two studies that objectively measured cough [11,12].

## Measuring cough sensitivity in children

The method in general has been outlined by Fuller (Chapter 6). In paediatrics, several tussive agents (acetic acid [21], capsaicin [90], citric acid [77]) and methods (astrograph, nebulizer with [90] and without dosimeter [77]) have been used. Cough receptors are unevenly distributed in the airways [9] and hence standardization of airway deposition is important for test validity. This is arguably more important in children who have smaller airways and who are less likely

to comply with complex respiratory manoeuvres like maintaining an open glottis throughout nebulizer delivery. For measurements to be interpretable, measures of repeatability within the laboratory are important. Inspiratory flow has been shown to influence repeatability of measurements of cough sensitivity [90] and hence should be regulated. Gender is known to influence cough sensitivity in adults but not in children [13]. Other influences on cough sensitivity are airway calibre and age [13]. A full description of a standardized reliable method of measuring cough sensitivity to capsaicin is available elsewhere [90].

The commonly used outcome measures for cough sensitivity are $C_2$ (the lowest concentration required to stimulate two or more coughs) and $C_5$ (the lowest concentration required to stimulate five or more coughs). Other outcome measures that have been described are number of coughs within a specific time period (e.g. 10 s) and cough latency. Unlike the $C_2$ and $C_5$ measurements, no repeatability studies have been performed on these other outcome measurements. Control solutions (diluent) should be used initially since hypo- and hyperosmolar solutions can stimulate cough, and doubling concentration of the chosen stimulant is then used. The coughs following the challenge should be objectively monitored or counted by an independent observer.

## Cough meters

The traditional method of recording cough is the audio tape recorder [32], which limits portability. The first ambulatory cough meter developed by the Brompton Unit used in adults [91] was also codeveloped in children [83]. Adopting the Brompton method, a cheaper alternative was described [82] and this was later utilized for an intervention study [30]. To date there have been no other studies that have objectively measured ambulatory cough frequency as an outcome, probably because of the time and expense in using this method. Until such meters become more assessable, their application will most likely be limited to research.

## Cough diary cards

Traditionally, in studies on children questionnaires and diary cards are parent-filled [32,92]. In quality of life questionnaires there is an increasing trend for children to fill their own questionnaires since child-completed

**Table 7.3** Verbal descriptive score for paediatric use. From [85].

| Cough score | | | | | | | |
|---|---|---|---|---|---|---|---|
| Day of month | 1st | 2nd | 3rd | 4th | 5th | 6th | 7th |
| Daytime score (0–5) | | | | | | | |

*Daytime score*

0 No cough during the day
1 Cough for one or two short periods only
2 Cough for more than two short periods
3 Frequent coughing which does not interfere with school or other daytime activities
4 Frequent coughing which does interfere with schoolwork or some daytime activities
5 Severe coughing that prevents most usual daytime activity

responses have been shown to be significantly different to those completed by parents [93]. In cough-specific diary cards, the difference in parent-completed vs. child-completed diary cards is small in subjects (children with recurrent cough) and moderate in controls [85].

Cough-specific diary cards can be related to cough severity in general (Likert scale, visual analogue scale) or categorical, based on limitation or effect on activity (verbal category descriptive score). In a study that compared these scores with objective monitoring, the most valid subjective method of scoring cough in children over 6 years old was the verbal category descriptive score completed by children with parental assistance. The verbal category descriptive score (Table 7.3) used was that modified from the diary described by the Brompton group [91]. Nocturnal cough diary cards have been repeatedly shown to be inaccurate and are hence invalid [32,85]. Indeed despite the wide use of cough as an outcome measure there is only one validated cough-specific diary card for children [85]. However, this study and others [32,91] comparing objective and subjective scores for cough assume that subjects and parents judge the severity of cough on the frequency of cough. However, it is possible that some parents may assess the severity of cough on the length of the paroxysms or the loudness of the cough, which would not necessarily correlate to the frequency of cough. Although the frequency of cough is forseeably the only objective ambulatory measurement available, it is likely that the severity of cough as defined on diary cards is not interchangeable with cough frequency measurements [85].

*Acknowledgement*
Dr I. Brent Masters is gratefully acknowledged for his critical review of the manuscript and for his valued mentorship.

# References

1 Clough JB, Williams JD, Holgate ST. Effect of atopy on the natural history of symptoms, peak expiratory flow, and bronchial responsiveness in 7- and 8-year-old children with cough and wheeze. *Am Rev Respir Dis* 1991; **143**: 755–60.

2 Ninan TK, Macdonald L, Russel G. Persistent nocturnal cough in childhood: a population based study. *Arch Dis Child* 1995; **73**: 403–7.

3 Robertson CF, Heycock E, Bishop J, Nolan T, Olinsky A, Phelan PD. Prevalence of asthma in Melbourne schoolchildren: changes over 26 years. *Br Med J* 1991; **302**: 1116–8.

4 Bush A. Paediatric problems of cough. *Pulm Pharmacol Ther* 2002; **15**: 309–15.

5 Chang AB, Asher MI. A review of cough in children. *J Asthma* 2001; **38**: 299–309.

6 Chung KF, Lalloo UG. Diagnosis and management of chronic persistent dry cough. *Postgrad Med J* 1996; **72**: 594–8.

7 Phelan PD, Olinsky A, Oswald H. Asthma: classification, clinical patterns and natural history. *Bailliere's Clin Paediatr* 1995; **3**: 307–18.

8 Irwin RS, Boulet LP, Cloutier MM *et al.* Managing cough as a defense mechanism and as a symptom. A consensus panel report of the American College of Chest Physicians. *Chest* 1998; **114**: 133S–81S.

9 Chang AB. State of the art: cough, cough receptors, and asthma in children. *Pediatr Pulmonol* 1999; **28**: 59–70.

10 Campanella SG, Asher MI. Current controversies: sinus disease and the lower airways. *Pediatr Pulmonol* 2001; **31**: 165–72.

11 Munyard P, Bush A. How much coughing is normal? *Arch Dis Child* 1996; **74**: 531–4.

12 Chang AB, Phelan PD, Robertson CF, Newman RG, Sawyer SM. Frequency and perception of cough severity. *J Paediatr Child Health* 2001; **37**: 142–5.

13 Chang AB, Phelan PD, Sawyer SM, Del Brocco S, Robertson CF. Cough sensitivity in children with asthma, recurrent cough, and cystic fibrosis. *Arch Dis Child* 1997; **77**: 331–4.

14 Chang AB, Phelan PD, Sawyer SM, Robertson CF. Airway hyperresponsiveness and cough-receptor sensitivity in children with recurrent cough. *Am J Respir Crit Care Med* 1997; **155**: 1935–9.

15 National Health Survey—summary of results. Canberra, Australia: Government Publishing Service, 1997: Catalog no. 4364.

16 Kogan MD, Pappas GYuSM, Kotelchuck M. Over-the-counter medication use among preschool-age children. *JAMA* 1994; **272**: 1025–30.

17 Grigg J, Riedler J, Robertson CF. Bronchoalveolar lavage fluid cellularity and soluble intercellular adhesion molecule-1 in children with colds. *Pediatr Pulmonol* 1999; **28**: 109–16.

18 Martinez FD, Taussig LM, Morgan WJ. Infants with upper respiratory illnesses have significant reductions in maximal expiratory flow. *Pediatr Pulmonol* 1990; **9**: 91–5.

19 Curley FJ, Irwin RS, Pratter MR, Stivers DH, Doern GV, Vernaglia PA, Larkin AB, Baker SP. Cough and the common cold. *Am Rev Respir Dis* 1988; **138**: 305–11.

20 O'Connell F, Thomas VE, Studham JM, Pride NB, Fuller RW. Capsaicin cough sensitivity increases during upper respiratory infection. *Respir Med* 1996; **90**: 279–86.

21 Shimizu T, Mochizuki H, Morikawa A. Effect of influenza A virus infection on acid-induced cough response in children with asthma. *Eur Respir J* 1997; **10**: 71–4.

22 Kelly YJ, Brabin BJ, Milligan PJM, Reid JA, Heaf D, Pearson MG. Clinical significance of cough and wheeze in the diagnosis of asthma. *Arch Dis Child* 1996; **75**: 489–93.

23 McKenzie S. Cough—but is it asthma? *Arch Dis Child* 1994; **70**: 1–2.

24 Thomson F, Masters IB, Chang AB. Persistent cough in children—overuse of medications. *J Paediatr Child Health* 2002; **38**: 578–81.

25 Siersted HC. Population based study of risk factors for underdiagnosis of asthma in adolescence: Odense schoolchild study. *Br Med J* 1998; **316**: 651–7.

26 Wright AL, Holberg CJ, Morgan WJ, Taussig L, Halonen M, Martinez FD. Recurrent cough in childhood and its relation to asthma. *Am J Respir Crit Care Med* 1996; **153**: 1259–65.

27 Gibson PG, Simpson JL, Chalmers AC, Toneguzzi RC, Wark PAB, Wilson A, Hensley MJ. Airway eosinophilia is associated with wheeze but is uncommon in children with persistent cough and frequent chest colds. *Am J Respir Crit Care Med* 2001; **164**: 977–81.

28 Powell CVE, Primhak RA. Stability of respiratory symptoms in unlabelled wheezy illness and nocturnal cough. *Arch Dis Child* 1996; **75**: 385–91.

29 Fitch PS, Brown V, Schock BC, Taylor R, Ennis M, Shields MD. Chronic cough in children: bronchoalveolar lavage findings. *Eur Respir J* 2000; **16**: 1109–14.

30 Chang AB, Phelan PD, Carlin J, Sawyer SM, Robertson CF. Randomised controlled trial of inhaled salbutamol and beclomethasone for recurrent cough. *Arch Dis Child* 1998; **79**: 6–11.

31 Davies MJ, Fuller P, Picciotto A, McKenzie SA. Persistent nocturnal cough: randomised controlled trial of high dose inhaled corticosteroid. *Arch Dis Child* 1999; **81**: 38–44.

32 Archer LNJ, Simpson H. Night cough counts and diary card scores in asthma. *Arch Dis Child* 1985; **60**: 473–4.

33 Finder JD. Primary bronchomalacia in infants and children. *J Paediatr* 1997; **130**: 59–66.

34 McFadden ER. Exertional dyspnea and cough as preludes to acute attacks of bronchial asthma. *N Engl J Med* 1975; **292**: 555–8.

35 Cloutier MM, Loughlin GM. Chronic cough in children: a manifestation of airway hyperreactivity. *Pediatrics* 1981; **67**: 6–12.

36 Stevens MW, Gorelick MH. Short-term outcomes after acute treatment of pediatric asthma. *Pediatrics* 2001; **107**: 1357–62.

37 Johnston SL, Pattemore PK, Sanderson G *et al.* Community study of role of viral infections in exacerbations of asthma in 9–11 year old children. *Br Med J* 1995; **310**: 1225–9.

38 Chang AB, Harrhy VA, Simpson JL, Masters IB. Gibson PG. Cough, airway inflammation and mild asthma exacerbation. *Arch Dis Child* 2002; **86**: 270–5.

39 Karlsson J-A, Sant'Ambrogio G, Widdicombe J. Afferent neural pathways in cough and reflex bronchoconstriction. *J Appl Physiol* 1988; **65**: 1007–23.

40 Chang AB, Gibson PG. Relationship between cough, cough receptor sensitivity and asthma in children. *Pulm Pharmacol Ther* 2001; **15**: 287–91.

41 Chang AB, Phelan PD, Robertson CF. Cough receptor sensitivity in children with acute and non-acute asthma. *Thorax* 1997; **52**: 770–4.

42 Lalloo UG, Barnes PJ, Chung FK. Pathophysiology and

clinical presentations of cough. *J Allergy Clin Immunol* 1996; **98**: S91–7.

43 Rosier MJ, Bishop J, Nolan T, Robertson CF, Carlin J, Phelan PD. Measurement of functional severity of asthma in children. *Am J Respir Crit Care Med* 1994; **149**: 1434–41.

44 Schwartz J, Timonen KL, Pekkanen J. Respiratory effects of environmental tobacco smoke in a panel study of asthmatic and symptomatic children. *Am J Respir Crit Care Med* 2000; **161**: 802–6.

45 Mertsola J, Ziegler T, Ruuskanen O, Vanto T, Koivikko A, Halonen P. Recurrent wheezy bronchitis and viral respiratory infections. *Arch Dis Child* 1991; **66**: 124–9.

46 Clough JB, Holgate ST. Episodes of respiratory morbidity in children with cough and wheeze. *Am J Respir Crit Care Med* 1994; **150**: 48–53.

47 Frischer T, Studnicka M, Neumann M, Gotz M. Determinants of airway response to challenge with distilled water in a population sample of children aged 7–10 years old. *Chest* 1992; **102**: 764–70.

48 Pattemore PK, Asher MI, Harrison AC, Mitchell EA, Rea HH, Stewart AW. The interrelationship among bronchial hyperresponsiveness, the diagnosis of asthma, and asthma symptoms. *Am Rev Respir Dis* 1990; **142**: 549–54.

49 Lombardi E, Morgan WJ, Wright AL, Stein RT, Holberg CJ, Martinez FD. Cold air challenge at age 6 and subsequent incidence of asthma. *Am J Respir Crit Care Med* 1997; **156**: 1863–9.

50 Johnston BT, Gideon RM, Castell DO. Excluding gastroesophageal reflux disease as the cause of chronic cough. *J Clin Gastroenterol* 1996; **22**: 168–9.

51 Ferrari M, Olivieri M, Sembenini C *et al*. Tussive effect of capsaicin in patients with gastroesophageal reflux without cough. *Am J Respir Crit Care Med* 1995; **151**: 557–61.

52 Laukka MA, Cameron AJ, Schei AJ. Gastroesophageal reflux and chronic cough: which comes first? *J Clin Gastroenterol* 1994; **19**: 100–4.

53 Treem WR, Davis PM, Hyams JS. Gastroesophageal reflux in the older child: presentation, response to treatment and long-term follow up. *Clin Pediatr* 1991; **30**: 435–40.

54 Lombardi E, Stein RT, Wright AL, Morgan WJ, Martinez FD. The relation between physician-diagnosed sinusitis, asthma, and skin test reactivity to allergens in 8-year-old children. *Pediatr Pulmonol* 1996; **22**: 141–6.

55 Diament MJ, Senac MO, Gilsanz V, Baker S, Gillespie T, Larsson S. Prevalence of incidental paranasal sinuses opacification in pediatric patients: a CT study. *J Comput Assist Tomogr* 1987; **11**: 426–31.

56 Shopfner CE, Rossi JO. Roentgen evaluation of the paranasal sinuses in children. *AJR* 1973; **118**: 176–86.

57 Nishino T, Hasegawa R, Ide T, Isono S. Hypercapnia enhances the development of coughing during continuous infusion of water into the pharynx. *Am J Respir Crit Care Med* 1998; **157**: 815–21.

58 Gormley PK, Colreavy MP, Patil N, Woods AE. Congenital vascular anomalies and persistent respiratory symptoms in children. *Int J Pediatr Otorhinolaryngol* 1999; **51**: 23–31.

59 Wood RE. Localised tracheomalacia or bronchomalacia in children with intractable cough. *J Pediatr* 1997; **116**: 404–6.

60 Grathwohl KW, Afifi AY, Dillard TA, Olson JP, Heric BR. Vascular rings of the thoracic aorta in adults. *Am Surg* 1999; **65**: 1077–83.

61 Stick S. Pediatric origins of adult lung disease. The contribution of airway development to paediatric and adult lung disease. *Thorax* 2000; **55**: 587–94.

62 Vedal S, Petkau J, White R, Blair J. Acute effects of ambient inhalable particles in asthmatic and nonasthmatic children. *Am J Respir Crit Care Med* 1998; **157**: 1034–43.

63 Wamboldt MZ, Wamboldt FS. Psychiatric aspects of respiratory syndromes. In: Taussig LM, Landau LI, eds. *Pediatric Respiratory Medicine*. St Louis: Mosby, Inc., 1999: 1222–34.

64 Rietveld SBI, Everaerd W. Psychological confounds in medical research: the example of excessive cough in asthma. *Behav Res Ther* 2000; **38**: 791–800.

65 Fuller P, Picciotto A, Davies M, McKenzie SA. Cough and sleep in inner-city children. *Eur Respir J* 1998; **12**: 426–31.

66 Wu-Williams AH, Samet JM. Environmental tobacco smoke: exposure–response relationships in epidemiologic studies. *Risk Anal* 1990; **10**: 39–48.

67 Couriel JM. Passive smoking and the health of children. *Thorax* 1994; **49**: 731–4.

68 Stott NC. Management and outcome of winter upper respiratory tract infections in children aged 0–9 years. *Br Med J* 1979; **1**: 29–31.

69 Mellis CM. Can we reduce acute asthma attendances to hospital emergency departments? *Aust NZ J Med* 1997; **27**: 275–6.

70 Galvez RA, McLaughlin FJ, Levison H. The role of the methacholine challenge in children with chronic cough. *J Allergy Clin Immunol* 1987; **79**: 331–5.

71 Paganin F, Seneterre E, Chanez P, Daures JP, Bruel JM, Michel FB, Bousquet J. Computed tomography of the lungs in asthma: influence of disease severity and etiology. *Am J Respir Crit Care Med* 1996; **153**: 110–4.

72 Strauch E, Neupert T, Ihorst G, Van's-Gravesande KS, Bohnet W, Hoeldke B, Karmaus W, Kuehr J. Bronchial hyperresponsiveness to 4.5% hypertonic saline indicates a past history of asthma-like symptoms in children. *Pediatr Pulmonol* 2001; **31**: 44–50.

73 Koh YY, Chae SA, Min KU. Cough variant asthma is associated with a higher wheezing threshold than classic asthma. *Clin Exp Allergy* 1993; **23**: 696–701.

74 McKenzie SA, Bridge PD, Healy MJ. Airway resistance and atopy in preschool children with wheeze and cough. *Eur Respir J* 2000; **15**: 833–8.

75 Klug B, Nielsen KG, Bisgaard H. Observer variability of lung function measurements in 2–6-yr-old children. *Eur Respir J* 2000; **16**: 472–5.

76 Mitsuhashi M, Mochizuki H, Tokuyama K, Morikawa A, Kuroume T. Hyperresponsiveness of cough receptors in patients with bronchial asthma. *Pediatrics* 1985; **75**: 855–8.

77 Riordan MF, Beardsmore CS, Brooke AM, Simpson H. Relationship between respiratory symptoms and cough receptor sensitivity. *Arch Dis Child* 1994; **70**: 299–304.

78 O'Connell F, Thomas VE, Pride NB, Fuller RW. Capsaicin cough sensitivity decreases with successful treatment of chronic cough. *Am J Respir Crit Care Med* 1994; **150**: 374–80.

79 Zimmerman B, Silverman FS, Tarlo SM, Chapman KR, Kubay JM, Urch B. Induced sputum: comparison of postinfectious cough with allergic asthma in children. *J Allergy Clin Immunol* 2000; **105**: 495–9.

80 Labbe A, Aublet-Cuvelier B, Jouaville L, Beaugeon G, Fiani L, Petit I, Ouchchane L, Doly M. Prospective longitudinal study of urinary eosinophil protein X in children with asthma and chronic cough. *Pediatr Pulmonol* 2001; **31**: 354–62.

81 Martinez FD. Context dependency of markers of disease. *Am J Respir Crit Care Med* 2000; **162**: 56S–57.

82 Chang AB, Newman RG, Phelan PD, Robertson CF. A new use for an old Holter monitor: an ambulatory cough meter. *Eur Respir J* 1997; **10**: 1637–9.

83 Munyard P, Busst C, Logan-Sinclair R, Bush A. A new device for ambulatory cough recording. *Pediatr Pulmonol* 1994; **18**: 178–86.

84 Ng-Man-Kwong G, Proctor A, Billings C, Duggan R, Das C, Whyte MK, Powell CV, Primhak R. Increasing prevalence of asthma diagnosis and symptoms in children is confined to mild symptoms. *Thorax* 2001; **56**: 312–4.

85 Chang AB, Newman RG, Carlin J, Phelan PD, Robertson CF. Subjective scoring of cough in children: parent-completed vs child-completed diary cards vs an objective method. *Eur Respir J* 1998; **11**: 462–6.

86 Brunekreef B, Groot B, Rijcken B, Hoek G, Steenbekkers A, de Boer A. Reproducibility of childhood respiratory symptom questions. *Eur Respir J* 1992; **5**: 930–5.

87 Clifford RD, Radford M, Howell JB, Holgate ST. Prevalence of respiratory symptoms among 7 and 11 year old schoolchildren and association with asthma. *Arch Dis Child* 1989; **64**: 1118–25.

88 Evald T, Munch EP, Kok-Jensen A. Chronic non-asthmatic cough is not affected by inhaled beclomethasone dipropionate. A controlled double blind clinical trial. *Allergy* 1989; **44**: 510–4.

89 Hutchings HA, Eccles R, Smith AP, Jawad MSM. Voluntary cough suppression as an indication of symptom severity in upper respiratory tract infections. *Eur Respir J* 1993; **6**: 1449–54.

90 Chang AB, Phelan PD, Roberts RGD, Robertson CF. Capsaicin cough receptor sensitivity test in children. *Eur Respir J* 1996; **9**: 2220–3.

91 Hsu JY, Stone RA, Logan-Sinclair RB, Worsdell M, Busst CM, Chung KF. Coughing frequency in patients with persistent cough: assessment using a 24 hour ambulatory recorder. *Eur Respir J* 1994; **7**: 1246–53.

92 van Essen-Zandvliet EE, Hughes MD, Waalkens HJ, Duiverman EJ, Kerrebijn KF, and the Dutch CNSLD Study Group. Remission of childhood asthma after long-term treatment with an inhaled corticosteroid (budesonide): Can it be achieved? *Eur Respir J* 1994; **7**: 63–8.

93 Juniper EF, Guyatt GH, Dolovich J. Assessment of quality of life in adolescents with allergic rhinoconjunctivitis: development and testing of a questionnaire for clinical trials. *J Allergy Clin Immunol* 1994; **93**: 413–23.

94 Weinberg G. 'Honking': psychogenic cough tic in children. *S Afr Med J* 1980; **57**: 198–200.

# 8 The quality of life in coughers

### Richard S. Irwin, Cynthia L. French & Kenneth E. Fletcher

## Introduction

The methods of assessing the impact of cough on patients have been categorized as subjective and objective [1]. Subjective measures such as health-related quality of life (HRQoL) instruments are likely to be the ones that best reflect the severity of cough from the patient's standpoint because a subjective response most likely integrates both cough frequency and intensity. We use the term HRQoL to define a patient's perception of the impact of health and disease on multiple domains of his or her life (e.g. physical function, psychosocial state). HRQoL can be distinguished from QoL in that it is primarily concerned with factors that fall under the responsibility or concerns of health care providers and health care systems. In this chapter, we review the state of the art regarding the HRQoL in patients who seek medical attention complaining of cough by posing and answering a series of questions.

## Does cough adversely affect the health-related quality of life?

While cough is an important defence mechanism that helps clear excessive secretions and foreign material from the airways, it also is a very common symptom. In fact, over the past decade, cough of undifferentiated duration has been the most common complaint for which patients have sought medical attention from primary care physicians in the US [2,3]. Moreover, referrals of patients with persistently troublesome chronic cough of at least 8 weeks' duration have been shown to

account for up to 38% of a pulmonologist's outpatient practice [4].

### Chronic cough

To better understand why patients with chronic cough seek medical attention so frequently, French et al. [5] performed a prospective study to determine whether chronic cough was associated with adverse psychosocial or physical effects on the HRQoL and to determine whether the elimination of chronic cough with specific therapy for the underlying cause(s) improved these adverse effects. Chronic cough has been defined as one that is persistently troublesome to the patient for at least 8 weeks in duration [6]. To characterize the complications of cough, the investigators used an adverse, cough-specific outcome survey (ACOS) that reflected physical and psychosocial complications of cough. The ACOS is a fixed-alternative, yes/no, self-administered, 29-item questionnaire. To assess the effects of cough on HRQoL, the sickness impact profile (SIP) was used. It had been previously shown to be a reliable and valid, generic (i.e. non-illness-specific) measure of health-related dysfunction in non-coughing disease states.

From this study, five important findings emerged. First, chronic cough was significantly associated with meaningful adverse psychosocial and physical effects on HRQoL. Second, successful treatment of chronic cough was associated with resolution of patients' deterioration in HRQoL. Third, the HRQoL induced by chronic cough was more likely to be psychosocial than physical in nature. While previous publications have emphasized the physical consequences of cough [7], this was the first study to highlight and show that pa-

**Table 8.1** Spectrum and frequency of cough-associated adverse occurrences before and after specific treatment in patients (*n*=28) cured of their coughs.

| Adverse occurrence | Before treatment (%) | After treatment (%) | *P* value |
|---|---|---|---|
| Needs reassurance nothing is serious | 75 | 19 | <0.001 |
| Concerned something is wrong | 68 | 11 | <0.001 |
| Frequent retching | 57 | 8 | <0.001 |
| Exhaustion | 61 | 15 | <0.001 |
| Others think something is wrong with me | 46 | 19 | 0.03 |
| Embarrassment | 46 | 11 | <0.004 |
| Self-consciousness | 46 | 14 | 0.01 |
| Difficulty speaking on the telephone | 43 | 22 | 0.10 |
| Hoarseness | 46 | 15 | 0.01 |
| Had to change lifestyle | 36 | 11 | 0.03 |
| Cannot sleep at night | 43 | 15 | 0.02 |
| Can no longer sing in church | 29 | 8 | <0.05 |
| Spouse cannot tolerate cough | 27 | 8 | 0.08 |
| Wetting pants | 32 | 7 | 0.02 |
| Concerned something is seriously wrong | 68 | 11 | <0.001 |
| Dizziness | 18 | 0 | 0.02 |
| Excessive sweating | 29 | 7 | 0.04 |
| Achiness | 21 | 0 | 0.01 |
| Hurts to breathe | 18 | 15 | 0.76 |
| Stopped going to movies | 18 | 4 | 0.09 |
| Headaches | 15 | 4 | 0.16 |
| Fear of AIDS or TB | 11 | 0 | 0.08 |
| Concern of cancer | 14 | 4 | 0.17 |
| Absences from school or work | 11 | 19 | 0.40 |
| Loss of appetite | 11 | 0 | 0.08 |
| Nausea or vomiting | 7 | 7 | 0.97 |
| Soiling of pants | 7 | 0 | 0.16 |
| Broken ribs | 7 | 0 | 0.16 |
| Loss of job | 4 | 4 | 0.97 |

AIDS, acquired immune deficiency syndrome; TB, tuberculosis.
In the 28 patients in whom before and after treatment data were available, $\chi^2$ analyses revealed a significant reduction in adverse occurrences. As shown above, 16 of the 29 adverse occurrences had significantly decreased; the reduction in an additional 4 approached significance. With successful treatment, the average (±SD) number of complaints had decreased from 8.6±4.8 to 1.9±3.2 (*P*<0.0001).

tients are most troubled by the psychosocial complications (Table 8.1). Fourth, the ACOS and SIP appeared to be valid tools in assessing the impact of chronic cough on patients. Fifth, based upon lack of correlation between adverse cough occurrences and the specific causes of chronic cough, it appeared that the adverse occurrences identified in this study were specific to chronic cough in general and not to chronic cough due to any specific disease. Because of this and because there was no difference in other characteristics of patients (e.g. the ages, gender distribution, duration and spectra and frequencies of the causes of chronic cough) in this study compared with the results of other prospective studies, it was concluded that the HRQoLs observed in this study could be generalized to other adult patients who seek medical attention complaining of cough.

Using a cough-specific HRQoL questionnaire, the CQLQ, French *et al.* [8] prospectively confirmed that chronic cough does indeed adversely affect the HRQoL of patients who seek medical attention because of this complaint. Before treatment, total CQLQ scores in chronic coughers were significantly higher (i.e. the higher the scores, the worse the HRQoL) than in the control group, which did not complain of cough. After specific treatment, the total CQLQ scores of chronic coughers had significantly decreased to the control group level.

## Acute cough

By studying acute coughers as well as chronic coughers in their study, French *et al.* [8] prospectively showed that acute cough as well as chronic cough adversely effects the HRQoL of subjects complaining of cough. Acute cough has been defined as cough that is troublesome to the patient for less than 3 weeks [6]. Using the CQLQ, it was demonstrated that the HRQoL of acute coughers was adversely affected overall and to a similar degree as for chronic coughers, and it was significantly more affected than the control group which did not complain of cough. A comparison of the six subscale and 28 individual item pretreatment scores revealed that acute coughers complained of similar adverse occurrences related to cough as chronic coughers.

## How should the health-related quality of life of coughers be measured?

In general, HRQoL instruments can be classified as disease- or symptom-specific, generic, or preference-based [9]. Disease-specific measures focus on the symptoms of the specific disease while generic measures assess how the varied aspects of patients' lives are affected. Because they focus on the symptoms of the specific disease, disease-specific instruments have the potential to be able to detect smaller, clinically important changes in health status than generic instruments. Moreover, compared with generic instruments, disease-specific meas-

ures may be more sensitive because they contain a higher percentage of directly relevant content to the specific disease being evaluated. On the other hand, disease-specific instruments are not as comprehensive in their approach as generic measures, and disease-specific instruments are not able to compare health status among different diseases as generic measures can. Unlike disease-specific and generic HRQoL instruments, preference-based measures can also gather information that reflects health benefits of interventions. This is because they can assess the willingness of subjects to undergo risk to reduce suffering.

While there is no general agreement about what QoL means and which class of measure is best [10], we contend that all will agree that the best instrument is one that has been shown to be reliable and valid by a battery of psychometric assessments. It should also be shown to have dimensionality, which means it is composed of subscales that assess the underlying dimensions of quality of life related to health problems. With respect to evaluating the HRQoL in coughers, only one instrument, the CQLQ, has been appropriately evaluated [8]. The CQLQ has been determined to have dimensionality that is consistent with a cough-specific HRQoL instrument. Moreover, it has been determined to be an internally consistent, reliable and valid instrument by which to assess the impact of HRQoL in chronic and acute coughers. It is a 28-item, symptom-specific, paper and pencil survey, scored on a 4-point Likert-type scale. There is an overall or total score, scores for six separate subscales, and 28 individual item scores. The lowest possible achievable total score indicating no adverse effects of cough on HRQoL is 28, the highest possible total score is 112. The six subscales were identified by factor analysis and named according to their content as follows: physical complaints (e.g. headache), psychosocial issues (e.g. family and/or close friends cannot tolerate it any more), functional abilities (e.g. prolonged absences from important activities such as work, school or volunteer services), emotional well-being (e.g. 'I have a fear that I might have AIDS or tuberculosis'), extreme physical complaints (e.g. 'I wet my pants'), and personal safety fears (e.g. 'I want to be reassured that I do not have anything seriously the matter with me'). While the ACOS and the SIP had been useful in determining the impact of chronic cough on the health status of patients, thereby demonstrating their construct validity, they have not been fully evaluated as HRQoL measures for cough.

## What have we learned by using the CQLQ?

To date, we have learned that the CQLQ can be used as an outcome measure to assess the severity of acute and chronic cough [8] and to assess the efficacy of cough therapies for chronic cough [8]. While the ability of the CQLQ to assess the efficacy of cough therapies in acute coughers has not yet been evaluated, the following reasons suggest that it will likely be shown to be a valid means of doing so in future studies: (i) the CQLQ was developed with data from both acute and chronic coughers [8]; (ii) it has been determined that pretreatment total CQLQ scores in acute coughers are similar to those of chronic coughers [8]; and (iii) a comparison of pretreatment subscale scores between acute and chronic coughers has revealed that both groups complain of similar types of adverse occurrences related to cough and both complain significantly more than a control group [8]. Therefore, it is reasonable to speculate that when cough goes away as a complaint, the CQLQ scores will drop in similar fashion, whether they reflect the impact of an acute or a chronic cough.

The CQLQ also has been used to better understand the reasons for the gender differences in patients complaining of cough [10,11]. Because past studies of patients with chronic cough have consistently established that more women than men seek medical attention, French *et al.* [10] sought to determine whether this difference was due to chronic cough more adversely affecting the HRQoL of women. Using a *post hoc* analysis of data collected prospectively from chronic coughers during the psychometric testing of the CQLQ, French *et al.* [8] have reported in abstract form that the HRQoL of women complaining of chronic cough is more adversely affected than men. Based upon their results, these investigators speculated that women were more adversely affected because they were more likely to suffer from physical complaints such as urinary stress incontinence and become embarrassed because of it. These same investigators then sought to determine if there were similar gender-specific data for women and men seeking medical attention complaining of acute cough. Using a *post hoc* analysis of data collected prospectively from acute coughers during the psychometric testing of the CQLQ [8] to which prospectively collected data from acute coughers were added to enhance their database, these investigators have reported in abstract form [11] that both genders

appeared to seek medical attention complaining of acute cough at approximately the same rate. Based upon their results, they concluded that the similar frequency was probably related to there being no difference in the overall effects of acute cough on HRQoL between the genders. In addition, they speculated that the differences in the few items (e.g. wetting of pants for women) had the potential to become much more important when the cough becomes persistent and chronic.

## Clinical and research implications

To optimally evaluate the impact of cough on patients and to assess the efficacy of cough-modifying agents, investigators ideally should use both subjective and objective methods because they have the potential to measure different aspects of cough. Subjective measures are likely to be the ones that will best reflect the severity of cough from the subject's perspective, because a subjective response most likely integrates both cough frequency and intensity. With respect to subjective methods, we believe that the 28-item CQLQ should be routinely used in adults because, to our knowledge, it has been shown, in adults, to be the only reliable, valid, simple, easy-to-use and easy-to-understand outcome measure that can be self-administered by patients in a matter of minutes. The only other reliable and validated subjective instrument that we are aware of has been developed by Faniran *et al.* [12] for use in children for measuring the prevalence, morbidity and risk factors of persistent cough in epidemiological studies.

## References

1 Irwin RS, French CT. Cough and gastroesophageal reflux: identifying cough and assessing the efficacy of cough-modifying agents. *Am J Med* 2001; **111** (8A): 45S–50S.
2 Schappert SM. National ambulatory medical care survey: 1991 Summary. *Vital Health Stat* 1993; **230**: 1–20.
3 Woodwell DA. National ambulatory medical care survey: 1998 Summary. *Vital Health Stat* 2000; **315**: 1–25.
4 Irwin RS, Curley FJ, French CL. Chronic cough. *Am Rev Respir Dis* 1990; **141**: 640–7.
5 French CL, Irwin RS, Curley FJ, Krikorian CJ. Impact of chronic cough on quality of life. *Arch Intern Med* 1998; **158**: 1657–61.

6 Irwin RS, Madison JM. The diagnosis and treatment of cough. *N Engl J Med* 2000; **343**: 1715–21.

7 Irwin RS. Cough. In: Irwin RS, Curley FJ, Grossman RF, eds. *Diagnosis and Treatment of Symptoms of the Respiratory Tract*. Armonk, NY: Futura Publishing Co., Inc., 1997: 1–54.

8 French CT, Irwin RS, Fletcher KE, Adams TM. Evaluation of a cough-specific quality-of-life questionnaire. *Chest* 2002; **121**: 1123–31.

9 Yusen RD. What outcomes should be measured in patients with COPD? *Chest* 2001; **119**: 327–8.

10 French C, Irwin RS, Fletcher K, Adams T. Gender differences in quality of life (QoL) in patients complaining of chronic cough. *Am J Respir Crit Care Med* 2001; **163**: A58.

11 French CL, Fletcher KL, Irwin RS. Gender differences in quality of life (QoL) in patients complaining of acute cough. *Am J Respir Crit Care Med* 2002; **165**: A460.

12 Faniran AO, Peat JK, Woolcock AJ. Measuring persistent cough in children in epidemiological studies: development of a questionnaire and assessment of prevalence in two countries. *Chest* 1999; **115**: 434–9.

# Clinical Conditions with Cough

# 9 Cough in lower airway infections

*Wee-Yang Pek & Homer A. Boushey*

## Introduction

Cough is a common manifestation of acute infections of the lower respiratory tract, and these infections are part of a continuum of acute respiratory infections common in all human populations. The continuum ranges from rhinosinusitis (the common cold) to laryngitis, tracheobronchitis, bronchiolitis and pneumonia. These infections are among the most common reasons for visits to primary care providers and for hospital admissions. In this chapter, 'acute lower airway infection' refers to acute tracheobronchitis, acute bronchiolitis and community-acquired pneumonia (CAP). From a clinical standpoint, it is sometimes difficult to distinguish these entities from each other, and one condition may progress into another. They may be due to the same microbiological agents and share many clinicopathological features. Cough is a common presenting feature of these conditions, but beyond generally localizing the infections to the respiratory tract, the symptom is non-specific, occurring with all conditions from rhinosinusitis (through postnasal drip) to pneumonia.

## Epidemiology and aetiology of lower airway infection

### Acute tracheobronchitis and bronchiolitis

Acute tracheobronchitis is commonly diagnosed in patients presenting with cough of recent onset. In the US, about a third of the 30 million visits for cough in 1997 were attributed to acute tracheobronchitis [1]. In the UK, the incidence of acute bronchitis is similarly high, ranging from 34.5 to 171.4 per 100 000 [2]. The rate is particularly high during the winter months, when acute infectious respiratory illnesses are most prevalent.

Acute tracheobronchitis refers to an acute inflammatory condition of the trachea and bronchi in which cough, with or without the production of sputum, is a predominant feature [3,4]. It is usually caused by acute respiratory infection. The infection is typically viral in origin, and is usually self-limited. All symptoms, including cough, usually resolve within 3 weeks.

Exceptions to this benign course are numerous, and may reflect differences in host or pathogen. An example of the importance of differences in the host is the difference in the clinical presentation of infection with respiratory syncytial virus (RSV) in infants and in older children or adults. In all but infants, infection with this organism typically causes nasopharyngitis frequently associated with acute bronchitis. In infants under the age of 2 years, it causes bronchiolitis. This acute inflammatory condition of the terminal, bronchiolar airways may be associated with respiratory distress from airway narrowing from oedema, smooth muscle contraction and mucus secretion. Viral bronchiolitis is one of the most common reasons for hospitalization in infancy [5–7], and RSV is its major cause, accounting for 45–75% of cases; parainfluenza virus is responsible for up to 30% [6]. Another potentially life-threatening respiratory infection due predominantly to parainfluenza virus (types 1, 2 and 3) and also RSV is acute laryngotracheobronchitis or croup [8,9]. These viruses cause inflammation and swelling of the subglottic tissues as well as the tracheal and bronchial mucosa resulting in upper airway narrowing and obstruction.

Table 9.1 Aetiological agents of acute tracheobronchitis.

| Viruses |
| --- |
| Influenza virus A and B |
| Rhinovirus |
| Parainfluenza virus |
| Respiratory syncytial virus |
| Adenovirus |
| Coronavirus |
| Coxsackievirus A21 |

| Bacteria |
| --- |
| *Mycoplasma pneumoniae* |
| *Chlamydia pneumoniae* |
| *Bordetella pertussis* |

The infection peaks in the second year of life and is associated with a hospitalization rate in up to a quarter of patients [10]. In addition to their importance as respiratory pathogens in infants and young children, RSV and parainfluenza viruses are also important respiratory pathogens in elderly adults, in whom they commonly cause moderate to severe acute inflammation of the lower respiratory tract [11,12]. Another respiratory pathogen, rhinovirus—the most common pathogen in humans—also causes different clinical presentations at the two extremes of age. Compared to the typically limited rhinorrhoea, sneezing and sore throat of common colds caused by rhinovirus infections in adolescents and in young and middle-aged adults, acute otitis media occurs much more commonly in children [13] and prolonged lower respiratory tract symptoms prompting physician consultation occur more commonly in people over 60 years of age [14].

Differences in the infecting pathogen also cause different clinical presentations. This is most infamously illustrated by influenza, which so characteristically provokes fever, rigors, myalgias and malaise in addition to cough and sputum production that 'the flu' has entered the English language as a generic term for an acute febrile respiratory illness with systemic symptoms. But influenza can also cause pneumonia, a complication thought to be responsible for deaths in the 1918 pandemic, which caused the greatest total mortality from any acute epidemic in human history [15,16]. The differences in rates of pneumonia and in mortality among influenza epidemics from year to year illustrate another cause of variation in clinical presen-

tation and consequence: genetic variations among strains of the same species of viruses.

The aetiological agents that cause acute tracheobronchitis are identified only in a minority of cases but are likely to be non-bacterial (Table 9.1). The supplementation of classical but insensitive techniques of viral culture with modern molecular techniques, like PCR (polymerase chain reaction), has shown that respiratory viruses account for more than 90% of acute respiratory illness in which an agent is identified [11,17,18].

The viruses identified include those that involve primarily the lower respiratory tract, like influenza A, influenza B, parainfluenza 3 and the respiratory syncytial virus. Other viruses like rhinovirus, adenovirus and coronavirus infections predominantly affect the upper respiratory tract, but also commonly involve the lower airways [11,17,19,20]. Because of the temperature dependence of some strains of rhinovirus, growing best in culture at 33 °C, rhinovirus infections were thought to be limited to the upper airways, causing lower airway symptoms only indirectly, through postnasal drip of inflammatory secretions. But rhinovirus has now been demonstrated by the *in situ* hybridization technique in bronchial mucosal biopsies from infected patients [21], proving that it can directly infect the subglottic, or 'lower' airways as well. While severe tracheobronchitis occurs in a smaller proportion of patients infected by rhinovirus than by influenza, parainfluenza and respiratory syncytial virus, the total number of infections by the >100 serotypes of rhinovirus is so great that this common virus likely contributes most to the overall burden of lower respiratory infection in the community [20,22], particularly in the elderly. In addition, rhinovirus infection is now recognized as the most common cause of exacerbations of asthma in people with the disease [23,24]. It is now also emerging as a major cause of acute exacerbations of chronic obstructive bronchitis (AECB) [25–27] and of cystic fibrosis [28].

Bacterial infections account for only about 5–10% of all cases of acute tracheobronchitis in previously healthy adults. Aetiological agents include *Bordetella pertussis, Mycoplasma pneumoniae* and *Chlamydia pneumoniae.* In recent years, infection with *B. pertussis* has been recognized as an important cause of acute but persistent tracheobronchitis. It has been identified in as many as 26% of cases presenting with prolonged cough [29,30]. The reasons for the apparent increase in the prevalence of *B. pertussis* include the waning of immunity in previously vaccinated individuals and an increased awareness of this infection in the adult population. The role of *C. pneumoniae* as an important aetiological agent in acute tracheobronchitis has been better defined in recent years, and is now thought to account for between 5 and 20% of cases of persistent cough [31,32]. Again, the use of PCR to detect this organism in airway biopsies and secretions is changing the appreciation of the organism's importance. The aetiological role of common bacterial causes of community-acquired pneumonia, like *Streptococcus pneumoniae*, *Haemophilus influenzae* and *Moraxella catarrhalis* in uncomplicated acute bronchitis in previously healthy patients remains uncertain.

The overwhelming predominance of viral infections in causing acute tracheobronchitis has not kept the condition from being an important reason for the inappropriate prescription of antibiotics. Despite the lack of evidence supporting their routine use, antibiotics are prescribed to a large majority of the patients with acute tracheobronchitis who present for care [33]. The Ambulatory Medical Care Survey in the US in 1992 showed that 66% of patients diagnosed as having bronchitis were treated with antibiotics [34]. The antibiotic prescription rate in patients diagnosed as having 'colds' or upper respiratory tract infections was slightly lower, at around 50%. The rate of antibiotic use by primary care physicians for patients with cough of recent onset has remained high, actually increasing from 1980 to 1994 [35]. This excessive use of antibiotics in outpatient respiratory infections is believed to be an important determinant of the recent rise in antibiotic resistance among common respiratory pathogens.

### Pneumonia

Community-acquired pneumonia (CAP) is one of the most common causes of hospitalization and death from infectious diseases in adults. About 4–6 million cases of CAP occur each year in the US, and up to 25% of these require hospital admission [36,37]. Most cases present with acute cough in association with other respiratory and systemic symptoms. Community-acquired pneumonia accounts for about 6% of all ambulatory visits with a chief complaint of cough [35].

The aetiology of CAP is identified in only half of all cases using currently available diagnostic methods

**Table 9.2** Microbial pathogens that cause pneumonia.

Viruses
  Influenza virus
  Cytomegalovirus
  Respiratory syncytial virus
  Measles virus
  Varicella zoster virus
  Hantavirus
Bacteria
  *Streptococcus pneumoniae*
  *Haemophilus influenzae*
  *Staphylococcus aureus*
  *Mycoplasma pneumoniae*
  *Chlamydia pneumoniae*
  *Chlamydia psittaci*
  *Legionella pneumophila*
  *Moraxella catarrhalis*
  Oral anaerobes
  Enteric aerobic Gram-negative bacilli
  *Pseudomonas aeruginosa*
  *Nocardia* spp.
  *Mycobacterium tuberculosis*
Fungi
  *Histoplasma*
  Coccidioides
  *Blastomyces* spp.

(Table 9.2). The most commonly identified organism is *Streptococcus pneumoniae*, followed by *Haemophilus influenzae* and *Staphylococcus aureus*. Viruses, *Chlamydia pneumoniae*, *Mycoplasma pneumoniae* and *Legionella* account for around a quarter of cases in which an aetiology is identified [38–40]. Enteric Gram-negative bacteria including *Pseudomonas aeruginosa* are not common in CAP but can be found more frequently in elderly patients, in patients with chronic lung diseases and in patients with underlying comorbidities that suppress immune function [41,42].

## Pathophysiology

The pathogenetic mechanism that gives rise to cough in acute airway infection is not well understood but is likely to result from one or more of the following (Table 9.3).

1 Infections limited to the upper airway, like many

Table 9.3 Possible mechanisms giving rise to cough in lower respiratory tract infections.

1 Irritation of nerve endings in the larynx and trachea from 'postnasal drip'.
2 Release of proinflammatory mediators at the site of viral replication.
3 Exposure of nerve endings secondary to damage and destruction of the airway epithelium.
4 Enhanced effect of neuropeptides such as substance P secondary to decrease in neutral endopeptidase on the epithelial cell surface.
5 Deformation of irritant receptors by accumulated secretion and debris.
6 Airway hyperresponsiveness and bronchospasm.

common colds with or without rhinosinusitis, often result in dripping of secretions rich in inflammatory mediators from the nasopharynx down onto the larynx or trachea ('postnasal drip'). Irritation of nerve endings at these sites commonly elicits coughing.

2 Proinflammatory mediators known to be released in response to rhinovirus infection of the airway mucosa include chemokines, cytokines, histamine, bradykinins and prostaglandins [43]. Cough can result from the stimulation of nerve endings in the lower airway mucosa by inflammatory mediators released directly from airway epithelial cells (the site of rhinovirus infection) or from inflammatory cells attracted to the site of infection by epithelial cell-derived chemokines, like interleukin-8 and eotaxin [44,45] (Fig. 9.1).

3 Damage and destruction of the airway epithelium in the lower respiratory tract is found in infection with influenza and RSV [46,47]. Necrosis and shedding of the epithelial layer of the bronchi could expose sensory nerve endings, like rapidly adapting irritant receptors, decreasing the cough threshold to environmental irritants and inflammatory secretions.

4 Studies of epithelial cells *in vitro* and of rats and guinea-pigs *in vivo* have suggested that some infections might lower the cough threshold by an indirect mechanism, through reduction in neutral endopeptidase on the epithelial cell surface [48,49]. This enzyme degrades neuropeptides released from adjacent afferent nerve endings, so a reduction in its concentration or activity might amplify the effects of stimulated release of neuropeptides. One of these effects, most clearly identified for substance P, is cough, and the administration of exogenous neutral endopeptidase has been shown to increase the cough threshold to inhalation of substance P in a guinea-pig model [50,51].

5 Together with the increase in mucus production, the impairment of mucociliary function during infection of the airways leads to accumulation of secretions and debris in the airway lumen. These secretions can mechanically deform irritant receptors in the adjacent bronchial mucosa, triggering cough as a defensive reflex for clearing the airways of excess secretions and foreign materials. The accumulation of secretions in the distal airways is also the mechanism likely to be responsible for cough in patients with pneumonia, as cough receptors are not present in the lung parenchyma.

6 Finally, cough in acute lower airway infection may be a manifestation of airway hyperresponsiveness and bronchospasm, as is associated with cough in asthma. The mechanism is presumed to be related to changes in smooth muscle tone, for bronchodilators are effective in relieving cough in patients with asthma [52] and in some patients with cough associated with tracheobronchitis [53–55]. In patients in whom acute infection of the lower airway is associated with abnormalities in pulmonary function, cough usually lasts for a longer period of time, and bronchodilator treatment is more likely to be effective [18,56].

## Clinical presentation

### Acute tracheobronchitis

Cough is so consistently present in patients with acute tracheobronchitis as to be a diagnostic criterion for the condition [3,4]. A review of 346 adults with self-diagnosed colds for 48 h or less (82% due to picornavirus infection) found that cough was reported by 75% within the first 2 days and by 25% on the 14th

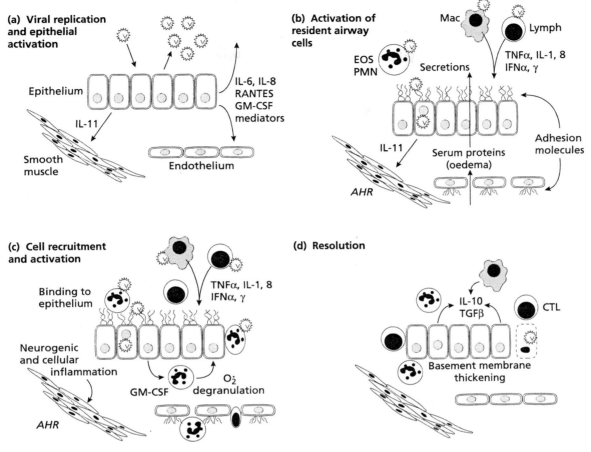

**Fig. 9.1** Cellular inflammatory responses to respiratory viral infection. (a) Respiratory viral infections are initiated when a virus enters a host epithelial cell, and viral replication causes the release of new infectious particles and activates secretion of cytokines, chemokines and mediators by the epithelial cells. (b) Viral particles released into the airway cause activation of resident cells in the airway, including macrophages, lymphocytes and granulocytes. Cytokines from epithelial cells and other resident airway cells increase adhesion molecule expression and increase airway responsiveness. (c) The combination of chemokine secretion and increased adhesion molecule expression causes recruitment and activation of additional leucocytes, which further add to airway inflammation and increased responsiveness. (d) Cytotoxic T cells kill virus-infected cells, and cytokines such as TGFβ and interleukin (IL) 10 are likely to play a role in the down-regulation of airway inflammation after viral infection. Increased numbers of airway lymphocytes and eosinophils may persist for weeks after the viral infection. The steps illustrated in this diagram can occur sequentially and/or in parallel, and the timing depends on factors related to both the host and virus. Abbreviations: EOS, eosinophil; IFN, interferon; PMN, polymorphonuclear leucocyte; Mac, macrophage; Lymph, lymphocyte; CTL, cytotoxic lymphocyte; $O_2^{\cdot}$, superoxide; AHR, airway hyperresponsiveness. Reproduced from: Folkerts G *et al*. Virus-induced airway hyperresponsiveness and asthma. *Am J Respir Crit Care Med* 1998; **157** (6 Part 1): 1708–20.

day. Cough was rated as moderate or severe by 44%, and as the most troubling symptom in 8% [57].

The symptom usually begins early and becomes more prominent as the illness progresses. Acute tracheobronchitis can begin as a severe cold or 'flu-like' illness with upper respiratory tract symptoms such as coryza and sore throat, but cough appears shortly afterwards, progressing to become the predominant complaint. Specific descriptors of cough in acute tracheobronchitis have not proven useful, but it is often described as 'chesty' and is productive of sputum in about 50% of cases. The sputum produced is typically mucoid at the outset, but more purulent in the later stages of illness. This purulence does not indicate a bacterial aetiology; it simply indicates the accumulation of inflammatory cells or sloughed mucosal epithelial cells in airway secretions [58]. Another common symptom of tracheal involvement in acute tracheobronchitis is retrosternal pain, typically worsened by respiration and coughing. Dyspnoea and cyanosis are not seen in healthy adults without underlying chronic lung disease.

Rhonchi and coarse rales may be heard on auscultation indicating the presence of loose intraluminal secretions. Wheezing may be heard but is infrequent except in patients with prior obstructive airway disease, or with a predisposition to asthma. Findings of lung consolidation are absent. Wheezing with otherwise unremarkable bouts of tracheobronchitis may be the first clue to a diagnosis of asthma. With the exception of influenza and adenovirus infection, fever is typically absent in acute tracheobronchitis due to viruses.

Although the cough in acute tracheobronchitis typically lasts less than 3 weeks, it may persist up to a month or longer in some patients [59]. Viral causes still predominate even in these patients, but the proportion attributable to *B. pertussis* and *C. pneumoniae* is increased [30,32,60,61]. In children, the first symptoms of pertussis are similar to those of a common cold with coryza: dry cough and mild fever. A week or two after this innocuous onset, coughing begins to occur in paroxysms lasting for a minute or even longer. The child may gasp for air between coughing paroxysms, with a characteristic 'whooping' sound. Coughing usually continues for at least 2 weeks and may persist for more than 3 months before gradually improving [62]. In contrast, adult pertussis usually presents with relatively mild respiratory complaints, as of simply prolonged 'postviral' cough without the classical paroxysms seen in children. No cluster of clinical features permits a specific diagnosis of pertussis in these patients, for no pattern of symptoms distinguishes it from other causes of acute tracheobronchitis [60,63].

## Acute bronchiolitis

Cough is usually not the predominant feature of this condition that affects primarily young children and infants. The key clinical features of viral bronchiolitis are acute respiratory illness with wheezing and concurrent fever, coryza or cough in a previously well infant. Auscultation of the lungs reveals bilateral crackles and expiratory wheezing. Severe cases can present with respiratory distress with intercostal retraction, hypoxia and respiratory failure. Viral bronchiolitis is most often due to RSV infection, and peaks in the winter months. Infants diagnosed with viral bronchiolitis have a higher rate of subsequent wheezing illness through childhood, with the increase over other children declining toward nil by about the age of 13 [64].

## Acute laryngotracheobronchitis

This is an important diagnosis to consider in young children in the second to third year of life. The classic signs of this condition — inspiratory stridor, hoarseness and a peculiar brassy or 'croupy' cough — arise from inflammation involving mainly the larynx and trachea. Most patients have an upper respiratory infection for several days before cough becomes apparent. Fever is common. With progressive compromise of the airway, stridor becomes continuous with a deepening cough. Suprasternal, infrasternal and intercostal retractions are frequently observed in severe cases. There may be diminished breath sounds, rhonchi and scattered crackles on auscultation. Nevertheless, most patients with croup have a relatively benign clinical course and only progress as far as stridor and slight dyspnoea before they start to recover [10]. The differential diagnosis includes other causes of upper airway obstruction in young children such as acute epiglottitis, aspiration of foreign body, diphtheria, and peritonsillar and retropharyngeal abscesses.

## Community-acquired pneumonia

Cough is present in about 80% of all cases of community-acquired pneumonia (CAP) and can be dry or productive [65]. Other associated features include fever, sputum production, dyspnoea and pleuritic chest pain. Elderly patients and patients with impaired immune response may have few or no respiratory symptoms. Physical findings on examination include tachypnoea, crackles, rhonchi and signs of consolidation. Dullness to percussion may suggest the presence of pleural effusion, but diagnosis often becomes apparent only on chest radiography. While many cases of CAP are due to viral infection, bacterial causes are much more prevalent than in tracheobronchitis or bronchiolitis [40].

## Evaluation

A wide variety of inflammatory and infectious conditions of the respiratory system can present as an acute cough illness. Most common causes of acute cough can usually be inferred from a detailed history and physical examination. Acute tracheobronchitis is essentially a clinical diagnosis characterized by the predominance of cough in the presence of other symptoms of upper respiratory tract infection such as sore throat and rhinorrhoea, which help differentiate it from other conditions. However, it is not possible to differentiate between bacterial and viral tracheobronchitis based on clinical presentation alone.

The most important objective in the evaluation of adults with acute cough illness is to exclude the presence of pneumonia. Other serious diseases that should be kept in mind include congestive heart failure, pulmonary embolism and aspiration. Various studies have been done to determine the accuracy of the patient's history and physical examination for diagnosing pneumonia in adults with acute cough in the outpatient and emergency room settings [66–69]. A recent review of these studies has concluded that in the absence of abnormalities in the vital signs and chest examination, further diagnostic work-up—as by chest radiography—in an otherwise healthy adult patient with acute cough is probably not necessary [70]. Nevertheless, the clinician is reminded of the atypical presentations of pneumonia in patients with comorbidities or immunosuppression, and in elderly patients whose presenting complaints may be of non-respiratory symptoms such as confusion or frequent falls [71].

In the initial evaluation of a patient with new acute respiratory symptoms, one has to take into account the patient's dermographic and epidemiological situation. *B. pertussis* infection has to be considered in any patient with a persistent cough when there is a history suggestive of a positive contact. Influenza should be considered a possible cause of acute febrile tracheobronchitis in the winter months or in outbreak settings. The presence of fever together with sore throat, headache and myalgia in adult patients presenting with acute cough illness during the flu season is sufficiently specific for the clinician to make a definitive diagnosis of influenza [72–74]. The early diagnosis of these two conditions is important, as specific antimicrobial therapy is available. The timely administration of antibiotics in patients with pertussis will help to reduce the transmission of this highly infectious disease in the community. In patients with influenza, the early administration of neuraminidase inhibitors such as oseltamivir and zanamivir will shorten the course of the illness.

Some patients presenting with acute cough illness due to acute tracheobronchitis may have underlying asthma. However, the diagnosis of asthma is difficult in the acute setting because a significant number of patients with otherwise uncomplicated tracheobronchitis have abnormal pulmonary function. These abnormalities are transient and include a bronchodilator-responsive decrease in $FEV_1$ and an increase in bronchial reactivity that can last up to 2 months [56,75]. It is therefore prudent to defer definitive diagnosis of asthma until at least 2 months after the onset of acute tracheobronchitis.

Radiographic examination of the chest is strongly recommended when pneumonia is suspected [36,37]. Standard posteroanterior and lateral chest radiographs are generally needed for all patients whose symptoms and physical examination suggest the possibility of pneumonia. The presence of lung infiltrates excludes uncomplicated acute tracheobronchitis as the cause of a patient's acute cough illness and greatly increases the possibility of bacterial infection.

Laboratory investigations are usually not helpful in the diagnosis of acute tracheobronchitis. The yield from a sputum culture is exceedingly low in this condition and neither Gram stain nor culture is recommended. The role of sputum Gram stain and culture in the evaluation of pneumonia is controversial. Some guidelines advocate the tests, whereas others discourage their routine use [36,37,76]. When the clinical suspicion of pertussis is high, a nasopharyngeal smear for direct fluorescent antibody test and culture for *B. pertussis* should be sent early in the illness. Serological tests for influenza and *B. pertussis* may be helpful in the setting of community or seasonal outbreaks. The availability of PCR-based testing for routine use in the future may shorten the time to detection of these infections.

Cough lasting more than 3 weeks is considered chronic. It is recommended that chest radiograph be obtained in all such cases. Irwin and colleague have developed recommendations for the evaluation of such cases [77]. The term 'postinfectious cough' is sometimes used to describe chronic cough developing after an upper or lower airway infection but should be reserved for those with a normal chest radiograph.

## Management

### Specific treatment of cough

#### Antibiotics in acute tracheobronchitis

Randomized controlled trials conducted in the last 20 years have repeatedly failed to demonstrate benefit from the routine use of antibiotic treatment in uncomplicated acute tracheobronchitis. This is not unexpected, as the majority of the cases of acute tracheobronchitis are caused by viral infections. While it is reasonable to expect that patients with acute tracheobronchitis from infection with bacteria such as *B. pertussis*, *M. pneumoniae* and *C. pneumoniae* would benefit from antibiotic treatment, it is impossible to differentiate bacterial from viral tracheobronchitis on clinical grounds, and no method currently allows prompt detection of bacterial causes of infection. Methods based on amplification of signature elements of bacterial DNA (e.g. PCR) may ultimately make this possible, but until they are developed, it will remain difficult to select patients who may potentially benefit from antibiotic therapy for treatment.

Trials of antibiotic treatment of uncomplicated acute tracheobronchitis have been done in sufficient numbers to permit meta-analyses of their findings. This approach has confirmed that the routine antibiotic treatment does not affect the duration of illness, limitation of activity or loss of work [78–82]. With regard to the specific symptoms of cough and sputum production, two meta-analyses have found a modest benefit in terms of shorter duration of these symptoms (by about half a day) in some patients treated with antibiotics [81,82]. Using improvement in the health-related quality of life as a primary outcome measure, a recent randomized double blind controlled trial using the broad-spectrum antibiotic azithromycin failed to demonstrate any beneficial effect in healthy adults with acute bronchitis [83]. Clinical practice guidelines with regard to appropriate antibiotic use have recently been published [84,85]. These guidelines recommend that the evaluation of adults with an acute cough illness or a presumptive diagnosis of uncomplicated acute bronchitis should focus on ruling out serious illness and the routine antibiotic treatment of uncomplicated acute bronchitis is not recommended, regardless of duration of cough. Patient satisfaction with care for acute bronchitis depends most on physician–patient communication than on whether an antibiotic is prescribed. Clinicians caring for patients with uncomplicated acute tracheobronchitis are encouraged to discuss with their patients the natural course of the disease and the lack of benefit of antibiotics in treating this condition.

#### Bronchodilators in acute tracheobronchitis

A few randomized controlled trials have indicated that the use of bronchodilator agents may be advantageous in selected patient with acute tracheobronchitis [53–55]. The use of $\beta_2$-agonists like albuterol has been shown to shorten the duration of cough in patients with bronchial hyperresponsiveness, wheezing or an $FEV_1 <$ 80% of predicted at the initial visit. No such benefit was seen in subjects without evidence of airflow limitation at presentation [53]. A recent Cochrane Database review of the literature concluded that there is no evidence to support the use of $\beta_2$-agonists in children with acute cough who do not have evidence of airflow obstruction. There is also little evidence to support their routine use in adults. While the risk of adverse effects from $\beta$-agonist use is small, it is not nil [86], and the selection of patients for bronchodilator treatment should rest on the use of objective, simple tests of lung function, like spirometry, when feasible. The duration of treatment needed in these patients is generally no longer than 1–2 weeks. In patients with $\beta$-agonist-responsive cough persisting for longer than 6 weeks, follow-up assessment of pulmonary function should be made.

#### Antihistamines in acute tracheobronchitis

Antihistamine decongestant therapy has been shown

to reduce postnasal drip and significantly decreases the severity of cough in patients with uncomplicated common colds [87]. The impact of this treatment in cases that have progressed to acute tracheobronchitis is unknown.

*Specific considerations*

*Pertussis.* The one possible exception to antibiotic use discussed above is when pertussis infection is suspected in patients with acute tracheobronchitis. Although studies have identified pertussis in up to 20% of patients with cough longer than 2–3 weeks, there is no specific clinical feature that identifies persistent cough due to pertussis [30,60,88]. This is especially true in adults where the classic features of whooping cough are not seen. In the setting of a familial or community outbreak of *B. pertussis* infection, a high index of suspicion is required and early institution of the appropriate antibiotics can shorten the duration of transmission of this highly infectious condition by decreasing the shedding of the organism. The most widely used antibiotic for this infection is erythromycin at 30–40 mg/kg every 6 h for 2 weeks. Nevertheless, there is no evidence to indicate that the natural course of pertussis, including the duration of cough, can be significantly altered when the treatment is started 7–10 days after the onset of illness [88–90].

*Influenza.* Specific antiviral agents are available for the treatment and prevention of acute tracheobronchitis due to influenza. Amantadine, rimantadine and the newer neuraminidase inhibitors such as oseltamivir and zanamivir have been shown to be effective in decreasing the duration as well as the severity of symptoms [72,73,91,92]. The caveat is that these agents in general must be started within 24–48 h to be effective. The accuracy of a clinical diagnosis of influenza in the setting of an outbreak is usually good, and laboratory confirmation may not be necessary before starting treatment [91]. This consideration is especially important for unvaccinated patients at high risk of complications of influenza infection. Outside of the period of influenza epidemics, however, diagnosing influenza as a cause of sporadic cases of acute tracheobronchitis on clinical grounds alone is difficult.

Antiviral agents effective against other common respiratory viruses, like rhinovirus, have been developed and tested, but are yet to be approved for clinical use [93]. When these agents are effective only against a particular family of viruses, the question is invited as to the necessity and cost of making a specific diagnosis early enough in the course of the illness for the therapy to make an impact.

*Acute bronchiolitis.* Treatment of RSV bronchiolitis is symptomatic, with emphasis primarily on adequate hydration and oxygenation. Aerosolized ribavirin has been approved to treat hospitalized infants and young children with severe lower respiratory infection due to RSV. Ribavirin is a guanosine analogue with good *in vitro* activity against a number of viruses, including RSV. However, aerosolized ribavirin is costly and the mode of delivery is elaborate requiring continuous administration with the use of a special nebulization device in a mist tent or hood. There is also concern about the effect of occupational exposure to ribavirin in health care workers of childbearing age, as this drug is known to be teratogenic and even embryocidal in most animal species. Most importantly, the clinical efficacy and benefit of this treatment remain uncertain despite its widespread use in the last two decades [94]. Consequently the American Academy of Pediatrics recommends its use only in patients in specific high-risk groups [95].

Some clinicians advocate the use of β-agonist bronchodilators, like albuterol, but evidence is lacking that it reduces admission rates or decreases length of hospitalization in children with acute bronchiolitis [96]. With regard to the use of corticosteroids, a meta-analysis using data from six randomized placebo-controlled trials of systemic corticosteroids in the treatment of patients hospitalized with RSV bronchiolitis reveals a statistically significant improvement of the clinical symptoms, length of stay and duration of symptoms [97]. However, two randomized control trials published later and not included in this meta-analysis show no evidence that corticosteroid treatment alters the course of the disease [98,99].

*Acute laryngotracheobronchitis.* Specific antiviral therapy is not available for the treatment of this infection. Administration of nebulized racemic epinephrine has been demonstrated to be effective in the treatment of airway obstruction in both outpatients and hospitalized patients with croup [100–103]. In patients with moderate to severe laryngotracheobronchitis, parenteral, oral and nebulized corticosteroids have been shown to lessen the symptoms and hospitalizations [104–109]. Oral dexamethasone at a dose of 0.15 mg/kg is also effective for outpatients with less severe disease [110].

*Pneumonia.* Most patients with community-acquired pneumonia are treated empirically with antibiotics initially. Pathogen-specific therapy may be possible in some patients when blood or sputum culture results become available. The initial choice of antibiotics is usually guided by relevant clinical factors that influence the likely aetiological pathogens. For example, in outpatients with no risk factors for drug-resistant *S. pneumoniae* or Gram-negative organisms, macrolide or tetracycline alone can be used. In patients with risk factors for these organisms, because of either underlying chronic lung diseases or immunosuppression, the choice is between a macrolide/β-lactam combination and an antipneumococcal fluoroquinolone alone. Detailed discussion of the treatment of community-acquired pneumonia is beyond the scope of this chapter and readers are referred to several guidelines published recently on this topic [36,37,76,111].

## Symptomatic treatment of cough

### Antitussive and protussive therapy
With the exception of pneumonia, the mainstay of treatment for patients with cough as a troublesome manifestation of acute lower airway infection will be the use of non-specific therapies aimed at suppressing cough or facilitating sputum mobilization and clearance. This is particularly true when specific treatment is not available, as in most patients with acute tracheobronchitis due to a viral origin.

Antitussive therapy—aimed at controlling or eliminating cough—is often prescribed for nocturnal use, for patients are often most bothered by cough interrupting sleep, but is also often prescribed for repeated use throughout the day, on an 'as needed' basis. Although inhibition of cough carries the theoretical risk of allowing accumulation of excessive respiratory secretions, thus predisposing to bacterial infection, no association of the use of antitussives and the development of secondary bacterial infections has been reported in the literature. The effectiveness of medications such as codeine, dextromethorphan and diphenhydramine has been demonstrated in random-

ized controlled trials to reduce cough in patients with bronchitis [77,112].

The use of protussive therapy is indicated when cough is deemed to perform a useful function and needs to be encouraged. Although there is some evidence that humidified air and guaifenesin are effective expectorants, there is a paucity of good-quality studies on the use of other protussive agents in the management of cough secondary to respiratory tract infection. The role of mucolytic and mucokinetic agents in acute tracheobronchitis remains unclear. While many of these agents are used widely in cough medications available over the counter, a recent systemic review of 15 randomized controlled trials involving 2166 adult patients with acute cough illness due to upper respiratory tract infections found no convincing evidence that over-the-counter cough preparations were helpful [113].

Although short courses of oral or inhaled corticosteroid have been given to patients in clinical practice in an attempt to shorten the duration of cough, there is no published report to suggest that this is effective in patients without underlying asthma.

## References

1 Schappert SM. Ambulatory care visits of physician offices, hospital outpatient departments, and emergency departments: United States, 1995. *Vital Health Stat 13* 1997; **129**: 1–38.
2 Ayres JG. Seasonal pattern of acute bronchitis in general practice in the United Kingdom 1976–83. *Thorax* 1986; **41** (2): 106–10.
3 Oeffinger KC, Snell LM, Foster BM, Panico KG, Archer RK. Diagnosis of acute bronchitis in adults: a national survey of family physicians. *J Fam Pract* 1997; **45** (5): 402–9.
4 Evan AS. Clinical syndromes in adults caused by respiratory infection. *Med Clin North Am* 1967; **51**: 803–18.
5 Shay DK, Holman RC, Newman RD, Liu LL, Stout JW, Anderson LJ. Bronchiolitis-associated hospitalizations among US children, 1980–96. *JAMA* 1999; **282** (15): 1440–6.
6 Henderson FW, Clyde WA Jr, Collier AM, Denny FW, Senior RJ, Sheaffer CI *et al.* The etiologic and epidemiologic spectrum of bronchiolitis in pediatric practice. *J Pediatr* 1979; **95** (2): 183–90.
7 Welliver RC, Wong DT, Sun M, McCarthy N. Parainfluenza virus bronchiolitis. Epidemiology and pathogenesis. *Am J Dis Child* 1986; **140** (1): 34–40.
8 Denny FW, Murphy TF, Clyde WA Jr, Collier AM,

Henderson FW. Croup: an 11-year study in a pediatric practice. *Pediatrics* 1983; **71** (6): 871–6.

9 Hall CB. Respiratory syncytial virus and parainfluenza virus. *N Engl J Med* 2001; **344** (25): 1917–28.

10 Sendi K, Crysdale WS, Yoo J. Tracheitis: outcome of 1,700 cases presenting to the emergency department during two years. *J Otolaryngol* 1992; **21** (1): 20–4.

11 Nicholson KG, Kent J, Hammersley V, Cancio E. Acute viral infections of upper respiratory tract in elderly people living in the community: comparative, prospective, population based study of disease burden. *Br Med J* 1997; **315** (7115): 1060–4.

12 Falsey AR, McCann RM, Hall WJ, Tanner MA, Criddle MM, Formica MA *et al.* Acute respiratory tract infection in daycare centers for older persons. *J Am Geriatr Soc* 1995; **43** (1): 30–6.

13 Pitkaranta A, Virolainen A, Jero J, Arruda E, Hayden FG. Detection of rhinovirus, respiratory syncytial virus, and coronavirus infections in acute otitis media by reverse transcriptase polymerase chain reaction. *Pediatrics* 1998; **102**: 291–5.

14 Nicholson KG, Kent J, Hammersley V, Cancio E. Risk factors for lower respiratory complications of rhinovirus infections in elderly people living in the community: prospective cohort study. *Br Med J* 1996; **313**: 1119–23.

15 Van Hartesveldt FR. *The 1918–1919 Pandemic of Influenza: the Urban Impact in the Western World*. Lewiston, NY: E. Mellen Press, 1992.

16 Crosby AW. *America's Forgotten Pandemic: the Influenza of 1918*. Cambridge, UK: Cambridge University Press, 1989.

17 Denny FW Jr. The clinical impact of human respiratory virus infections. *Am J Respir Crit Care Med* 1995; **152**: S4–12.

18 Boldy DA, Skidmore SJ, Ayres JG. Acute bronchitis in the community: clinical features, infective factors, changes in pulmonary function and bronchial reactivity to histamine. *Respir Med* 1990; **84** (5): 377–85.

19 Monto AS. Viral respiratory infections in the community: epidemiology, agents and interventions. *Am J Med* 1995; **99**: 24S–27S.

20 Monto AS, Sullivan KM. Acute respiratory illness in the community. Frequency of illness and the agents involved. *Epidemiol Infect* 1993; **110** (1): 145–60.

21 Gern JE, Galagan DM, Jarjour NN, Dick EC, Busse WW. Detection of rhinovirus RNA in lower airway cells during experimentally induced infection. *Am J Respir Crit Care Med* 1997; **155** (3): 1159–61.

22 Monto AS, Fendrick AM, Sarnes MW. Respiratory illness caused by picornavirus infection: a review of clinical outcomes. *Clin Ther* 2001; **23** (10): 1615–27.

23 Johnston SL, Pattemore PK, Sanderson G, Smith S, Lampe F, Josephs L *et al.* Community study of role of viral infections in exacerbations of asthma in 9–11 year old children. *Br Med J* 1995; **310**: 1225–9.

24 Nicholson KG, Kent J, Ireland DC. Respiratory viruses and exacerbations of asthma in adults. *Br Med J* 1993; **307**: 982–6.

25 Seemungal TA, Harper-Owen R, Bhowmik A, Jeffries DJ, Wedzicha JA. Detection of rhinovirus in induced sputum at exacerbation of chronic obstructive pulmonary disease. *Eur Respir J* 2000; **16** (4): 677–83.

26 Wedzicha JA. Exacerbations: etiology and pathophysiologic mechanisms. *Chest* 2002; **121** (5 Suppl.): 136S–41S.

27 Greenberg SB, Allen M, Wilson J, Atmar RL. Respiratory viral infections in adults with and without chronic obstructive pulmonary disease. *Am J Respir Crit Care Med* 2000; **162** (1): 167–73.

28 Smyth AR, Smyth RL, Tong CY, Hart CA, Heaf DP. Effect of respiratory virus infections including rhinovirus on clinical status in cystic fibrosis. *Arch Dis Child* 1995; **73** (2): 117–20.

29 Mink CM, Cherry JD, Christenson P, Lewis K, Pineda E, Shlian D *et al.* A search for *Bordetella pertussis* infection in university students. *Clin Infect Dis* 1992; **14** (2): 464–71.

30 Nennig ME, Shinefield HR, Edwards KM, Black SB, Fireman BH. Prevalence and incidence of adult pertussis in an urban population. *JAMA* 1996; **275** (21): 1672–4.

31 Grayston JT, Kuo CC, Wang SP, Altman J. A new *Chlamydia psittaci* strain, TWAR, isolated in acute respiratory tract infections. *N Engl J Med* 1986; **315** (3): 161–8.

32 Wright SW, Edwards KM, Decker MD, Grayston JT, Wang S. Prevalence of positive serology for acute *Chlamydia pneumoniae* infection in emergency department patients with persistent cough. *Acad Emerg Med* 1997; **4** (3): 179–83.

33 Gonzales R, Malone DC, Maselli JH, Sande MA. Excessive antibiotic use for acute respiratory infections in the United States. *Clin Infect Dis* 2001; **33** (6): 757–62.

34 Gonzales R, Steiner JF, Sande MA. Antibiotic prescribing for adults with colds, upper respiratory tract infections, and bronchitis by ambulatory care physicians. *JAMA* 1997; **278** (11): 901–4.

35 Metlay JP, Stafford RS, Singer DE. National trends in the use of antibiotics by primary care physicians for adult patients with cough. *Arch Intern Med* 1998; **158** (16): 1813–18.

36 Niederman MS, Mandell LA, Anzueto A, Bass JB, Broughton WA, Campbell GD *et al.* Guidelines for the management of adults with community-acquired pneumonia. Diagnosis, assessment of severity, antimicrobial therapy, and prevention. *Am J Respir Crit Care Med* 2001; **163** (7): 1730–54.

37 Bartlett JG, Breiman RF, Mandell LA, File TM Jr. Community-acquired pneumonia in adults: guidelines for management. The Infectious Diseases Society of America. *Clin Infect Dis* 1998; **26** (4): 811–38.

38 Macfarlane JT, Finch RG, Ward MJ, Macrae AD. Hospital study of adult community-acquired pneumonia. *Lancet* 1982; **2**: 255–8.

39 Ostergaard L, Andersen PL. Etiology of community-acquired pneumonia. Evaluation by transtracheal aspiration, blood culture, or serology. *Chest* 1993; **104** (5): 1400–7.

40 Bartlett JG, Mundy LM. Community-acquired pneumonia. *N Engl J Med* 1995; **333** (24): 1618–24.

41 Ruiz M, Ewig S, Marcos MA, Martinez JA, Arancibia F, Mensa J et al. Etiology of community-acquired pneumonia: impact of age, comorbidity, and severity. *Am J Respir Crit Care Med* 1999; **160** (2): 397–405.

42 Ruiz M, Ewig S, Torres A, Arancibia F, Marco F, Mensa J et al. Severe community-acquired pneumonia. Risk factors and follow-up epidemiology. *Am J Respir Crit Care Med* 1999; **160** (3): 923–9.

43 Gwaltney JM Jr. Rhinovirus infection of the normal human airway. *Am J Respir Crit Care Med* 1995; **152**: S36–9.

44 Halperin SA, Eggleston PA, Hendley JO, Suratt PM, Groschel DH, Gwaltney JM Jr. Pathogenesis of lower respiratory tract symptoms in experimental rhinovirus infection. *Am Rev Respir Dis* 1983; **128** (5): 806–10.

45 Folkerts G, Busse WW, Nijkamp FP, Sorkness R, Gern JE. Virus-induced airway hyperresponsiveness and asthma. *Am J Respir Crit Care Med* 1998; **157**: 1708–20.

46 Loosli CG, Stinson SF, Ryan DP, Hertweck MS, Hardy JD, Serebrin R. The destruction of type 2 pneumocytes by airborne influenza PR8-A virus; its effect on surfactant and lecithin content of the pneumonic lesions of mice. *Chest* 1975; **67** (2 Suppl.): 7S–14S.

47 Aherne W, Bird T, Court SD, Gardner PS, McQuillin J. Pathological changes in virus infections of the lower respiratory tract in children. *J Clin Pathol* 1970; **23** (1): 7–18.

48 Borson DB, Brokaw JJ, Sekizawa K, McDonald DM, Nadel JA. Neutral endopeptidase and neurogenic inflammation in rats with respiratory infections. *J Appl Physiol* 1989; **66** (6): 2653–8.

49 Jacoby DB, Tamaoki J, Borson DB, Nadel JA. Influenza infection causes airway hyperresponsiveness by decreasing enkephalinase. *J Appl Physiol* 1988; **64** (6): 2653–8.

50 Kohrogi H, Nadel JA, Malfroy B, Gorman C, Bridenbaugh R, Patton JS et al. Recombinant human enkephalinase (neutral endopeptidase) prevents cough induced by tachykinins in awake guinea pigs. *J Clin Invest* 1989; **84** (3): 781–6.

51 Nadel JA, Borson DB. Modulation of neurogenic inflammation by neutral endopeptidase. *Am Rev Respir Dis* 1991; **143**: S33–6.

52 Corrao WM, Braman SS, Irwin RS. Chronic cough as the sole presenting manifestation of bronchial asthma. *N Engl J Med* 1979; **300** (12): 633–7.

53 Melbye H, Aasebo U, Straume B. Symptomatic effect of inhaled fenoterol in acute bronchitis: a placebo-controlled double-blind study. *Fam Pract* 1991; **8** (3): 216–22.

54 Hueston WJ. A comparison of albuterol and erythromycin for the treatment of acute bronchitis. *J Fam Pract* 1991; **33** (5): 476–80.

55 Hueston WJ. Albuterol delivered by metered-dose inhaler to treat acute bronchitis. *J Fam Pract* 1994; **39** (5): 437–40.

56 Williamson HA Jr. Pulmonary function tests in acute bronchitis: evidence for reversible airway obstruction. *J Fam Pract* 1987; **25** (3): 251–6.

57 Witek TJ, Doyle C, Hayden FG. The incidence of 'post viral cough' following natural colds in a community setting. *Am J Respir Crit Care Med* 2002; **165**: 8 (2): A130.

58 Robertson AJ. Green sputum. *Lancet* 1952; **1**: 12–15.

59 Williamson HA Jr. A randomized, controlled trial of doxycycline in the treatment of acute bronchitis. *J Fam Pract* 1984; **19** (4): 481–6.

60 Wright SW, Edwards KM, Decker MD, Zeldin MH. Pertussis infection in adults with persistent cough. *JAMA* 1995; **273** (13): 1044–6.

61 He Q, Viljanen MK, Arvilommi H, Aittanen B, Mertsola J. Whooping cough caused by *Bordetella pertussis* and *Bordetella parapertussis* in an immunized population. *JAMA* 1998; **280** (7): 635–7.

62 Feigin RD, Cherry JD. Pertussis. In: Bralow L, ed. *Textbook of Pediatric Infectious Diseases*, 3rd edn. Pennsylvania: W.B. Saunders, 1992: 1211–12.

63 Yaari E, Yafe-Zimerman Y, Schwartz SB, Slater PE, Shvartzman P, Andoren N et al. Clinical manifestations of *Bordetella pertussis* infection in immunized children and young adults. *Chest* 1999; **115** (5): 1254–8.

64 Stein RT, Sherrill D, Morgan WJ, Holberg CJ, Halonen M, Taussig LM et al. Respiratory syncytial virus in early life and risk of wheeze and allergy by age 13 years. *Lancet* 1999; **354**: 541–5.

65 Marrie TJ. Community-acquired pneumonia. In: Niederman MS, ed. *Respiratory Infections: a Scientific Basis for Management*. Philadelphia: W.B. Saunders, 1994: 125–38.

66 Heckerling PS, Tape TG, Wigton RS, Hissong KK, Leikin JB, Ornato JP et al. Clinical prediction rule for pulmonary infiltrates. *Ann Intern Med* 1990; **113** (9): 664–70.

67 Diehr P, Wood RW, Bushyhead J, Krueger L, Wolcott B, Tompkins RK. Prediction of pneumonia in outpatients

with acute cough—a statistical approach. *J Chronic Dis* 1984; **37** (3): 215–25.

68 Singal BM, Hedges JR, Radack KL. Decision rules and clinical prediction of pneumonia: evaluation of low-yield criteria. *Ann Emerg Med* 1989; **18** (1): 13–20.

69 Gennis P, Gallagher J, Falvo C, Baker S, Than W. Clinical criteria for the detection of pneumonia in adults: guidelines for ordering chest roentgenograms in the emergency department. *J Emerg Med* 1989; **7** (3): 263–8.

70 Metlay JP, Kapoor WN, Fine MJ. Does this patient have community-acquired pneumonia? Diagnosing pneumonia by history and physical examination. *JAMA* 1997; **278** (17): 1440–5.

71 Metlay JP, Schulz R, Li YH, Singer DE, Marrie TJ, Coley CM *et al.* Influence of age on symptoms at presentation in patients with community-acquired pneumonia. *Arch Intern Med* 1997; **157** (13): 1453–9.

72 Monto AS, Fleming DM, Henry D, de Groot R, Makela M, Klein T *et al.* Efficacy and safety of the neuraminidase inhibitor zanamivir in the treatment of influenza A and B virus infections. *J Infect Dis* 1999; **180** (2): 254–61.

73 Hayden FG, Osterhaus AD, Treanor JJ, Fleming DM, Aoki FY, Nicholson KG *et al.* Efficacy and safety of the neuraminidase inhibitor zanamivir in the treatment of influenzavirus infections. Gg167 Influenza Study Group. *N Engl J Med* 1997; **337** (13): 874–80.

74 Dolin R, Reichman RC, Madore HP, Maynard R, Linton PN, Webber-Jones J. A controlled trial of amantadine and rimantadine in the prophylaxis of influenza A infection. *N Engl J Med* 1982; **307** (10): 580–4.

75 Melbye H, Kongerud J, Vorland L. Reversible airflow limitation in adults with respiratory infection. *Eur Respir J* 1994; **7** (7): 1239–45.

76 BTS Guidelines for the Management of Community Acquired Pneumonia in Adults. *Thorax* 2001; **56** (Suppl. 4): IV1–64.

77 Irwin RS, Boulet LP, Cloutier MM, Fuller R, Gold PM, Hoffstein V *et al.* Managing cough as a defense mechanism and as a symptom. A consensus panel report of the American College of Chest Physicians. *Chest* 1998; **114** (2 Suppl. Managing): 133S–181S.

78 Fahey T, Stocks N, Thomas T. Quantitative systematic review of randomised controlled trials comparing antibiotic with placebo for acute cough in adults. *Br Med J* 1998; **316**: 906–10.

79 Orr PH, Scherer K, Macdonald A, Moffatt ME. Randomized placebo-controlled trials of antibiotics for acute bronchitis: a critical review of the literature. *J Fam Pract* 1993; **36** (5): 507–12.

80 MacKay DN. Treatment of acute bronchitis in adults without underlying lung disease. *J Gen Intern Med* 1996; **11** (9): 557–62.

81 Smucny JJ, Becker LA, Glazier RH, McIsaac W. Are antibiotics effective treatment for acute bronchitis? A meta-analysis. *J Fam Pract* 1998; **47** (6): 453–60.

82 Bent S, Saint S, Vittinghoff E, Grady D. Antibiotics in acute bronchitis: a meta-analysis. *Am J Med* 1999; **107** (1): 62–7.

83 Evans AT, Husain S, Durairaj L, Sadowski LS, Charles-Damte M, Wang Y. Azithromycin for acute bronchitis: a randomised, double-blind, controlled trial. *Lancet* 2002; **359**: 1648–54.

84 Snow V, Mottur-Pilson C, Gonzales R. Principles of appropriate antibiotic use for treatment of acute bronchitis in adults. *Ann Intern Med* 2001; **134** (6): 518–20.

85 Gonzales R, Bartlett JG, Besser RE, Cooper RJ, Hickner JM, Hoffman JR *et al.* Principles of appropriate antibiotic use for treatment of uncomplicated acute bronchitis: background. *Ann Intern Med* 2001; **134** (6): 521–9.

86 Smucny J, Flynn C, Becker L, Glazier R. Beta2-agonists for acute bronchitis. *Cochrane Database Syst Rev* 2001; (1): CD001726.

87 Curley FJ, Irwin RS, Pratter MR, Stivers DH, Doern GV, Vernaglia PA *et al.* Cough and the common cold. *Am Rev Respir Dis* 1988; **138** (2): 305–11.

88 Bergquist SO, Bernander S, Dahnsjo H, Sundelof B. Erythromycin in the treatment of pertussis: a study of bacteriologic and clinical effects. *Pediatr Infect Dis J* 1987; **6** (5): 458–61.

89 Sprauer MA, Cochi SL, Zell ER, Sutter RW, Mullen JR, Englender SJ *et al.* Prevention of secondary transmission of pertussis in households with early use of erythromycin. *Am J Dis Child* 1992; **146** (2): 177–81.

90 Wirsing von Konig CH, Postels-Multani S, Bogaerts H, Bock HL, Laukamp S, Kiederle S *et al.* Factors influencing the spread of pertussis in households. *Eur J Pediatr* 1998; **157** (5): 391–4.

91 Randomised trial of efficacy and safety of inhaled zanamivir in treatment of influenza A and B virus infections. The MIST (Management of Influenza in the Southern Hemisphere Trialists) Study Group. *Lancet* 1998; **352**: 1877–81.

92 Jefferson T, Demicheli V, Deeks J, Rivetti D. Neuraminidase inhibitors for preventing and treating influenza in healthy adults. *Cochrane Database Syst Rev* 2000; (2): CD001265.

93 Rotbart HA. Treatment of picornavirus infections. *Antiviral Res* 2002; **53** (2): 83–98.

94 Randolph AG, Wang EE. Ribavirin for respiratory syncytial virus infection of the lower respiratory tract. *Cochrane Database Syst Rev* 2000; (2): CD000181.

95 American Academy of Pediatrics. Hemophilus influenza type b and respiratory syncytial virus. In: Peter G, ed. *Red Book: Report of the Committee on Infectious Diseases,*

24th edn. Elk Grove Village, IL: American Academy of Pediatrics, 1997: 443–7.

96 Flores G, Horwitz RI. Efficacy of beta2-agonists in bronchiolitis: a reappraisal and meta-analysis. *Pediatrics* 1997; **100**: 233–9.

97 Garrison MM, Christakis DA, Harvey E, Cummings P, Davis RL. Systemic corticosteroids in infant bronchiolitis: a meta-analysis. *Pediatrics* 2000; **105** (4): E44.

98 Cade A, Brownlee KG, Conway SP, Haigh D, Short A, Brown J *et al*. Randomised placebo controlled trial of nebulised corticosteroids in acute respiratory syncytial viral bronchiolitis. *Arch Dis Child* 2000; **82** (2): 126–30.

99 Bulow SM, Nir M, Levin E, Friis B, Thomsen LL, Nielsen JE *et al*. Prednisolone treatment of respiratory syncytial virus infection: a randomized controlled trial of 147 infants. *Pediatrics* 1999; **104** (6): e77.

100 Ledwith CA, Shea LM, Mauro RD. Safety and efficacy of nebulized racemic epinephrine in conjunction with oral dexamethasone and mist in the outpatient treatment of croup. *Ann Emerg Med* 1995; **25** (3): 331–7.

101 Waisman Y, Klein BL, Boenning DA, Young GM, Chamberlain JM, O'Donnell R *et al*. Prospective randomized double-blind study comparing l-epinephrine and racemic epinephrine aerosols in the treatment of laryngotracheitis (croup). *Pediatrics* 1992; **89** (2): 302–6.

102 Fitzgerald D, Mellis C, Johnson M, Allen H, Cooper P, Van Asperen P. Nebulized budesonide is as effective as nebulized adrenaline in moderately severe croup. *Pediatrics* 1996; **97** (5): 722–5.

103 Wright RB, Pomerantz WJ, Luria JW. New approaches to respiratory infections in children. Bronchiolitis and croup. *Emerg Med Clin North Am* 2002; **20** (1): 93–114.

104 Super DM, Cartelli NA, Brooks LJ, Lembo RM, Kumar ML. A prospective randomized double-blind study to evaluate the effect of dexamethasone in acute laryngotracheitis. *J Pediatr* 1989; **115** (2): 323–9.

105 Geelhoed GC, Macdonald WB. Oral dexamethasone in the treatment of croup: 0.15 mg/kg versus 0.3 mg/kg versus 0.6 mg/kg. *Pediatr Pulmonol* 1995; **20** (6): 362–8.

106 Klassen TP, Feldman ME, Watters LK, Sutcliffe T, Rowe PC. Nebulized budesonide for children with mild-to-moderate croup. *N Engl J Med* 1994; **331** (5): 285–9.

107 Johnson DW, Jacobson S, Edney PC, Hadfield P, Mundy ME, Schuh S. A comparison of nebulized budesonide, intramuscular dexamethasone, and placebo for moderately severe croup. *N Engl J Med* 1998; **339** (8): 498–503.

108 Klassen TP, Craig WR, Moher D, Osmond MH, Pasterkamp H, Sutcliffe T *et al*. Nebulized budesonide and oral dexamethasone for treatment of croup: a randomized controlled trial. *JAMA* 1998; **279** (20): 1629–32.

109 Ausejo M, Saenz A, Pham B, Kellner JD, Johnson DW, Moher D *et al*. Glucocorticoids for croup. *Cochrane Database Syst Rev* 2000; (2): CD001955.

110 Geelhoed GC, Turner J, Macdonald WB. Efficacy of a small single dose of oral dexamethasone for outpatient croup: a double blind placebo controlled clinical trial. *Br Med J* 1996; **313**: 140–2.

111 Heffelfinger JD, Dowell SF, Jorgensen JH, Klugman KP, Mabry LR, Musher DM *et al*. Management of community-acquired pneumonia in the era of pneumococcal resistance: a report from the Drug-Resistant Streptococcus pneumoniae Therapeutic Working Group. *Arch Intern Med* 2000; **160** (10): 1399–408.

112 Irwin RS, Curley FJ. The treatment of cough. A comprehensive review. *Chest* 1991; **99** (6): 1477–84.

113 Schroeder K, Fahey T. Systematic review of randomised controlled trials of over the counter cough medicines for acute cough in adults. *Br Med J* 2002; **324**: 329–31.

# 10 Cough and gastro-oesophageal reflux

*Alvin J. Ing*

## Gastro-oesophageal reflux

The primary event in gastro-oesophageal reflux (GOR) is the movement of acid, pepsin and other noxious substances from the stomach into the oesophagus [1]. In healthy individuals, reflux is a normal, mostly asymptomatic event. Gastro-oesophageal reflux disease (GORD) is defined as occurring when reflux leads to symptoms or physical complications. In most patients this occurs when there is excessive exposure of the distal oesophageal mucosa to refluxed gastric contents resulting in heartburn, epigastric or retrosternal discomfort and chest pain [2]. Prolonged exposure can lead also to oesophagitis, oesophageal ulceration and its complications such as bleeding or stricture formation. However, oesophageal reflux symptoms can also occur without oesophagitis, and there can be significant reflux without classical symptoms [3].

GOR has long been associated with pulmonary symptoms and diseases, many of which present with cough. These range from bronchopulmonary dysplasia in the newborn, bronchial asthma, chronic persistent cough, chronic bronchitis and diffuse pulmonary fibrosis, through to the pulmonary aspiration syndromes, including lung abscess, bronchiectasis, aspiration pneumonitis, recurrent pneumonia and eventually respiratory failure [4]. Pulmonary complications may result from either direct micro- and/or macroaspiration, as well as from both local and centrally mediated reflex mechanisms.

As a cause of chronic cough, GORD has been documented in many series to be one of the most common aetiologies, across all age groups [5–7].

## The normal antireflux barrier

The lower oesophageal sphincter (LOS), the crural diaphragm and the phreno-oesophageal ligament are considered to be the anatomical structures that play a major role in the normal antireflux barrier [1]. The intraluminal pressure at the gastro-oesophageal junction reflects the strength of the antireflux barrier, and reflux only occurs when this pressure is reduced.

The lower oesophageal sphincter is 2.5–3.5 cm in length, and is probably part intra-abdominal and part intrathoracic. It consists of a zone of thickened muscle with evidence of higher neuronal density than that of the adjacent oesophagus in animals. The end expiratory pressure at the gastro-oesophageal junction at rest is due to the smooth muscle activity of the LOS, but the LOS pressure can also fluctuate with the migrating motor activity of the stomach. The circular muscle of the LOS can generate tonic activity, which is influenced by neurogenic, hormonal and myogenic factors [8,9].

The crural diaphragm, phreno-oesophageal ligament and LOS form an anatomical and physiological antireflux barrier which prevents GOR under both resting conditions and when increased intra-abdominal pressure occurs. The transdiaphragmatic pressure ($P_{di}$) or the pressure difference between the stomach and the oesophagus is +4–6 mmHg during tidal volume expiration, while it is +10–18 mmHg during tidal volume expiration. During maximal inspiratory efforts, e.g. to total lung capacity, the $P_{di}$ can reach values of 60–80 mmHg [1]. However, GOR does not result from raised transdiaphragmatic pressure alone. This is because as $P_{di}$ increases during inspiration, oesophagogastric junction pressure increases due to contraction of the crural diaphragm. For GOR to occur, therefore, there must be significant defects in the normal antireflux barrier since increases in $P_{di}$ and intra-abdominal pressures are effectively counteracted by intact antireflux mechanisms.

### Pathogenesis of gastro-oesophageal reflux disease

It is currently thought that LOS dysfunction is the major cause of defective gastro-oesophageal competence and thus reflux, with non-sphincteric mechanisms having a secondary role [2]. The majority of patients with GORD have normal basal LOS tone. Reflux occurs, however, because of transient relaxation of this tone, a phenomenon termed transient lower oesophageal sphincter relaxation (TLOSR) by Dent *et al.* [10].

Simultaneous measurements of oesophageal pH and motility have found that, under resting conditions, LOS sphincter pressure has to be absent for reflux to occur in normal subjects, both adults and children [10–12]. In the majority of reflux episodes this is due to TLOSR, with only a minority of episodes due to chronic absence of LOS pressure, or reduced basal LOS tone. TLOSR is likely to be neurally mediated, and triggered by gastric distension, and perhaps pharyngeal activity [13]. There are also non-sphincteric factors related to occurrence of pathological gastro-oesophageal reflux. Of particular interest in patients with chronic persistent cough is increased $P_{di}$ during the inspiratory phase of cough, and raised intra-abdominal pressure during the compressive and expiratory phases of cough. In healthy subjects, increased $P_{di}$ provokes GOR only if basal LOS pressure is less than or equal to 4 mmHg [14], normal resting pressure being 10–26 mmHg. Reflux was not demonstrated when LOS was normal, and only occurred in the presence of raised $P_{di}$ when there was TLOSR or swallowing [10].

The relationship between cough and oesophageal reflux, with regard to mechanisms by which cough may aggravate or precipitate reflux episodes, is not known. There is no doubt that raised transdiaphragmatic pressure occurs as a result of chronic cough, but this alone is not sufficient to produce reflux on a background of normal basal lower esophageal sphincter tone [1,10]. Possible mechanisms by which cough may precipitate reflux include cough stimulating either TLOSR or swallow-induced sphincter relaxation; as yet neither has been proven, although some animal studies are suggestive.

## Chronic persistent cough

Chronic persistent cough has been the most widely studied entity in the investigation of the role of GORD in the pathogenesis of cough. It is defined as cough persisting for at least 3 weeks in patients with a normal chest X-ray and not on angiotensin-converting enzyme inhibitors. In multiple series, GOR has been documented to be a cause of chronic persistent cough (either solely or in combination with bronchial asthma and postnasal drip) in 38–82% of patients [3,5–7,15–17]. GORD, bronchial asthma and postnasal drip account either singly or in combination for over 90% of patients with chronic persistent cough. As a consequence, using evidence-based guidelines, the American College of Chest Physicians have published a consensus statement on the management of cough, including an algorithm on the evaluation of chronic cough in immunocompetent adults (Fig. 10.1) [18]. At the heart of this algorithm is the principle that, in patients with chronic persistent cough with a normal chest X-ray, the possibility of postnasal drip, bronchial asthma and GORD should be evaluated in that order to determine the underlying aetiology of cough.

### Role of GOR in the pathogenesis of cough

Chronic cough secondary to GOR has been associated with a wide range of disease entities. These can be categorized based on the pathogenesis of the cough.

Gross aspiration or macroaspiration has been documented in many pathologies including recurrent aspiration pneumonia, pulmonary abscess, pulmonary fibrosis including progressive systemic sclerosis and cryptogenic fibrosing alveolitis, bronchiectasis and obliterative bronchiolitis in heart–lung transplant recipients.

Microaspiration has been documented in patients with laryngeal inflammation (especially posterior laryngitis), chronic bronchitis and sinusitis.

Vagally mediated distal oesophageal–tracheobronchial reflex mechanisms have been documented in patients with chronic persistent cough with otherwise asymptomatic reflux [19], and patients with bronchial asthma [20].

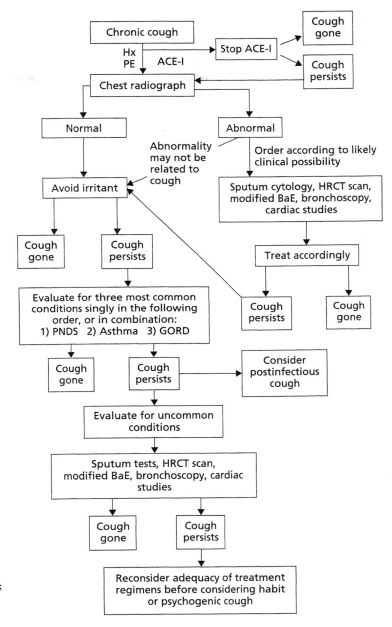

**Fig. 10.1** Guidelines for evaluating chronic cough in immunocompetent adults. ACE-I, angiotensin-converting enzyme inhibitor; BaE, barium examination; GORD, gastro-oesophageal reflux disease; HRCT scan, high-resolution computed tomographic scan; Hx, history; PE, physical examination; PNDS, postnasal drip syndrome. From [18].

In patients with chronic persistent cough whose cough is unexplained after a standard diagnostic evaluation, including history and examination, chest X-rays, laryngoscopy, paranasal sinus X-rays, lung function testing, bronchial provocation testing and home peak flow monitoring, cough is commonly associated with GOR [18]. In this setting, cough has been shown to be a result of gastric acid stimulating a distal oesophageal tracheobronchial reflex mechanism with no evidence of microaspiration or proximal oesophageal reflux [19,21]. The afferent pathway is inhibited by the oesophageal instillation of local anaesthetic (4% topical lidocaine), while the efferent pathway is inhibited by nebulized ipratropium bromide [19]. This reflex arc is the likely mechanism by which GOR leads to cough in these patients, although intraoesophageal acid may not be the sole mediator [21].

The nature of this reflex arc has not been fully elucidated in patients with cough, although in patients with bronchial asthma there is evidence that GOR may initiate airway inflammation from the oesophagus via axonal reflexes [22]. Axonal reflexes are mediated by nociceptive afferent nerves that release neurotransmitters which act to trigger an inflammatory response. Tachykinins including substance P and neurokinin A are associated with nociceptive afferent nerves and are potent mediators of bronchospasm and mucus secretion. Whether local axonal reflexes such as this have a role in the pathogenesis of cough associated with GOR is unknown, although it is likely to play a role in the development of cough secondary to GOR in patients with asthma.

There is also growing evidence that central nervous reflexes may be important in the pathogenesis of GOR-induced cough in patients with chronic persistent cough. An animal model has been developed using Wistar rats, showing that stimulation of their oesophagus by acid and pepsin resulted in an increase in c-Fos immunoreactivity in brainstem regions [23,24]. In a randomized controlled fashion, Suwanprathes et al. [24] perfused the oesophagus of 10 rats with 0.1 mol/L HCl and pepsin (3200–4500 IU/mL). The brainstem was then processed immunohistochemically for detection of c-Fos protein, an immediate-early gene with low basal CNS expression, which is detected maximally in CNS neurones 30–45 min after stimulation. This study found that c-Fos immunoreactivity was significantly increased in a number of brainstem regions in rats including the nucleus of the solitary tract, medial part (mNTS), Kolliker–Fuse nucleus (KF), central amygdala nucleus (CeC), nucleus ambiguus (Amb), retroambigualis nucleus (RA) and paratrigeminal nucleus (PTN). These areas represent the dorsomedial medulla (mNTS), dorsolateral medulla (PTN), ventrolateral medulla (Amb and RA) and forebrain (CeC). Other studies have found that vagal efferent pathways originate from the RA and Amb, and that the PTN is the initial processing centre for afferent signals, with a subpopulation of secondary neurones projecting onto the NTS and then onto the RA and Amb which possibly represent the cough efferent centre [25,26]. These stud-

ies therefore suggest that acid and pepsin in the distal oesophagus may stimulate afferent pathways which project to the brainstem 'cough centre' (including the PTN, NTS, Amb and RA), which in turn may activate cough efferent pathways. The applicability of this in humans remains unknown.

### The cough–reflux self-perpetuating cycle

GOR precipitates cough via the mechanisms described above. A number of investigators have proposed a self-perpetuating positive feedback cycle between cough and oesophageal reflux, whereby cough from any cause may precipitate further reflux [18,19,25]. The mechanisms by which GOR is worsened or triggered by cough are still unknown. Evidence for the existence of this cycle is found in studies showing that the antitussive action of antireflux therapy is prolonged and is present long after the antireflux therapy has ceased [27,28].

## Clinical presentation

Apart from cough, the clinical presentation in adults is very much dependent on the underlying aetiology. The most common clinical syndrome is due to distal oesophageal–tracheobronchial reflex mechanisms, and in such patients GOR symptoms such as heartburn, waterbrash and acid regurgitation are unusual. Between 50 and 77% of patients have no reflux symptoms [15,29], while the remainder have symptoms only after the development of cough, suggesting cough as the initiating event in the cough–reflux cycle. In one study, cough was the sole presenting manifestation of GOR in nine patients [3]. The cough occurs predominantly during the day, with minimal nocturnal symptoms, as reflux occurs generally in the upright position. This is as a result of the preservation of the normal reflex which suppresses TLOSR when supine.

The cough may be productive or non-productive and is generally longstanding with a mean duration of 13–58 months [3,15,29], the majority of patients recalling its onset after an upper respiratory tract infection. Often the cough has not responded to either non-specific or specific trials of therapy, and investigations including chest X-rays, lung function testing, bronchial provocation testing and laryngoscopy have been unhelpful. GOR in this situation needs to be suspected and initial empirical therapy is appropriate and

cost-effective [18]. There is also evidence to suggest that chronic cough from any cause may precipitate GOR via the cough–reflux self-perpetuating cycle, and thus GOR should be considered as a contributory cause of cough in any patients with persistent symptoms despite a specific diagnosis and specific therapy. Chronic cough has been documented to have multiple causes in over 25% of patients [18].

In patients with microaspiration, symptoms of GOR are more prominent and may predate the onset of cough, implying that cough may not be the initiating event in this group. Laryngeal symptoms such as dysphonia, hoarseness and a sore throat are also prominent, and laryngoscopy may be abnormal. Posterior vocal cord inflammation is suggestive of microaspiration, but not diagnostic.

## Diagnosis

GOR should be considered if there are typical symptoms or if cough remains unexplained after standard investigations. This should include history, examination, chest X-ray, pulmonary function studies and laryngoscopy. The diagnosis of GORD is usually made on the basis of clinical grounds. There is evidence that if cough remains unexplained after the above investigations, and in particular if postnasal drip and bronchial asthma have been excluded, then an empirical trial of

antireflux therapy is justified [18] (Fig. 10.2). If empirical therapy fails, it cannot be assumed that GORD has been excluded as a cause of chronic cough, as empirical therapy may have been inadequate or medical therapy may have failed. In such a situation, objective investigation for GORD is recommended, and specifically 24-h ambulatory oesophageal pH monitoring while on antireflux therapy. Twenty-four-hour ambulatory oesophageal pH monitoring is well recognized as the most sensitive and specific investigation for GORD, since significant and/or symptomatic reflux can occur in the absence of macroscopic mucosal damage at endoscopy, and patients may have significant reflux without symptoms other than chronic cough. It is recommended that pH monitoring should be performed during therapy if there is failure of cough to respond to empirical antireflux treatment, since the presence of significant acid reflux will indicate inadequate therapy, while the absence of acid reflux would suggest that GOR is not the cause of the chronic cough.

The other advantages of pH monitoring of the oesophagus are that it may demonstrate a temporal relationship between cough and reflux, as well as quantifying the degree of reflux present (Fig. 10.3). It may be the only method of diagnosing GOR in up to 32% of patients with cough [5]. There is evidence that conventionally used diagnostic indices of GORD, such as those proposed by De Meester [30], may be misleadingly normal in patients with chronic cough, and

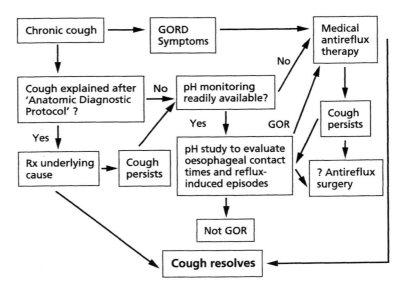

**Fig. 10.2** Suggested guidelines for the evaluation of a patient with chronic cough and suspected gastro-oesophageal reflux disease (GORD).

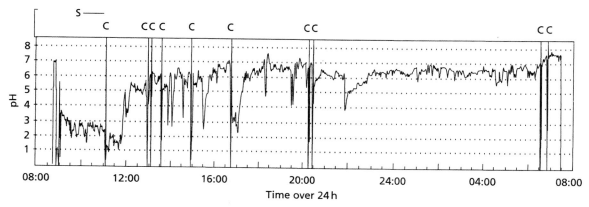

**Fig. 10.3** Twenty-four-hour ambulatory oesophageal pH trace in a patient with cough and gastro-oesophageal reflux disease. Note temporal association between reflux episodes and cough events (C).

analysis of the temporal relationship between cough episodes and reflux events may be a more sensitive indicator [3].

Oesophageal pH monitoring is also indicated in patients with chronic cough with a proven aetiology, and when there is a poor response to specific therapy, since GOR may complicate chronic cough of any cause [8].

Upper gastrointestinal endoscopy, while necessary to document oesophagitis, may miss GORD without mucosal changes, and the presence of oesophagitis by itself does not lead to the establishment of this as a cause of the cough. For this to occur, a temporal relationship between cough and reflux should be demonstrated. Upper gastrointestinal endoscopy should, however, be performed if there are typical GOR symptoms, or when the clinical suspicion of GORD is high, to document the presence of oesophagitis and to exclude concomitant pathology such as strictures or Barrett's oesophagus.

In patients with microaspiration, laryngoscopy may be abnormal with posterior vocal cord inflammation. However, a diagnosis of proximal GOR is best made on 24-h ambulatory oesophageal pH monitoring with both distal (5 cm above LOS) and proximal (20 cm above LOS) oesophageal pH probes [31]. Upper gastrointestinal tract endoscopy, although often performed to exclude complications of GORD, is less specific for proximal oesophageal or laryngeal acid reflux.

There is also evidence that proximal oesophageal reflux and laryngeal reflux may be assessed accurately utilizing fibreoptic endoscopic evaluation of swallow-

ing and sensory testing (FEESST) [32,33]. This technique uses the delivery of a calibrated air pulse administered to the larynx via a specifically manufactured laryngoscope. This air pulse stimulates the laryngeal adductor reflex (LAR), with the normal threshold for this reflex being 2.5–4.0 mmHg air pressure. In patients with proximal GOR, the threshold for eliciting the LAR is increased to above 5.0 mmHg, and is often greater than 10.0 mmHg.

Patients with gross aspiration should be investigated with upper gastrointestinal endoscopy to document the presence and degree of oesophagitis, as well as to exclude strictures, Barrett's oesophagus and achalasia. Oesophageal motility studies should be performed to investigate motility disorders, with standard water-perfused manometry being most accurate. Although techniques for 24-h ambulatory oesophageal motility monitoring have been reported, their role is predominantly in the diagnosis of atypical chest pain.

## Therapy

Therapeutic trials of medical antireflux therapy in patients with chronic persistent cough and proven GOR are summarized in Table 10.1. Most of these trials are uncontrolled, unblinded descriptive studies, and report response rates of between 64.5% and 100%. Early studies investigated the role of lifestyle measures and histamine $H_2$-receptor antagonists ($H_2$-antagonists), with only one of these studies being a randomized controlled study. Treatment regimes using $H_2$-antagonists

**Table 10.1** Summary of therapeutic trials of antireflux therapy in patients with cough and gastro-oesophageal reflux, not including proton pump inhibitor trials (see text). From [18].

| Study | Intervention | No. of patients | Study design | Response rate (%) | Evidence grade |
|---|---|---|---|---|---|
| Irwin *et al. Am Rev Respir Dis* 1981; **123**: 413–7 | Antacid Cimetidine | 5 | PUU | 100 | Descriptive grade II-3 |
| Irwin *et al. Am Rev Respir Dis* 1989; **140**: 294–300 | Metoclopramide $H_2$-antagonists | 9 | PUU | 100 | Descriptive grade II-3 |
| Fitzgerald *et al. Can Med Assoc J* 1989; **140**: 520–4 | Metoclopramide Cimetidine | 20 | PUU | 70 | Descriptive grade II-3 |
| Irwin *et al. Am Rev Respir Dis* 1990; **141**: 640–7 | Metoclopramide $H_2$-antagonists | 28 | PUU | 100 | Descriptive grade II-3 |
| Ing *et al. Am Rev Respir Dis* 1992; **144**: A11 | Ranitidine | 25 | PBC | 84 | Grade I |
| Dordal *et al. Allerg Immunol* 1994; **26**: 53–8 | Cisapride Domperidone | 55 | PUU | 64.5 | Descriptive grade II-3 |
| Waring *et al. Dig Dis Sci* 1995; **40**: 1093–7 | PPI $H_2$-antagonists | 25 | PUU | 80 | Descriptive grade II-3 |
| Smyrnios *et al. Chest* 1995; **108**: 991–7 | Prokinetics Antagonists | 20 | PUU | 97 | Descriptive grade II-3 |

PUU, prospective, unrandomized, uncontrolled; PBC, prospective, blind, controlled; PPI, proton pump inhibitor.

report response rates of 80–100%, with no correlation between 24-h ambulatory oesophageal pH monitoring results and response. There are also no important differences on pH monitoring between partial and complete responders.

The antitussive and antireflux effects of $H_2$-antagonists are prolonged, with both cough symptoms and reflux parameters as measured by repeat 24-h oesophageal pH monitoring being significantly suppressed for more than 6 weeks after the drug is ceased. This implies that $H_2$-antagonists break the cough–reflux self-perpetuating cycle in patients with cough due to distal oesophageal–tracheobronchial reflex mechanisms [28].

There have been two published randomized, controlled, blinded trials of the effect of proton pump inhibitors in patients with chronic persistent cough and GOR. Ours *et al.* [34] studied 17 patients with chronic persistent cough and proven GOR on ambulatory oesophageal pH monitoring. They randomized 8 patients to omeprazole 40 mg p.o. b.d. and 9 patients to placebo for 12 weeks. They reported that 1 of 8 patients receiving omeprazole and 0 of 9 patients on placebo responded. After 12 weeks, all 17 patients received

omeprazole 40 mg p.o. b.d. for another 4 weeks (open label medication). The authors then reported that 1 of 8 patients in the initial active treatment group responded, and 5 of 9 in the initial placebo group responded. There were no differences noted between the active and placebo groups and between the responders and non-responders for any GOR parameter (including all oesophageal pH indices), cough duration or GOR symptoms. All patients who responded did so within 2 weeks of commencing active therapy. Ours *et al.* concluded that empirical high-dose proton pump inhibitor therapy for 2 weeks in all patients with chronic persistent cough not secondary to asthma or postnasal drip syndrome was a 'practical and simple approach' [34].

Kiljander *et al.* [27] investigated 29 patients with chronic persistent cough and proven GOR: 21 of 29 patients completed a randomized, double-blind, placebo-controlled crossover trial of omeprazole 40 mg p.o. daily. Each treatment period was for 8 weeks with a 2-week washout period. In the group receiving omeprazole in the first period there was a marked reduction in cough scores when compared with baseline, and this reduction was maintained in the second or placebo period. In the group receiving omeprazole in the second period there was a marked reduction in cough scores when compared to baseline and when compared to the initial placebo period. Kiljander *et al.* [27] concluded that omeprazole 40 mg p.o. daily for 8 weeks relieved GOR-related cough and that the reduction in cough continued after the treatment period. Maximal response in cough occurred after antireflux therapy was ceased, and Kiljander *et al.* [27] concluded that this supported the existence of a cough–reflux positive feedback cycle.

An empirical trial of proton pump inhibitors would therefore be appropriate in patients with chronic persistent cough, after asthma and postnasal drip have been excluded. The duration of therapy, however, remains unclear, with some authors recommending a minimum therapeutic trial of 4 weeks.

Table 10.2 summarizes the studies investigating the role of antireflux surgery in patients with chronic persistent cough and GOR. Unfortunately all series are non-randomized, uncontrolled descriptive studies, though most are prospective. The definitions of response rates for cough are variable, and range from 84% to 100%. One of the more recent series was reported by Novitsky *et al.* [35]. They investigated 21 patients with cough proven to be secondary to GOR. Cough was the sole presentation in 53% and persisted despite intensive medical therapy including high-dose proton pump inhibitors and antireflux diet. After fundoplication, 62% of patients reported complete resolution of cough, and another 24% reported significant improvement in cough.

Irwin *et al.* [36] reported a subgroup of 8 of the initial 21 patients that had persistent cough despite total or near-total acid suppression using proton pump inhibitors, prokinetic agents and antireflux diet (omeprazole 20–80 mg p.o. daily and cisapride 40–80 mg p.o. daily). These 8 patients had 24-h ambulatory oesophageal pH monitoring while on medical therapy, and in all patients the percentage of 24 h spent at $pH < 4.0$ was zero or near zero. Despite this, all 8 patients underwent antireflux surgery with marked reduction in cough scores after surgery (as measured by visual analogue scale and Adverse Cough Outcome Survey), which was maintained after 12 months of follow-up.

These descriptive studies investigating the effect of antireflux surgery on cough in patients with proven GOR suggest that surgery may improve cough that is resistant to medical therapy, and that the improvement is sustained. In addition, there is a suggestion that acid reflux disease in patients with cough and GORD may be a misnomer since non-acid reflux may be responsible for cough in some patients (volume reflux with gastric enzymes, bile salts, etc.).

It is unclear at present if antireflux surgery should be offered to all patients with cough and proven GOR who fail intensive medical therapy. In the series published by Novitsky *et al.* [35], 14% of patients (3 of

Table 10.2 Summary of trials of antireflux surgery in patients with chronic cough and gastro-oesophageal reflux.

| Study | Intervention | No. of patients | Study design | Response rate (%) | Evidence grade |
|---|---|---|---|---|---|
| Pellegrini *et al. Surgery* 1979; **86:** 110–19 | Fundoplication | 5 | PUU | 100 | Descriptive grade II-3 |
| De Meester *et al. Ann Surg* 1990; **211** (3): 337–45 | Fundoplication | 17 | PUU | 100 | Descriptive grade II-3 |
| Giudicelli *et al. Ann Chir* 1990; **44** (7): 552–4 | Fundoplication | 13 | PUU | 84.6 | Descriptive grade II-3 |
| Thoman *et al. J Gastrointest Surg* 2002; **6** (1): 17–21 | Fundoplication | 37 | RUU | 91 | Descriptive grade II-3 |
| Novitsky *et al. Surg Endosc* 2002; **16** (4): 567–71 | Fundoplication | 21 | PUU | 86 | Descriptive grade II-3 |
| Irwin *et al. Chest* 2002; **121** (4): 1132–40 | Fundoplication | 8 | PUU | 100 | Descriptive grade II-3 |

PUU, prospective, unrandomized, uncontrolled; RUU, retrospective, unrandomized, uncontrolled.

21) had no response. The reasons are unclear, but failure to address multiple aetiologies remains possible. There have been no randomized controlled studies on antireflux surgery in patients with chronic persistent cough and GORD, and as a result evidence-based guidelines for management of refractory cough are lacking.

A recent development that may help predict response to surgery is the technique of endoscopic implantation of biopolymer into the LOS. This involves the injection of a biopolymer such as Enteryx (ethylene vinyl alcohol) into the muscle of the gastric cardia. Although not reported in patients with cough and GORD, there have been reports of its efficacy in patients with GORD in general. Deviere [37] reported 15 patients with proven GORD on long-term proton pump inhibitors. After biopolymer injection, LOS pressure increased in 13 of 15 patients at 1 month, and this was sustained for a median of 6 months. Patients were able to cease proton pump inhibitors, though 4 of 15 resumed this therapy eventually. This technique has the potential of being used to predict the response of patients with cough and GORD to antireflux surgery, but requires further evaluation in this specific group.

## Summary

1 GORD along with bronchial asthma and postnasal drip syndrome is one of the three most common causes of chronic persistent cough.
2 Cough may be the only symptom of GORD.
3 GORD most commonly causes chronic cough via an oesophageal–bronchial reflex mechanism with both local and central nervous reflexes likely to be important.
4 Other components of gastric refluxate apart from acid are likely to be important in the pathogenesis of cough.
5 Empirical medical antireflux therapy including proton pump inhibitors is likely to be successful in treating the cough in over 80% of patients.
6 Patients who do not respond to empirical medical therapy should have 24-h ambulatory oesophageal pH monitoring while on therapy.
7 Antireflux surgery may be useful in patients refractory to medical treatment, even if acid reflux is not demonstrated on follow-up oesophageal pH monitoring.

## References

1 Mittal RK. Current concepts of the antireflux barrier. *Gastroenterol Clin North Am* 1990; **19** (3): 501–17.
2 Dent J. Recent views on the pathogenesis of gastro-oesophageal reflux disease. *Bailliere's Clinical Gastroenterol* 1987; **1** (4): 727–45.
3 Irwin RS, Zawacki JK, Curley FJ, French CL, Hoffman PJ. Chronic cough as the sole presenting manifestation of gastro-oesophageal reflux. *Am Rev Respir Dis* 1989; **140** (5): 294–300.
4 Mansfield LE. Gastro-esophageal reflux and respiratory disorders: a review. *Ann Allergy* 1989; **62**: 158–63.
5 Irwin RS, Curley FJ, French CL. Chronic cough. The spectrum and frequency of causes, key components of the diagnostic evaluation and outcomes of specific therapy. *Am Rev Respir Dis* 1990; **141**: 640–7.
6 Palombi BC, Villanova CAC, Gastal OL, Stolz DP. A pathogenic triad in chronic cough: asthma, post nasal drip syndrome, and gastro-oesophageal reflux disease. *Chest* 1999; **116**: 279–84.
7 McGarvey LP, Forsythe P, Heaney LG, McMahon J, Ennis M. Bronchoalveolar lavage findings in patients with chronic nonproductive cough. *Eur Respir J* 1999; **13** (1): 59–65.
8 Liebermann-Meffert D, Allgower M, Schmid P. Muscular equivalent of the lower esophageal sphincter. *Gastroenterology* 1979; **76**: 31–8.
9 Tottrup A, Forman A, Uldbjerg N *et al.* Mechanical properties of isolated human esophageal smooth muscle. *Am J Physiol* 1990; **21**: G329–37.
10 Dent J, Dodds WJ, Friedman RH *et al.* Mechanisms of gastro-oesophageal reflux in recumbent asymptomatic human subjects. *J Clin Invest* 1980; **65**: 256–67.
11 Mittal RK, McCallum RW. Characteristics of transient lower esophageal sphincter relaxation in humans. *Am J Physiol* 1987; **252**: G636.
12 Dent J, Holloway RH, Toouli J, Dodds WJ. Mechanisms of lower esophageal sphincter incompetence in patients with symptomatic gastro-esophageal reflux. *Gut* 1988; **29**: 1020–8.
13 Holloway RH, Dent J. Pathophysiology of gastro-esophageal reflux: lower esophageal sphincter dysfunction in gastroesophageal reflux disease. *Gastroenterol Clin North Am* 1990; **19** (3): 517–35.
14 Stanciu C, Bennett JR. Esophageal acid clearing: One factor in production of reflux oesophagitis. *Gut* 1974; **15**: 852–7.
15 Ing AJ, Ngu MC, Breslin ABX. Chronic persistent cough and gastro-oesophageal reflux. *Thorax* 1991; **46**: 479–83.
16 Irwin RS, Corrao WM, Pratter MR. Chronic persistent cough in the adult. The spectrum and frequency of causes

and successful outcome of specific therapy. *Am Rev Respir Dis* 1981; **123**: 413–7.

17 Poe RH, Harder RV, Israel RH, Kallay MC. Chronic persistent cough: experience in diagnosis and outcome using an anatomic diagnostic protocol. *Chest* 1989; **95**: 723–8.

18 American College of Chest Physicians. Managing cough as a defence mechanism and as a symptom—a consensus panel report of the American College of Chest Physicians. *Chest* 1998; **114** (2): 133S–181S.

19 Ing AJ, Ngu MC, Breslin ABX. Pathogenesis of chronic persistent cough associated with gastro-esophageal reflux. *Am J Respir Crit Care Med* 1994; **149**: 160–7.

20 Harding SM. The role of gastro-oesophageal reflux in chronic cough and asthma. *Chest* 1997; **111**: 1389–402.

21 Irwin RS, French CL, Curley FJ, Zawacki JK, Bennett FM. Chronic cough due to gastro-oesophageal reflux. Clinical, diagnostic and pathogenetic aspects. *Chest* 1993; **104** (5): 1511–17.

22 Canning BJ. Role of nerves in asthmatic inflammation and potential influence of gastro-oesophageal reflux disease. *Am J Med* 2001; **111** (Suppl. 8A): 13S–17S.

23 Suwanprathes P, Hunt G, Breslin A, Ing AJ, Ngu MC. Identification of brainstem regions involved with coughing: a study using c-Fos immunohistochemistry. *Am J Respir Crit Care Med* 2000; **161** (8): Abstract B52.

24 Suwanprathes P, Hunt G, Seow F, Ing AJ, Ngu MC. Cough and gastro-oesophageal reflux: evidence for a common centre in the brainstem. *Am J Respir Crit Care Med* 2001; **163** (8): Abstract F57.

25 Bieger D. Muscarinic activation of rhombencephalic neurones controlling oesophageal peristalsis in the rat. *Neuropharmacology* 1984; **23**: 1451–64.

26 Bieger D, Hopkins DA. Viscerotopic representation of the upper alimentary tract in the medulla oblongata in the rat: the nucleus ambiguus. *J Comp Neurol* 1987; **262**: 546–62.

27 Kiljander TO, Salomaa ERM, Hietanen EK, Terho EO. Chronic cough and gastro-oesophageal reflux: a double blind placebo controlled study with omeprazole. *Eur Respir J* 2000; **16**: 633–8.

28 Ing AJ. Cough and gastro-oesophageal reflux. *Am J Med* 1997; **103** (5A): 91–6.

29 Ing AJ, Ngu MC, Breslin ABX. Chronic persistent cough and clearance of oesophageal acid. *Chest* 1992; **102**: 1668–71.

30 Johnson LF, De Meester TR. Development of the 24-hour intra-oesophageal pH monitoring composite scoring system. *J Clin Gastroenterol* 1986; 8 (Suppl. 1): 52–8.

31 Paterson WG, Murat BW. Combined ambulatory oesophageal manometry and dual-probe pH-metry in evaluation of patients with chronic unexplained cough. *Dig Dis Sci* 1994; **39** (5): 1117–25.

32 Phua SY, McGarvey LPA, Peters MJ, Breslin ABX, Ing AJ. Assessing laryngeal sensitivity of patients with chronic cough and gastro-oesophageal reflux using fibreoptic endoscopic evaluation of laryngeal sensitivity. *Am J Respir Crit Care Med* 2002; **165** (8): A406.

33 Aviv JE, Parides M, Fellowes J, Close LG. Endoscopic evaluation of swallowing as an alternative to 24-hour pH monitoring for diagnosis of extra-oesophageal reflux. *Ann Otol Rhinol Laryngol* 2000; **184** (Suppl.): 25–7.

34 Ours TM, Kavuru MS, Schilz RJ, Richter JE. A prospective evaluation of oesophageal testing and a double blind, randomized study of omeprazole in a diagnostic and therapeutic algorithm for chronic cough. *Am J Gastroenterol* 1999; **94**: 3131–8.

35 Novitsky YW, Zawacki JK, Irwin RS, French CT, Hussey VM, Callery MP. Chronic cough due to gastro-oesophageal reflux disease: efficacy of antireflux surgery. *Surg Endosc* 2002; **16** (4): 567–71.

36 Irwin RS, Zawacki JK, Wilson MM, French CT, Callery MP. Chronic cough due to gastro-oesophageal reflux disease: failure to resolve despite total/near total elimination of oesophageal acid. *Chest* 2002; **121**: 1132–40.

37 Deviere J, Pastorelli A, Louis H, de Maertelaer V, Lehman G, Cicala M, Le Moine O, Silverman D, Costamagna G. Endoscopic implantation of a biopolymer in the lower oesophageal sphincter for gastro-oesophageal reflux: a pilot study. *Gastrointest Endosc* 2002; **55** (3): 335–41.

# 11 Cough in postnasal drip, rhinitis and rhinosinusitis

*Bruno C. Palombini & Elisabeth Araujo*

## Introduction

In 1998 the *Consensus Panel Report* of the American College of Chest Physicians (ACCP) stated that 'the most common causes of chronic cough in non-smokers are postnasal drip syndrome (PNDS), asthma and/or gastro-oesophageal reflux disease (GORD), whether or not the cough is described as dry or productive' [1–4].

The incidence of PNDS in chronic cough is disputed, with published values ranging from 2 to 57% It seems far more common in the US than in Europe [5]. The reasons for this variation may be social or semantic. Few studies were randomized, and selection of patients might depend on the reputation and interests of the investigator. In almost none of the studies was cough measured, either subjectively or objectively, or even defined to distinguish between true cough and huff.

## Postnasal drip syndrome

According to the ACCP [3], the diagnosis of PNDS largely rests on the patient reporting certain symptoms or sensations. Since PNDS is a syndrome, and since there are no pathognomonic findings to prove its presence, the diagnosis of postnasal drip-induced cough is best determined by considering a combination of criteria, including symptoms, physical examination, radiographic findings, and ultimately, response to specific therapy.

A favourable response to specific therapy for PNDS with resolution of cough is a crucial step in confirming that PNDS was present and that it was the aetiology of the cough.

Cough initiated at the upper respiratory tract is usually produced by stimulation of pharyngeal branch nerve endings (vagal branches). It is speculated that the cough in PNDS may be caused by chemical or mechanical irritation of receptors located in the larynx and/or pharynx [1,2], Proctor [6] claims that, in patients with purulent rhinosinusitis, secretions are aspirated into the trachea and bronchi during the night, a process which is further stimulated by the reduction in mucociliary activity. Bucca *et al.* [7] have demonstrated an increase in the extrathoracic reactivity of airways mediated by pharyngobronchial reflexes following drainage of upper airway secretions.

Clinical studies suggest that the pathogenesis of cough from PNDS is due to mechanical or chemical stimulation of the afferent limb of the cough reflex in the upper airway. This stimulation is secondary to secretions emanating from the nose and/or sinuses dripping down into the hypopharynx. A number of conditions can cause PNDS. The differential diagnosis includes seasonal allergic rhinitis, perennial allergic rhinitis, perennial non-allergic rhinitis, vasomotor rhinitis, postinfectious rhinitis, chronic (bacterial) rhinosinusitis, allergic fungal rhinosinusitis, non-allergic rhinitis due to medication abuse or environmental irritants, and non-allergic rhinitis associated with pregnancy [6–8].

In addition to this clinical presentation, there is usually a history of rhinosinopathy. These clinical findings are relatively sensitive, but not specific for diagnostic purposes [3,4]. In addition to cough (which is productive in 50% of cases), Villanova *et al.* [8,9] have found that throat-clearing (66.7%) and pharyngeal aspiration (26.7%) are the two most common clinical manifestations in PNDS patients [3,4,8,9].

When chronic cough results from a multicausal association, diagnosis is usually based on the recently described pathogenic triad of chronic cough (asthma, PNDS and gastro-oesophageal reflux (GOR)) [9,10].

The clinical presentation of patients with PNDS, in addition to cough, commonly involves complaints of a sensation of something dripping into the throat (drainage in posterior pharynx), a need to clear the throat, a tickle in the throat or nasal congestion and/or nasal discharge [6]. Patients sometimes complain of hoarseness. Cough can also occur with talking, but this is a non-specific complaint associated with essentially all causes of cough. A history of upper respiratory illness (a cold) is often present. A history of wheeze is also common. Most patients with PND-induced cough will have symptoms or evidence of one or more of the following: drainage in posterior pharynx, throat-clearing, nasal discharge, cobblestone appearance of the oropharyngeal mucosa and mucus in the oropharynx. These clinical findings are relatively sensitive, but they are not specific. They are also found in many patients with cough due to other causes [1–4].

## Pharyngeal aspiration and throat-clearing

PNDS has been described and discussed in several studies and publications. It is caused by disorders affecting the nasal fossae, pharynx and paranasal sinuses. Cough in PNDS may be triggered by numerous stimuli, and in most cases the aetiopathogenesis is clear. Cough is undoubtedly associated with certain conditions such as bronchopneumonia, bronchiectasis, bronchial cancer, tuberculosis, use of angiotensin-converting enzyme (ACE) inhibitors, lung fibrosis and asthma. However, cases with multiple or obscure aetiopathogenesis pose a challenge. For these situations, it is useful to discuss some recent advances [9,10].

One of the characteristics of non-productive cough is that it is not associated with expectoration and does not present the clinical signs of pharyngeal aspiration (PA) or throat-clearing (TC).

On the other hand, chronic productive cough is frequently observed in smokers, since smoking is often associated with both emphysema and chronic bronchitis.

However, this type of productive cough does not present signs of PA, since there is little association between smoking and chronic rhinosinusitis. In turn, signs of TC are frequently found in smokers with productive cough.

Inspiratory signs of PA, even when present in smokers, do not present a cause-and-effect association with smoking. Signs of PA strongly suggest the presence of chronic suppurative foci in the upper airway. In other words, since smoking does not prevent smokers from having rhinosinusitis, some smokers may simultaneously present signs of PA (due to rhinosinusitis) and signs of TC (secondary to chronic smoker's bronchitis). Figure 11.1 shows cinematography images of pharyngeal aspiration and throat-clearing.

Preliminary results of research concerning the meaning of these clinical signs have already become available. Recent studies in Brazil have employed injection of barium contrast in the nasal fossae followed by pharyngeal aspiration and throat-clearing with simultaneous radioscopy with digital subtraction [11]. Concerning the drainage of upper airway secretions, preliminary impressions suggest that the pharynx may act as a pump, with inspiration and expiration movements, and its lumen may go from expanded dimensions (inspiration) to a small volume (expiration) (see Fig. 11.1).

Another major characteristic associated with the basic physiopathogenic mechanism of PA and TC is the possibility of airway vibration, also found in other PND manoeuvres in general. The physical characteristics of such vibration and its role in clearing the airways are still uncertain.

One of the objectives of the present chapter is to provide tools to general practitioners, pneumologists and paediatricians to support the diagnosis of chronic cough using simple rules. Basically, the objective is to provide further knowledge regarding PA and TC. Figure 11.1 shows the results of radiological studies with forced inspiration, characterizing signs of PA, and forced expiration, constituting signs of TC. The clinical recognition of these signs is easy, and they have great diagnostic value, dispensing with expensive diagnostic procedures that often delay treatment (for example, computed tomography (CT) of paranasal sinuses and pharynx and/or fibreoptic nasal endoscopy).

Therefore, the need to train resident physicians to perform the differential diagnosis of chronic productive cough is underscored, highlighting the dif-

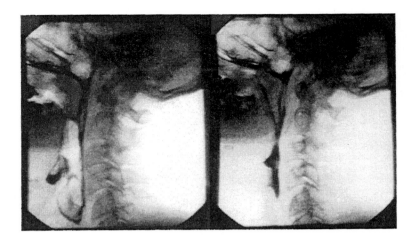

**Fig. 11.1** Cinematography images obtained through digital subtraction fluoroscopy and schematic illustrations: pharyngeal aspiration and 'throat-clearing'.

ference between a strong indication of rhinosinusitis (manifested as signs of PA), and an indication of chronic bronchitis, suggested mainly by the presence of signs of TC.

Figure 11.2 shows the most common causes of chronic cough according to clinical presentation, with emphasis on the signs of PA and of TC.

The signs of PA are the most frequent inspiratory/vibratory manoeuvres observed in patients with chronic suppuration of paranasal sinuses, especially rhinosinusitis. The soft palate is dislocated backwards and the patient, taking a deep breath, makes it vibrate, causing the secretions in this recess to pass into the oropharynx where they are swallowed or expectorated.

The expiratory/vibratory signs of TC correspond to an expiratory clearing of the hypopharynx and larynx, with dislocation of secretions from either the lower respiratory tract (for example, in chronic bronchitis and bronchiectasis) or the upper respiratory tract (rhinosinusitis and its variants). The resulting action is similar to that of a 'force pump.' After a throat-clearing manoeuvre, the individual swallows the secretions, either through the nasal cavities or through the mouth (Fig. 11.1).

It is important to keep in mind that expiratory signs of TC are typical of smokers with chronic bronchitis and/or bronchiectasis. However, this sign is also detectable in cases of cough secondary to isolated rhinosinusitis or rhinosinusitis associated with chronic bronchitis and bronchiectasis.

It is not clear why some individuals presenting with PNDS have chronic cough and others do not. It is possible that patients who cough also present lesions that cause hypersensitivity in the afferent limbs of the cough reflex.

Since a recent publication demonstrates that an aetiopathogenic triad must be considered in cases of chronic cough of unknown origin (rhinosinusitis, GOR and bronchial hyperreactivity), it is important to rely on laboratory tests for diagnostic purposes in this case also [9,10].

As discussed above, PNDS is associated with inflammatory processes such as rhinitis, rhinosinusitis and adenoids, and also with anatomical alterations such as infected concha bullosa [1–3]. GOR, asthma and smoking may also lead to PNDS due to the irritating effect of the reflux on the pharynx [8–14].

In our hospital, we follow some diagnostic guidelines aimed at helping respiratory disease physicians, general practitioners and paediatricians diagnose PNDS:

1 most patients with chronic productive cough associated with signs of PA have rhinosinusitis;

2 most patients with chronic productive cough associated with signs of TC have chronic bronchitis (with or without rhinosinusitis);

3 most patients with productive cough associated with signs of TC and of PA have rhinosinusitis alone or rhinosinusitis associated with bronchitis;

4 patients with non-productive or mildly productive cough associated with signs of TC may have GOR;

5 patients with wheezy non-productive cough may have cough-variant asthma.

**109**

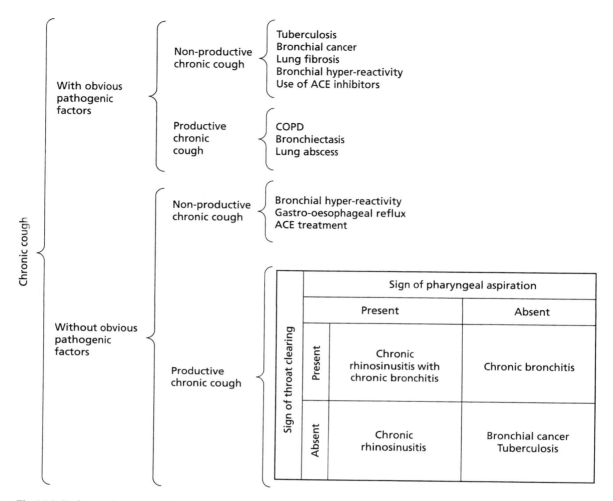

**Fig. 11.2** Pathogenetic routes of the most common types of chronic cough and some accompanying signs.

These clinical findings are relatively sensitive, but not specific for diagnostic purposes [3,4]. In addition to chronic cough (which was productive in 50% of cases of chronic cough, in adults), Villanova *et al.* [8,9] have found that the signs of TC were positive in 66.7% and signs of PA in 26.7%. These were the two most common clinical manifestations in patients with PNDS.

## Rhinitis

The concept of rhinitis implies inflammation of the nasal mucosa. Clinical diagnosis is based on the pres-

ence of the following symptoms: pruritus, sneezing, rhinorrhoea and nasal obstruction.

Patients with rhinitis can be divided into 'sneezers with a runny nose' and those with a 'stuffy nose.' Cough is more frequently associated with increased secretion, especially thicker secretion with posterior drainage. The presence of secretion with inflammatory mediators results in stimulation of receptors present in the nasal mucosa that are innervated by the trigeminus and of receptors found in the posterior pharynx innervated by the glossopharyngeus.

Infectious rhinitis is the most common cause of acute cough. Viral infections due to rhinovirus, influenza and parainfluenza induce the activation of several types of cells, including nasal epithelial cells, and the release of several types of cytokines. The frequency of cough is higher in the first 48 h, when it is detected in 83% of the patients [3], and decreases gradually to 26% on the 14th day. Cough associated with viral infections starts out 'short', dry and infrequent; its intensity and frequency may increase quickly. With evolution of the viral status, clear and mucoid secretion may appear, with the cough becoming gradually thicker and assuming a whitish or yellowish colour until spontaneous resolution. Infectious rhinitis is the most common form of rhinitis. It is caused by the proliferation of microorganisms in the nasal mucosa alone or in association with other forms of rhinitis. Bacteria such as *Streptococcus pneumoniae* and *Haemophilus influenzae* are the most common. About 11–25% of the patients complain of cough more than 3 weeks after upper airway infections; this is known as postinfectious cough [3].

Allergic rhinitis is induced by IgE-mediated inflammation. It may be reversed spontaneously or with treatment. It may also be subdivided into intermittent or persistent types. Allergic rhinitis is characterized by nasal obstruction, rhinorrhoea, sneezing, nasal pruritus and postnasal drip. It is important to identify the exposure to allergens. There may be a history of exposure to specific allergens, such as pollen or animal fur. The association of cough with feather pillows, rooms with curtains or carpeting, and the presence of cats and dogs must be investigated.

Some situations of cough associated with postnasal drip result in occupational rhinitis from inhalation of allergens in work settings.

A careful investigation may reveal rhinitis medicamentosa (drug-induced rhinitis), which may be caused by misuse of the medication employed to treat rhinitis [15]. The overuse of topical vasoconstrictors or systemic drugs (especially aspirin and other non-steroidal antihypertensive agents (such as reserpine, methyldopa or guanethidine, and nifedipine) can cause rhinitis and persistent dry cough, possibly because these drugs interfere with α-adrenergic activity [16].

In endocrinological or hormonal rhinitis, nasal symptoms result from alterations in the nasal blood flow and/or in glandular reactivity in conditions such as pregnancy, menopause, puberty or hypothyroidism [17,18]. The cough usually disappears after delivery or after hormonal stabilization.

Irritant rhinitis is caused by exposure of the nasal mucosa to harmful substances such as tobacco smoke or sulphur dioxide; it can also be induced by exposure of the nasal mucosa to cold dry air, with the release of chemical basophil mediators. Irritant rhinitis is characterized by clear rhinorrhoea, postnasal drip with nasal congestion and minimal sneezing. The duration and intensity of the cough associated with irritant rhinitis depends on the inflammatory response, with activation of mast cells and occurrence of late-phase reaction. In children, passive smoking may exacerbate chronic cough.

Idiopathic rhinitis is characterized by nasal symptoms caused by vasomotor/secretory instability in the absence of a well-defined cause. It may be associated with either vasoconstriction or enhanced secretion [12,13]. Non-specific nasal hyperreactivity may be associated with pharyngeal hyperreactivity, causing cough due to nasopharyngeal irritation.

Persistent non-allergic rhinitis in association with eosinophilia is a heterogeneous syndrome consisting of at least two categories: non-allergic rhinitis with eosinophilia syndrome, and aspirin intolerance. It is often characterized by the presence of nasal eosinophilia and perennial symptoms, such as sneezing, itching, rhinorrhoea, postnasal drip, signs of PA and nasal obstruction, without allergy [19].

## Evaluation

The clinical presentation of patients with rhinitis-associated cough includes non-specific signs and symptoms. Whenever the aetiology of rhinitis is not clear, and in cases of persistent cough or signs of PA, patients must undergo laboratory investigation. Laboratory assessment is performed in order to determine atopic status and to identify the probable aetiological agent as well as other conditions frequently associated with allergic rhinitis [20]. The presence of specific IgE antibodies should be demonstrated by means of *in vivo* (skin testing) and/or *in vitro* (radioallergosorbent test, RAST) testing. Nasal endoscopy using rigid or flexible fibreoptic endoscopes certainly constitutes an important diagnostic tool, and should be performed prior to CT, since they are complementary procedures [18].

## Treatment

The objective of clinical rhinitis treatment is to restore nasal function in order to maintain the functional integrity of the entire airway. Treatment must be individualized and extended to associated infectious and mechanical complications. Important points include cleanliness of physical environment, pharmacotherapy and specific immunotherapy.

The drugs used to treat allergic rhinitis-associated cough include antihistamines, oral and topical vaso-constrictors, ipratropium bromide, disodium chromoglycate, nedochromil sodium, and oral and topical corticosteroids. These drugs can be used either in isolation or in association [13].

## Rhinosinusitis

As previously mentioned, rhinosinusitis is caused by inflammation of the mucosa lining the nasal cavity and PNS. Rhinitis may occur in isolation, but cases of sinusitis without associated rhinitis are rare.

Rhinosinusitis is a major public health problem, affecting approximately 14% of the worldwide adult population, and this prevalence has been increasing [12].

### Diagnosis

Acute rhinosinusitis is one of the most common reasons for medical appointments. Between 0.5% and 5% of the viral infections affecting the upper airways result in acute rhinosinusitis. A differential diagnosis with viral infection is often difficult, since most symptoms (nasal obstruction, rhinorrhoea, hyposmia, facial pressure, PND, signs of PA, cough and fever) are non-specific. Certain symptoms, such as fever, halitosis and hyposmia, considered as minor symptoms in adults, might be the sole indication of rhinosinusitis in children [13].

In chronic rhinosinusitis, chronic cough (lasting longer than 3 weeks) and purulent or mucopurulent expectoration, as well as signs of PA, are common findings, without evidence of suppurative foci in the lower airways [9,10]. The time of the day in which the cough appears is also an important indication for its origin. Productive cough appearing at night and on waking up indicates rhinosinusitis. Between 18 months and 6 years of age, rhinosinusitis is the most frequent cause of chronic cough. Between 6 and 16 years, it is associated with asthma-variant cough and psychogenic cough as the most common causes of chronic cough.

For adults with chronic cough due to PND, rhinosi-

nusitis is the cause in 30–60% of cases. Less frequent causes are some forms of rhinitis, such as allergic, postinfectious, vasomotor, perennial, non-allergic and drug-induced rhinitis [12].

In non-allergic and non-infectious rhinosinusitis, the common cold (acute coryza) deserves special attention. Primary symptoms include mouth dryness and nasal pruritus/itch, followed by dryness and pain in the throat, sneezing, watery coryza and constitutional symptoms (febricula, indisposition). After 2 or 3 days, a secondary infection occurs, with nasal obstruction and purulent secretions, non-productive cough, febricula and muscle pain lasting for 5–10 days [13].

When chronic cough results from a multicausal association, diagnosis is usually based on the recently described [8–10] pathogenic triad of chronic cough (asthma, PND, GOR) (Fig. 11.3). Over 50% of the cases of chronic cough are related to this triad. In order to recognize this condition, in addition to CT of the PNS, oesophageal pH-metry (detection of oesophageal reflux) and spirometry with or without bronchoprovocation testing (diagnosis of asthma without wheezing) should be performed [9,10].

Traditional nasal evaluation with a frontal light source and nasal speculum provides only limited information. Rigid and flexible fibreoptic endoscopes allow for a direct and systematic evaluation of nose areas. Endoscopy must be considered whenever the patient presents with severe and persistent cough, despite clinical treatment [17]. The presence of cough is often related to drainage of purulent secretions in the nasopharynx

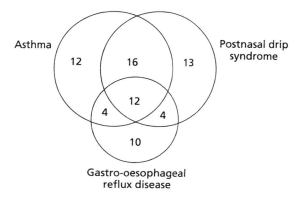

**Fig. 11.3** Aetiological factor in 78 cases of chronic cough: 15.4% of the patients had three simultaneous causes; 26% had two causes; 35% had one single cause. From [8].

originating at the draining ostia of the maxillary, ethmoid and sphenoid sinuses. In such situations, our experience has shown the presence of thick pharyngeal secretion at endoscopy, despite the fact that some patients refer to having dry cough.

Generally, the diagnostic relevance of simple radiographs is controversial, since radiological abnormalities in the ethmoid and sphenoid sinuses, frontal recess and osteomeatal complex may go unnoticed. A normal result in a simple radiograph is not sufficient to rule out the presence of rhinosinusitis. In children, it is important to underscore that the younger they are the greater the radiological limitations imposed [17,18].

CT is the preferred method for assessing PNS because it clearly shows the relationship between soft tissues and bones. CT allows for a specific diagnosis and for the identification and systematic evaluation of anatomical areas that are inaccessible to conventional radiological tests (Fig. 11.4) [18,19].

Approximately 70% of the cases of acute rhinosinusitis are caused by *Streptococcus pneumoniae* and *Haemophilus influenzae*. In chronic rhinosinusitis, bacteriological studies demonstrate a predominance of polymicrobial flora and anaerobes, due to the reduced oxygen concentration in the PNS. Fungi (*Aspergillus, Candida albicans* and *Alternaria*) are isolated in 3–10% of cases of chronic rhinosinusitis [20].

The main aetiological agent of infection in the airways is *S. pneumoniae*. Recent studies show that approximately 20% of the strains present intermediate resistance to penicillin; high resistance was observed in approximately 1%. With regard to other microorganisms, β-lactamase was found in approximately 10% of *H. influenzae* strains and in more than 90% of *Moraxella catarrhalis* [15,16].

A favourable response to specific therapy, with resolution of cough, is a crucial stage in confirming the association of bacteria with cough.

Cases of chronic cough caused by chronic rhinosinusitis or sinusitis resistant to treatment should be referred to an otorhinolaryngologist for investigation of structural abnormalities of the osteomeatal complex, hypertrophy of adenoids, septal deviation and dental abscess [15].

## References

1 Irwin RS. Cough. In: Irwin RS, Curley FJ, Grossman RF, eds. *Diagnosis and Treatment of Symptoms of the Respiratory Tract*. New York: Futura Publishing Co., 1997: 1–54.

2 Irwin RS, Madison JM. The diagnosis and treatment of cough. *N Engl J Med* 2000; **343**: 1715–21.

3 Irwin RS, Boulet LP, Cloutier MM, Fuller R, Gold PM, Hoffstein V *et al*. Managing cough as a defense mechanism and as a symptom—a consensus panel report of the American College of Chest Physicians. *Chest* 1998; **114** (2 Suppl. Managing): 133S–81S.

4 Irwin RS, Curley FJ, French CL. The spectrum and frequency of causes, key components of the diagnostic evaluation and outcome of specific therapy. *Am Rev Respir Dis* 1990; **141**: 640–7.

5 Morice AH. Epidemiology of cough. *Pulm Pharmacol Ther* 2002; **15**: 253–60.

6 Proctor DF. Nasal physiology and defense of the lung. *Am Rev Respir Dis* 1977; **115**: 97–102.

7 Bucca C, Rolla G, Scappaticci E, Chiampo F, Bugiani M, Magnano M *et al*. Extrathoracic and intrathoracic airway responsiveness in sinusitis. *J Allergy Clin Immunol* 1995; **95**: 52–9.

8 Villanova CA, Palombini BC, Pereira EA, Stolz DP, Gastal OL, Alt DC *et al*. Post-nasal drip syndrome as a cause of chronic cough: its place among other conditions. *Am J Respir Crit Care Med* 1996; **153**: A517.

9 Palombini BC, Villanova CA, Araújo E, Gastal OL, Alt DC, Stolz DP *et al*. A pathogenic triad in chronic cough—asthma, postnasal drip syndrome, and gastroesophageal reflux disease. *Chest* 1999; **116** (2): 279–84.

10 Palombini BC, Villanova CA, Araújo E, Gastal OL, Alt

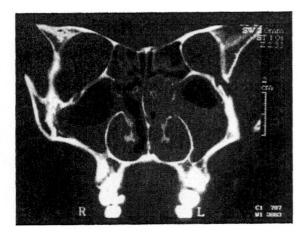

Fig. 11.4 Computed tomography section (coronal view) showing bilateral ethmoid and maxillary opacification, with obstruction of the aorta.

DC, Stolz DP *et al.* A pathogenic triad in chronic cough—asthma, post-nasal drip syndrome, and gastroesophageal reflux disease. *Chest* 1999; **116** (2): 279–84. (Quotation in the Journal Watch (General), *N Engl J Med* 1999; **19** (19): 155.)

11 Irion KL, Porto NS, Palombini BC, Letti N, Pereira EA, Fraga JC *et al.* Documentação radiológica da falência eventual dos mecanismos supostamente capazes de evitar aspiração para traquéia das secreções faríngeas durante as manobras da tosse, da aspiração faríngea e do pigarrear [abstract]. *J Pneumologia* 1992; **18** (1): 33.

12 Madison JM, Irwin RS. Cough. In: Albert R, Spiros S, Jett J, eds. *Comprehensive Respiratory Medicine.* London: Mosby, 1999: 15.1.

13 Mitchel D. Rhinitis and sinusitis. In: Albert R, Spiros S, Jett J, eds. *Comprehensive Respiratory Medicine.* London: Mosby, 1999: 31.1.

14 Palombini BC, Pereira EA, Alves MR, Irion KL. The need to recognize new and accurate symptoms and signs in the diagnosis of sinobronchitis: the qualification of their

sensitivity and specificity [abstract]. *Am Rev Respir Dis* 1992; **145** (4): 301.

15 Brandileone MC, Di Fabio JL, Vieira VS, Zanella RC, Casagrande ST, Pignatari AC *et al.* Geographic distribution of penicillin resistance of *Streptococcus pneumoniae* in Brazil: genetic relatedness. *Microb Drug Resist* 1998; **4** (3): 209–17.

16 Naclerio RM, Proud D, Togias AG, Adkinson NF Jr, Meyers DA, Kagey-Sobotka A *et al.* Inflammatory mediators in late-phase antigen-induced rhinitis. *N Engl J Med* 1985; **313**: 6570.

17 McCaffrey TV. *Rhinologic Diagnosis and Treatment.* New York: Thieme, 1997.

18 Mackay I, ed. *Rhinitis—Mechanisms and Management.* London: Royal Society of Medicine, 1989.

19 Kennedy DW. International conference on sinus disease: terminology staging therapy. *Ann Otol Rhinol Laryngol* 1995; **104** (10).

20 Mackay IS, Durham SR. Perennial rhinitis. *Br Med J* 1998; **316**: 917–20.

# 12 Cough and airway hyperresponsiveness

*Paul M. O'Byrne*

## Introduction

Asthma is a disease which is identified by the presence of characteristic symptoms and by the demonstration of variable airflow obstruction, either spontaneously, or improving as a result of treatment. The symptoms of asthma are dyspnoea, wheezing, chest tightness and, in many patients with persistent asthma, troublesome cough. Cough has been recognized as a symptom of asthma since the earliest descriptions of the disease. Persistent cough in asthma is often, but not always, associated with the presence of airflow obstruction, and associated with other asthma symptoms. The presence of persistent cough, with or without sputum production, even when the only asthma symptom, is an indication of poor asthma control [1].

## Airway inflammation and asthma

Asthma is an airway inflammatory disease, with inflammation present even when asthma is stable and well controlled. This has been shown in studies which have provided information on airway cell populations in mild stable asthmatics with ongoing and persistent airway hyperresponsiveness [2,3]. Common findings in all of these studies are the presence of increased numbers of inflammatory cells such as eosinophils, lymphocytes and mast cells compared with normal control subjects with normal airway responsiveness. The eosinophils have shown signs of activation, as indicated by increased airway levels of granular proteins, major basic protein (MBP) [4] and eosinophil cationic protein (ECP) [5]. In the bronchial mucosa the eosinophils have shown morphological features of activation as indicated by heterogeneity of the granular structure or as eosinophil granules released from eosinophils lying free in the mucosal interstitium [6]. Increased numbers of activated T lymphocytes have also been shown in several studies [7], together with increased number of mast cells in the airway mucosa exhibiting various stages of degranulation [8]. The extent and severity of the airway inflammation increases at times when asthma is unstable and poorly controlled, with increased numbers of airway eosinophils and/or neutrophils [9]. As will be discussed later, the presence of persistent airway inflammation is likely to be responsible not only for asthma symptoms, including cough, but also for the structural changes and the associated physiological abnormalities of asthma.

## Airway hyperresponsiveness in asthma

Airway responsiveness is a term which describes the ability of the airways to narrow after exposure to constrictor agonists. Airway hyperresponsiveness is an increased ability to develop this response and consists of the ability of a smaller concentration of an agonist needed to initiate the bronchoconstrictor response (increased sensitivity of the airways), a steeper slope of the dose–response curve (increased reactivity of the airways), as well as a greater maximal response to the agonist (Fig. 12.1). The initial description of an increased responsiveness of asthmatic airways was made by Alexander and Paddock in 1921 [10], who demonstrated an 'asthmatic breathing' in asthmatic subjects, but not normals, after subcutaneous administration of the

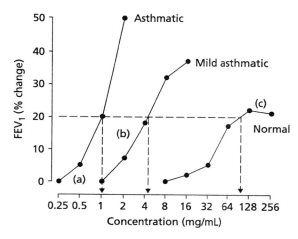

**Fig. 12.1** The change in $FEV_1$ vs. baseline, induced by increasing doses of a bronchoconstrictor stimulus (methacholine) in mild, moderate and severe asthmatics vs. healthy individuals. The $PC_{20}$ value is calculated by interpolating a 20% fall in $FEV_1$ to the log–linear dose–response curve for each individual. Asthmatic subjects have a reduced threshold response (a), indicating increased sensitivity of the airways; an increased slope (b), indicating increased reactivity of the airways; and an increased maximal response (c).

cholinergic agonist pilocarpine. This observation was confirmed by Weiss *et al.* [11], who reported that asthmatic subjects, but not normals, developed bronchoconstriction after being given intravenous histamine. Later Curry [12] described an increased bronchoconstrictor response to histamine that occurred with intramuscular, intravenous and nebulized histamine, again only in asthmatic subjects. Tiffeneau and Beauvallet [13] were the first to describe the use of acetylcholine inhalation tests to determine the degree of airway responsiveness in asthmatics. Airway hyperresponsiveness is often considered to be non-specific, in that asthmatic subjects will develop bronchoconstriction after exposure to many different chemical stimuli such as histamine [14], the cholinergic agonists methacholine [15] and carbachol [16], cysteinyl leukotrienes (LT) $C_4$ and $D_4$ [17], and prostaglandins (PG) $D_2$ [18] and $PGF_{2\alpha}$ [19]. This is to contrast the *specific* airway responses that develop when subjects inhale substances, such as allergens [20] or occupational sensitizing agents [21], to which they have become sensitized. The term non-specific airway hyperresponsiveness can, however, be misleading. It suggests that a common mechanism exists by which these pharmacological or physical stimuli cause bronchoconstriction. This is clearly not the case, as most of the pharmacological agents act on specific receptors in the airways, and the mechanisms by which receptor activation causes bronchoconstriction are different for different agents. However, as each of these chemical bronchoconstrictors activates specific receptors, they are considered to be 'direct-acting' stimuli. In addition, some stimuli such as exercise [22], hyperventilation of cold, dry air [23], both hypotonic and hypertonic solutions [24], and mannitol [25] also cause bronchoconstriction in asthmatics. In contrast to the direct-acting stimuli, these cause release of bronchoconstrictor mediators, such as histamine [26] and cysteinyl leukotrienes [27], in the airways, and therefore are called 'indirect-acting' stimuli.

In studies of populations of asthmatic patients, the severity of airway hyperresponsiveness has been shown to correlate with the severity of asthma [14] and with the amount of treatment needed to control symptoms [28]. A variety of methods of measuring airway responsiveness have been reported, and the clinical significance and the effects of antiasthma medications on these measurements, and the pathophysiology and pathogenesis of airway hyperresponsiveness in asthmatic patients have been extensively studied. As a result of this research, the methods of its measurement have been standardized, and are widely accepted. Almost all patients with symptomatic asthma have airway hyperresponsiveness [14], and for this reason the absence of airway hyperresponsiveness in a patient with symptoms suggestive of asthma should result in an alternative diagnosis being considered.

## Mechanisms of airway hyperresponsiveness

Studies of monozygotic and dizygotic twins have suggested that there is a genetic basis for the development of airway hyperresponsiveness, but that environmental factors are more important [29]. Also measurements of airway hyperresponsiveness in young infants have indicated that airway hyperresponsiveness can be present very early in life, and that a family history of asthma and parental smoking were risk factors for its development [30]. More recently, reports of genetic linkage of airway hyperresponsiveness have been published. One study has identified genetic linkage between histamine airway hyperresponsiveness and several genetic markers on chromosome 5q, near a locus that regulates serum IgE levels [31]. Another study has identified linkage between a highly polymorphic marker of the B subunit of the high-affinity IgE receptor on chromosome 11q and methacholine airway hyperresponsiveness, even in patients with non-atopic asthma [32]. One specific gene polymorphism (Glu 27) of the nine identified for the $\beta_2$-adrenoceptor has also been associated with increased methacholine airway hyperresponsiveness [33], while another polymorphism (Gly 16) was associated with the presence of nocturnal asthma [34]. Thus, a genetic basis for airway hyperresponsiveness seems very likely; however, the genetic linkage studies need to be confirmed by other investigators in different patient populations.

In addition to a possible genetic basis causing airway hyperresponsiveness in asthma, airway inflammatory processes are thought to be important (Fig. 12.2). Mediators released from airway eosinophils have

been suggested to cause many of the tissue changes seen in the disease, including epithelial damage and thickening of the basement membrane. Eosinophils also produce cysteinyl leukotrienes which cause airway smooth muscle contraction [35] and exudation of plasma [36], resulting in thickening of the airway wall. It is likely that airway wall thickening, which has been described in asthmatics of varying degrees of severity, could explain some of the differences in airway hyperresponsiveness between normal individuals and asthmatic patients. The thickness of the airway wall from autopsy specimens is greater in fatal asthmatics than in patients with milder disease and in non-asthmatics [37]. It is not exactly clear which tissue contributes mostly to airway wall thickening in asthma. One factor that may be involved is the subepithelial thickening seen in bronchial biopsy specimens from most asthmatics. Furthermore, bronchial smooth muscle has a larger volume in asthmatics [38]. Lastly, exudation of

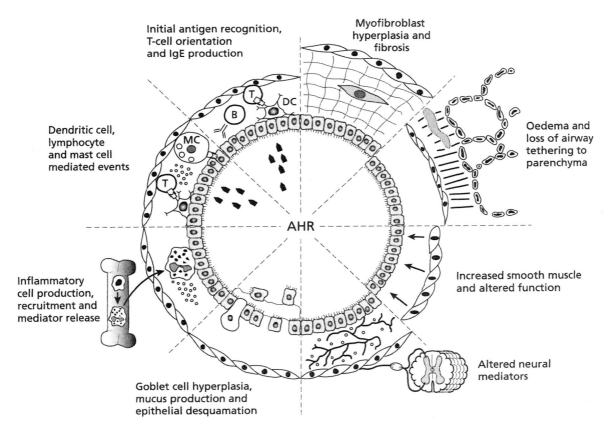

Fig. 12.2 Potential mechanisms for the development of airway hyperresponsiveness in asthma.

plasma can cause oedema, and thus thickening, of the airway wall. Together these factors may, by geometric mechanisms, enhance the airway luminal resistance induced by a certain degree of airway smooth muscle shortening. Another feature of the asthmatic airway that correlates with the degree of airway hyperresponsiveness is loss of epithelial structure [6]. Possibly the partial loss of the epithelial barrier allows greater amounts of bronchoconstrictor mediators to reach the smooth muscle or other cells which amplify the bronchoconstricting effect of the inhaled mediators. Alternatively, the release of bronchodilating substances from the epithelium could be reduced by epithelial damage, which could enhance bronchial smooth muscle contraction [39]. Indeed, it is possible that a number of these different mechanisms interact to produce airway hyperresponsiveness, but it is also likely that different mechanisms are involved in causing different components of airway hyperresponsiveness. Thus, while airway structural changes appear to be responsible for the underlying persisting airway hyperresponsiveness in asthmatic patients, other mechanisms cause the variable changes in airway hyperresponsiveness seen in asthmatic subjects during the course of the disease.

Variable airway hyperresponsiveness can last days or weeks after experimental allergen inhalation [40], or during a seasonal allergen exposure [41]. These changes are temporally related to increases in airway inflammatory cells, particularly eosinophils and basophils [42]. In addition, the release of cysteinyl leukotrienes, likely from these cells, is partially responsible for allergen-induced airway hyperresponsiveness. This has been confirmed by the demonstration that leukotriene receptor antagonists, such as montelukast [43] or pranlukast [44], partially attenuate allergen-induced airway hyperresponsiveness, but not the persistent airway hyperresponsiveness of asthma.

## Cough-variant asthma

Cough-variant asthma was initially described as a clinical entity in 1979 [45]. It was identified in six patients who had chronic persistent cough, without airflow obstruction, but who did have methacholine airway hyperresponsiveness. These authors argued that the presence of airway hyperresponsiveness, together with even one symptom of asthma, established the diagnosis

of asthma. In all subjects, the cough improved with regular inhaled bronchodilators. Subsequently, the term cough-variant asthma was used to indicate a 'forme fruste' of asthma [46]. However, it is now recognized that in some patients with asthma, cough is the main, and indeed sometimes the only, symptom and that variable airflow obstruction may not accompany the symptom of cough. Koh et al. [47] have suggested that it is the level of maximal airway response to inhaled methacholine, rather than the degree of airway hypersensitivity, that may be an important risk factor for the eventual development of wheezing in patients who initially present with cough as the only symptom of asthma. It has become clear that cough-variant asthma is rather not a 'forme fruste' of asthma, but a clinical manifestation of (usually mild) asthma, with similar pathological changes in the airway wall [48]. Consistent with this view, Niimi et al. [49] have described that serum eosinophil cationic protein level and the percentage of eosinophils in bronchoalveolar lavage (BAL) fluid and in bronchial biopsy specimens were elevated and comparable to those found in patients with classic asthma associated with wheeze. The same group found an increased thickness of the bronchial basement membrane in patients with cough-variant asthma, indicating that a similar process of airway wall remodelling as observed in classic asthma was present [48].

## Eosinophilic bronchitis without airway hyperresponsiveness

Another clinical entity, identified in 1989 by Gibson et al. [50], is the presence of troublesome persistent cough, associated with airway inflammation, as measured by increased numbers of eosinophils in induced sputum, but without airway hyperresponsiveness (Fig. 12.3). This was called eosinophilic bronchitis, to indicate a clinical condition separate from asthma. One study has suggested that eosinophilic bronchitis is the cause of troublesome cough in 13% of patients presenting to a speciality clinic [51], and has been described in an occupational setting [52]. The cough associated with eosinophilic bronchitis responds to treatment with inhaled corticosteroids [53], associated with resolution of the eosinophilic airway inflammation. In the majority of the patients described in the original clinical description, the cough did not return after treatment. However, occasionally, the cough did not fully improve

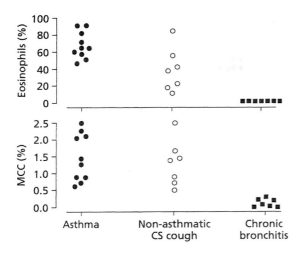

**Fig. 12.3** Numbers of eosinophils and metachromatic cells in either spontaneous or induced sputum in patients with asthma (●), eosinophilic bronchitis (○) or chronic bronchitis (■). Reproduced from [50].

with even high doses of inhaled corticosteroids, and required oral corticosteroids for benefit. Interestingly, in one case report, inadequately treated eosinophilic bronchitis resulted in symptomatic asthma, with partially fixed, irreversible airflow obstruction [54]. The pathological features of eosinophilic bronchitis have been compared to asthma in airway biopsies [55]. These studies have shown that the main differences demonstrated were an increased number of mast cells present in the airway smooth muscle in asthma. Gibson and colleagues [56] found that sputum cells obtained from patients with chronic cough, who had normal spirometry and normal airway responsiveness, and whose cough responded to inhaled corticosteroids, expressed interleukin-5 (IL-5) and granulocyte–macrophage colony-stimulating factor (GM-CSF) mRNA by *in situ* hybridization. These patients would fit into the category of eosinophilic bronchitis, and such expression has also been observed in patients with asthma indicating that both diseases may be caused by eosinophils.

## Airway hyperresponsiveness and cough sensitivity

The lack of relationship between airway hyperre-sponsiveness and capsaicin cough response has been highlighted by a study of Fujimura and colleagues [57]. They described two groups of patients with chronic non-productive cough: those with methacholine airway hyperresponsiveness, but with a normal capsaicin cough threshold, whose cough was responsive to bronchodilator therapy; and those had normal airway responsiveness with a hypertussive response to capsaicin whose coughs responded to inhaled corticosteroids or antihistamines. Furthermore, these patients did not demonstrate any BAL eosinophilia, but had only a small number of eosinophils in the subepithelium of the tracheal and bronchial biopsies [58] and in induced sputum [59]. Thus, it appears that what Fujimura called 'atopic' cough may be part of 'eosinophilic bronchitis' or at least at one spectrum of this condition. In addition, atopic cough, as with eosinophilic bronchitis, is responsive to inhaled corticosteroid therapy with a reduction in the capsaicin tussive response [60].

This lack of concordance between airway responsiveness and capsaicin cough response [61] has not been confirmed by other investigators. Doherty *et al.* [62] described a cohort of asthmatic patients, who as a group showed enhanced capsaicin cough response when compared to a cohort of non-asthmatic volunteers and capsaicin cough sensitivity was related to symptomatic cough as measured by diary card score. Thus, capsaicin cough response may be increased in some patients with asthma, since some patients may have a persistent dry cough, even though other asthma symptoms are well controlled on adequate therapy. Cough receptor sensitivity in children with uncontrolled asthma, who have troublesome cough, is increased, but decreases when asthma is controlled to levels similar to those in children with asthma without cough [63].

## Mechanisms of cough in asthma

The mechanisms of cough in asthma are similar to those causing other symptoms; that is, a consequence of airway inflammation. In some instances, cough may occur as a direct result of airway obstruction and increased mucus production that occurs during an asthma exacerbation. As described above, some asthmatics have also been demonstrated to have an increased cough reflex as measured by capsaicin inhalation [64], which suggests that axonal reflexes, the stimulation of airway C fibres and substance P release in the airways may be abnormal in asthmatics [65]. Sensitization of the cough response by mediators such as $PGE_2$ or by bradykinin may occur [66,67]. In addition to peripheral sensitization, central sensitization pathways have been proposed by integration from various sensory nerve subtypes in the central nervous system to initiate exaggerated reflexes and sensation, and substance P has been proposed as an important central mechanism for sensitization of the cough reflex, and its persistence [68]. Interestingly, recent studies have shown that allergen inhalation in atopic asthmatic subjects caused increases in eosinophilic airway inflammation and airway hyperresponsiveness, but not in capsaicin sensitivity [69]. This suggests that cough receptor sensitivity to capsaicin is not associated with airway eosinophilic inflammation, at least in patients with allergic asthma. By contrast, Weinfeld *et al.* [70] described increased capsaicin sensitivity in allergic asthmatic patients to be increased during allergen exposure as during the birch pollen season, and argued that allergic inflammation in the lower and/or upper airways may trigger neurogenic mechanisms of significant clinical importance. However, the best evidence for an involvement of airway inflammation, in particular eosinophils, in cough is the observation that cough associated with eosinophilic inflammation such as asthma, cough-variant asthma and an eosinophilic bronchitis responds to corticosteroid therapy which also inhibits eosinophilic inflammation.

## Management of cough in asthma

The management of cough in asthma is, generally, the same as the management of other asthma symptoms [1]. This means treating airway inflammation, which is done most effectively with inhaled corticosteroids and inhaled $\beta_2$-agonists as needed. Inhaled $\beta_2$-agonists will be particularly and rapidly effective if the cough is a result of airflow obstruction. The clinical effectiveness of inhaled corticosteroids will take days to weeks to achieve the maximal benefit. Other treatment options that have been considered for asthmatic cough include inhaled ipratropium bromide or sodium cromoglycate. Ipratropium bromide has been shown to reduce capsaicin-induced bronchoconstriction [64], while cromoglycate reduces angiotensin-converting enzyme-induced cough [71]. However, only inhaled corticosteroids have been shown to improve the cough

threshold in asthmatics [72], while neither cromoglycate [64], nor leukotriene receptor antagonists [73] have this effect.

## Conclusions

Cough is an important symptom in asthmatic patients. It is often, but not always, associated with airflow obstruction. Occasionally, cough is the only symptom of asthma, and the diagnosis is established by demonstrating the presence of airway hyperresponsiveness. More commonly, persistent cough as the only respiratory symptom is caused by eosinophilic bronchitis, where airway hyperresponsiveness is absent, but is associated with eosinophils as in asthma. Some asthmatics have an enhanced cough reflex as measured by capsaicin inhalation, likely as a consequence of airway inflammation. The treatment of cough in patients with asthma or eosinophilic bronchitis is the same as with asthma, with inhaled corticosteroids, with or without inhaled $\beta_2$-agonists.

## References

1 Global Initiative for Asthma. *Global Strategy for Asthma Management and Prevention*, 2002. NIH Publication 02–3659.

2 Kirby JG, Hargreave FE, Gleich GJ, O'Byrne PM. Bronchoalveolar cell profiles of asthmatic and nonasthmatic subjects. *Am Rev Respir Dis* 1987; **136**: 379–83.

3 Beasley R, Roche WR, Roberts JA, Holgate ST. Cellular events in the bronchi in mild asthma and after bronchial provocation. *Am Rev Respir Dis* 1989; **139**: 806–17.

4 Gleich GJ, Frigas E, Loegering DA, Wassom DL, Steinmuller D. Cytotoxic properties of the eosinophil major basic protein. *J Immunol* 1979; **123**: 2925–7.

5 Venge P, Bystrom J. Eosinophil cationic protein (ECP). *Int J Biochem Cell Biol* 1998; **30** (4): 433–7.

6 Jeffery PK, Wardlaw AJ, Nelson FC, Collins JV, Kay AB. Bronchial biopsies in asthma. An ultrastructural, quantitative study and correlation with hyperreactivity. *Am Rev Respir Dis* 1989; **140**: 1745–53.

7 Robinson DS, Hamid Q, Ying S, Tsicopoulos A, Barkans J, Bentley AM *et al.* Predominant TH-2 like bronchoalveolar T-lymphocyte populations in atopic asthma. *N Engl J Med* 1992; **326**: 298–304.

8 Jeffery PK. Comparative morphology of the airways in asthma and chronic obstructive pulmonary disease. *Am J Respir Crit Care Med* 1997; **150**: S6–S13.

9 Turner MO, Hussack P, Sears MR, Dolovich J, Hargreave FE. Exacerbations of asthma without sputum eosinophilia. *Thorax* 1995; 50: 1057–61.

10 Alexander HL, Paddock R. Bronchial asthma: response to pilocarpine and epinephrine. *Arch Intern Med* 1921; 27: 184–91.

11 Weiss S, Robb GP, Ellis LB. The systematic effects of histamine in man. *Arch Intern Med* 1932; 49: 360–96.

12 Curry JJ. Comparative action of acetyl-beta-methyl choline and histamine on the respiratory tract in normals, patients with hay fever and subjects with bronchial asthma. *J Clin Invest* 1947; 26: 430–8.

13 Tiffeneau R, Beauvallet P. Epreuve de bronchoconstriction et de bronchodilation par aerosols. *Bull Acad Med* 1945; 129: 165–8.

14 Cockcroft DW, Killian DN, Mellon JJ, Hargreave FE. Bronchial reactivity to inhaled histamine: a method and clinical survey. *Clin Allergy* 1977; 7: 235–43.

15 Juniper EF, Frith PA, Dunnett C, Cockcroft DW, Hargreave FE. Reproductibility and comparison of responses to inhaled histamine and methacholine. *Thorax* 1978; 33: 705–10.

16 Sotomayor H, Badier M, Vervloet D, Orehek J. Seasonal increase of carbachol airway responsiveness in patients allergic to grass pollen. Reversal by corticosteroids. *Am Rev Respir Dis* 1984; 130: 56–8.

17 Adelroth E, Morris MM, Hargreave FE, O'Byrne PM. Airway responsiveness to leukotrienes C4 and D4 and to methacholine in patients with asthma and normal controls. *N Engl J Med* 1986; 315: 480–4.

18 Hardy CC, Robinson C, Tattersfield AE, Holgate ST. The bronchoconstrictor effect of inhaled prostaglandin D2 in normal and asthmatic men. *N Engl J Med* 1984; 311: 209–13.

19 Thomson NC, Roberts R, Bandouvakis J, Newball H, Hargreave FE. Comparison of bronchial responses to prostaglandin F2 alpha and methacholine. *J Allergy Clin Immunol* 1981; 68: 392–8.

20 O'Byrne PM, Dolovich J, Hargreave FE. Late asthmatic responses. *Am Rev Respir Dis* 1987; 136: 740–51.

21 Chan-Yeung M, Malo JL. Occupational asthma. *N Engl J Med* 1995; 333: 107–12.

22 McFadden ER Jr, Gilbert IA. Exercise-induced asthma. *N Engl J Med* 1994; 330: 1362–7.

23 O'Byrne PM, Ryan G, Morris M, McCormack D, Jones NL, Morse JL *et al.* Asthma induced by cold air and its relation to nonspecific bronchial responsiveness to methacholine. *Am Rev Respir Dis* 1982; 125: 281–5.

24 Anderson SD, Schoeffel RE, Finney M. Evaluation of ultrasonically nebulised solutions for provocation testing in patients with asthma. *Thorax* 1983; 38: 284–91.

25 Anderson SD, Brannan J, Spring J, Spalding N, Rodwell LT, Chan K *et al.* A new method for bronchial-provocation testing in asthmatic subjects using a dry powder of mannitol. *Am J Respir Crit Care Med* 1997; 156: 758–65.

26 Anderson SD, Brannan JD. Exercise-induced asthma: is there still a case for histamine? *J Allergy Clin Immunol* 2002; 109 (5): 771–3.

27 Manning PJ, Watson RM, Margolskee DJ, Williams VC, Schwartz JI, O'Byrne PM. Inhibition of exercise-induced bronchoconstriction by MK-571, a potent leukotriene D4-receptor antagonist. *N Engl J Med* 1990; 323: 1736–9.

28 Juniper EF, Frith PA, Hargreave FE. Airway responsiveness to histamine and methacholine: relationship to minimum treatment to control symptoms of asthma. *Thorax* 1981; 36: 575–9.

29 Hopp RJ, Bewtra A, Biven R, Nair NM, Townley RG. Bronchial reactivity pattern in nonasthmatic parents of asthmatics. *Ann Allergy* 1988; 61: 184–6.

30 Young S, Le Souef PN, Geelhoed GC, Stick SM, Turner KL, Landau LI. The influence of a family history of asthma and parental smoking on airway responsiveness in early infancy. *N Engl J Med* 1991; 324: 1168–73.

31 Postma DS, Bleeker ER, Amelung PJ, Holroyd KJ, Xu J, Panhysen CIM *et al.* Genetic susceptibility to asthma-bronchial hyperresponsiveness coinherited with a major gene for atopy. *N Engl J Med* 1995; 333: 894–900.

32 van Herwerden L, Harrap SB, Wong ZY, Abramson MJ, Kutin JJ, Forbes AB *et al.* Linkage of high-affinity IgE receptor gene with bronchial hyperreactivity, even in the absence of atopy. *Lancet* 1995; 346: 1262–5.

33 Hall IP, Wheatley A, Wilding P, Liggett SB. Association of Glu 27 beta 2-adrenoceptor polymorphism with lower airway reactivity in asthmatic subjects. *Lancet* 1995; 345: 1213–4.

34 Turki J, Pak J, Green SA, Martin RJ, Liggett SB. Genetic polymorphism of the beta-2 adrenergic receptor in nocturnal and nonnocturnal asthma. Evidence that Gly 16 correlates with the nocturnal phenotype. *J Clin Invest* 1995; 95: 1635–41.

35 Dahlen SE, Hedqvist P, Hammarstrom S, Samuelsson B. Leukotrienes are potent constrictors of human bronchi. *Nature* 1980; 288: 484–6.

36 Cui ZH, Pullerits T, Linden A, Skoogh BE, Lotvall J. Attenuation of early phase airway response and plasma exudation due to reduction of leukotrienes production after repeated allergen exposure. *J Allergy Clin Immunol* 2000; 105 (1): S294.

37 Carroll N, Elliot J, Morton A, James AL. The structure and function of large and small airways in nonfatal and fatal asthma. *Am Rev Respir Dis* 1993; 147: 405–10.

38 Dunnill MS, Massarell GR, Anderson JA. A comparison of the quantitive anatomy of the bronchi in normal subjects, in status asthmaticus, in chronic bronchitis and in emphysema. *Thorax* 1969; 24: 176–9.

39 Manning PJ, Jones GL, Otis J, Daniel EE, O'Byrne PM. The inhibitory influence of tracheal mucosa mounted in close proximity to canine trachealis. *Eur J Pharmacol* 1990; **178**: 85–9.

40 Cartier A, Thomson NC, Frith PA, Roberts R, Hargreave FE. Allergen-induced increase in bronchial responsiveness to histamine: relationship to the late asthmatic response and change in airway caliber. *J Allergy Clin Immunol* 1982; **70**: 170–7.

41 Monteseirin J, Guardia P, Delgado J, Llamas E, Palma J, Conde A *et al.* Peripheral-blood T-lymphocytes seasonal bronchial asthma. *Allergy* 1995; **50** (2): 152–6.

42 Gauvreau GM, Watson RM, O'Byrne PM. Kinetics of allergen-induced airway eosinophilic cytokine production and airway inflammation. *Am J Respir Crit Care Med* 1999; **160**: 640–7.

43 Leigh R, Vethanayagam D, Yoshida M, Watson RM, Rerecich T, Inman MD *et al.* Effects of montelukast and budesonide on airway responses and airway inflammation in asthma. *Am J Respir Crit Care Med* 2002; **166** (9): 1212–7.

44 Hamilton AL, Faiferman I, Stober P, Watson RM, O'Byrne PM. Pranlukast, a leukotriene receptor antagonist, attenuates allergen-induced early and late phase bronchoconstriction and airway hyperresponsiveness in asthmatic subjects. *J Allergy Clin Immunol* 1998; **102**: 177–83.

45 Corrao WM, Braman SS, Irwin RS. Chronic cough as the sole presenting manifestation of bronchial asthma. *N Engl J Med* 1979; **300** (12): 633–7.

46 Tokuyama K, Shigeta M, Maeda S, Takei K, Hoshino M, Morikawa A. Diurnal variation of peak expiratory flow in children with cough variant asthma. *J Asthma* 1998; **35** (2): 225–9.

47 Koh YY, Park Y, Kim CK. The importance of maximal airway response to methacholine in the prediction of wheezing development in patients with cough-variant asthma. *Allergy* 2002; **57** (12): 1165–70.

48 Niimi A, Matsumoto H, Minakuchi M, Kitaichi M, Amitani R. Airway remodelling in cough-variant asthma. *Med J Aust* 2000; **356** (9229): 564–5.

49 Niimi A, Amitani R, Suzuki K, Tanaka E, Murayama T, Kuze F. Eosinophilic inflammation in cough variant asthma. *Eur Respir J* 1998; **11** (5): 1064–9.

50 Gibson PG, Dolovich J, Denburg J, Ramsdale EH, Hargreave FE. Chronic cough: eosinophilic bronchitis without asthma. *Lancet* 1989; **1**: 1346–8.

51 Brightling CE, Ward R, Goh KL, Wardlaw AJ, Pavord ID. Eosinophilic bronchitis is an important cause of chronic cough. *Am J Respir Crit Care Med* 1999; **160** (2): 406–10.

52 Lemiere C, Efthimiadis A, Hargreave FE. Occupational eosinophilic bronchitis without asthma: an unknown occupational airway disease. *J Allergy Clin Immunol* 1997; **100** (6): 852–3.

53 Gibson PG, Hargreave FE, Girgis-Gabardo A, Morris M, Denburg JA, Dolovich J. Chronic cough with eosinophilic bronchitis: examination for variable airflow obstruction and response to corticosteroid. *Clin Exp Allergy* 1995; **25**: 127–32.

54 Brightling CE, Woltmann G, Wardlaw AJ, Pavord ID. Development of irreversible airflow obstruction in a patient with eosinophilic bronchitis without asthma. *Eur Respir J* 1999; **14** (5): 1228–30.

55 Brightling CE, Bradding P, Symon FA, Holgate ST, Wardlaw AJ, Pavord ID. Mast-cell infiltration of airway smooth muscle in asthma. *N Engl J Med* 2002; **346** (22): 1699–705.

56 Gibson PG, Zlatic K, Scott J, Sewell W, Woolley K, Saltos N. Chronic cough resembles asthma with IL-5 and granulocyte–macrophage colony-stimulating factor gene expression in bronchoalveolar cells. *J Allergy Clin Immunol* 1998; **101** (3): 320–6.

57 Fujimura M, Kamio Y, Hashimoto T, Matsuda T. Cough receptor sensitivity and bronchial responsiveness in patients with only chronic non-productive cough: in view of effect of bronchodilator therapy. *J Asthma* 1994; **31**: 463–72.

58 Fujimura M, Ogawa H, Yasui M, Matsuda T. Eosinophilic tracheobronchitis and airway cough hypersensitivity in chronic non-productive cough. *Clin Exp Allergy* 2000; **30** (1): 41–7.

59 Fujimura M, Songur N, Kamio Y, Matsuda T. Detection of eosinophils in hypertonic saline-induced sputum in patients with chronic nonproductive cough. *J Asthma* 1997; **34** (2): 119–26.

60 Brightling CE, Ward R, Wardlaw AJ, Pavord ID. Airway inflammation, airway responsiveness and cough before and after inhaled budesonide in patients with eosinophilic bronchitis. *Eur Respir J* 2000; **15** (4): 682–6.

61 Fujimura M, Kamio Y, Hashimoto T, Matsuda T. Airway cough sensitivity to inhaled capsaicin and bronchial responsiveness to methacholine in asthmatic and bronchitic subjects. *Respirology* 1998; **3**: 267–72.

62 Doherty MJ, Mister R, Pearson MG, Calverley PMA. Capsaicin responsiveness and cough in asthma and chronic obstructive pulmonary disease. *Thorax* 2000; **55** (8): 643–9.

63 Chang AB, Phelan PD, Robertson CF. Cough receptor sensitivity in children with acute and non-acute asthma. *Thorax* 1997; **52** (9): 770–4.

64 Fuller RW, Dixon CM, Barnes PJ. Bronchoconstrictor response to inhaled capsaicin in humans. *J Appl Physiol* 1985; **58** (4): 1080–4.

65 Millqvist E, Bende M, Lowhagen O. Sensory hyperreactivity—a possible mechanism underlying cough and asthma-like symptoms. *Allergy* 1998; **53** (12): 1208–12.

66 Fox AJ, Lalloo UG, Belvisi MG, Bernareggi M, Chung KF,

Barnes PJ. Bradykinin-evoked sensitization of airway sensory nerves: a mechanism for ACE-inhibitor cough. *Nature Med* 1996; **2** (7): 814–7.

67 Nichol GM, Nix A, Barnes PJ, Chung KF. Enhancement of capsaicin-induced cough by inhaled prostaglandin F2a: modulation by beta-adrenergic agonist and anticholinergic agent. *Thorax* 1990; **45**: 694–8.

68 Undem BJ, Hunter DD, Liu M, Haak-Frendscho M, Oakragly A, Fischer A. Allergen-induced sensory neuroplasticity in airways. *Int Arch Allergy Immunol* 1999; **118**: 150–3.

69 Minoguchi H, Minoguchi K, Tanaka A, Matsuo H, Kihara N, Adachi M. Cough receptor sensitivity to capsaicin does not change after allergen bronchoprovocation in allergic asthma. *Thorax* 2003; **58**: 19–22.

70 Weinfeld D, Ternesten-Hasseus E, Lowhagen O, Millqvist E. Capsaicin cough sensitivity in allergic asthmatic patients increases during the birch pollen season. *Ann Allergy Asthma Immunol* 2002; **89** (4): 419–24.

71 Hargreaves MR, Benson MK. Inhaled sodium cromoglycate in angiotensin-converting enzyme inhibitor cough. *Lancet* 1995; **345**: 13–6.

72 Di Franco A, Dente FL, Giannini D, Vagaggini B, Conti I, Macchioni P *et al.* Effects of inhaled corticosteroids on cough threshold in patients with bronchial asthma. *Pulm Pharmacol Ther* 2001; **14** (1): 35–40.

73 Dicpinigaitis PV, Dobkin JB. Effect of zafirlukast on cough reflex sensitivity in asthmatics. *J Asthma* 1999; **36** (3): 265–70.

**123**

# 13

# Cough in chronic obstructive pulmonary disease

*Kian Fan Chung & Peter M.A. Calverley*

## Introduction

Chronic obstructive pulmonary disease (COPD) is a leading cause of death and disability throughout the world, and it is predicted that COPD will increase from the twelfth to become the fifth most prevalent disease and from the sixth to become the third most common cause of death in the world [1]. In the UK, hospital admissions for COPD amounted to just over 200 000 in 1994, with an average hospital stay of 10 days, and the estimated total direct and indirect costs were £846 million in 1996. Currently, in the US, there are 16 million patients with COPD, and the estimated direct and indirect costs are $30 billion per year.

COPD is a term that encompasses many conditions including emphysema and chronic obstructive bronchitis characterized by progressive airflow limitation that is not substantially reversed by bronchodilators, usually resulting from an abnormal response of the lungs to noxious particles or gases [2]. The resulting endogenous inflammatory response is likely to be the driving cause for the loss of airway function. The most common cause of COPD is tobacco smoke, with its composition of noxious gases and particles. The causes of airflow limitation in COPD include a combination of airways inflammation and remodelling, bronchospasm, mucus hypersecretion and loss of elastic lung recoil. In this chapter, we will overview the pathophysiology, clinical presentation and treatment of COPD, with emphasis particularly on the importance of cough and the mechanisms underlying cough.

## Cough and COPD — clinical aspects

Before the Global Initiative for Chronic Obstructive Lung Disease (GOLD) definition of COPD was agreed, chronic persistent coughing was recognized among clinicians as a hallmark of at least the early stages of this illness. This led to the clinical concept of chronic bronchitis, with its associated sputum production, as a marker for future ill health and possibly mortality. When this was tested by the epidemiological studies of Fletcher and colleagues in the 1970s it became clear that airflow obstruction and not cough and sputum production was the best predictor of subsequent mortality [3]. Indeed, inclusion of the data about cough productive of sputum did not add further to the mortality prediction [4].

This led many clinicians to discount cough in COPD as being of any importance, apart from its perceived nuisance value. However this view is now changing again as further data have accumulated. There is now better evidence that people who have cough regularly productive of sputum are more likely to develop pneumonic complications during COPD exacerbations and subsequently die [5]. Patients spirometrically diagnosed as having COPD are more likely to report any form of exacerbation if they regularly cough and produce sputum [6]. Even in early COPD there are now data suggesting that those with persistent infection, associated as it is with regular cough, will have a more rapid decline in $FEV_1$ than those who do not experience this problem [7]. This small effect is independent of the effects of tobacco smoke but its mechanism remains to be explained.

Thus, there is renewed interest in cough in COPD.

Clinically cough does contribute independently to the reduction in quality of life (better described as health status) which is typical of patients affected by COPD [8]. Chronic bronchitis is now recognized as being a very common complaint reported by over 5 million people in the US and often associated with undiagnosed airflow obstruction [9]. This has led the GOLD initiative to propose persistent coughing even without airflow obstruction as a warning sign of the individual's potential for developing COPD [2]. This may not be accurate, at least as judged in other population data sets [10], but it does serve to raise public awareness that a persistent cough is not something that should be simply ignored or rationalized as being the result of cigarette smoking and of no consequence.

## Aetiological factors and amplifying mechanisms

Much thinking has gone into the fact that, although tobacco smoking induces airway and lung inflammation in all smokers, only 15% of smokers develop COPD, indicating that there are either host or environmental factors (or both) that may determine the onset of progressive airflow limitation. Genetic factors are likely to be important as illustrated by the development of emphysema in non-smokers, and with accelerated development of emphysema in smokers associated with a severe deficiency of $\alpha_1$-protease inhibitor, a major circulating inhibitor of serine protease [11,12]. Other aetiological or interacting factors with cigarette smoke may be environmental pollution, bacterial or viral infections, nutritional factors, low birth weight and bronchial hyperresponsiveness. A growing area of investigation is that of the innate host response factors to external environmental factors such as viruses and bacteria, as well as components of these infective organisms such as viral DNA and bacterial lipopolysaccharides, and environmental pollutants.

It has been proposed that latent adenoviral genes may act as an enhancing transcription factor to enhance the inflammatory response of cigarette smoke exposure [13]. Furthermore, the propensity of bacterial and viral mucosal infections leading to exacerbations of COPD may themselves damage the epithelial barrier and enhance the chronic inflammation. Finally, defence mechanisms of the airways may be impaired primarily, to allow continuing damage such as the reduction in the production of secretory IgA in the epithelium of patients with COPD [14], and the impairment of mucociliary clearance in smokers and chronic bronchitis [15].

### The inflammatory process

The close association between tobacco smoking and the development of emphysema, chronic bronchitis and the full spectrum of COPD has been known for many years. Increased numbers of neutrophils, macrophages and natural killer lymphocytes as compared with values in smokers without airflow obstruction has been described, and each variable inversely correlated with $FEV_1$ [16]. The association of inflammation and COPD is very complex. Cigarette smoking-induced inflammation is present in the lungs of all smokers, including those with normal lung function. In the minority of smokers that develop COPD, the inflammatory process is more pronounced. Airway and parenchymal inflammation are consistently found in COPD, and the airways of patients with airflow limitation contain a higher number of inflammatory cells than do airways of patients with normal $FEV_1$ [16]. However, the inflammation can persist for a long time after smoking cessation [17].

The inflammatory process in the airways involves neutrophils, macrophages, $CD8^+$ T cells and epithelial alterations. The role of overexpressed cytokines and chemokines is particularly important in the initiation and maintenance of the inflammatory process [18]. Macrophages can be activated by cigarette smoke to release inflammatory mediators such as tumour necrosis factor-$\alpha$ (TNF$\alpha$), interleukin-8 (IL-8) and leukotriene B$_4$ (LTB$_4$). These mediators are likely to contribute to the recruitment of neutrophils to the lungs. There is also an increase in the number of macrophages in patients with COPD, and macrophages are localized to the sites of alveolar wall destruction in patients with emphysema [19], and in the epithelium of small airways [20]. Part of the inflammatory process or altered tissue repair can lead to large and small airway wall thickening, together with epithelial squamous and mucous cell metaplasia, excessive matrix deposition, hypertrophy of the submucosal glands, and an increased airway smooth muscle mass in large and small airways.

Neutrophils are increased in the airways of smokers

and of patients with COPD, especially those with chronic bronchitis [21], and this is related to the severity of airflow obstruction [16]. Increased neutrophil elastase activity has been measured in both blood and lavage from patients with emphysema [22], and in smokers compared with non-smokers [23]. Other potential effects of neutrophils include the actions of neutrophil elastase in causing mucus secretion, epithelial damage and slowing of ciliary beat frequency [24,25].

Increased numbers of CD8+ T cells in the central and peripheral airways and lung parenchyma of smokers with COPD negatively correlated with the degree of airflow obstruction [26]. These T cells appear activated, expressing surface activation markers IL-2R and VLA-1 (very late antigen-1) [27]. Interestingly, once established, the number of CD8+ T cells and the expression of these activation markers do not change on cessation of smoking for up to 1 year [28]. These CD8+ T cells coexpress interferon-γ (IFNγ) and the chemokine receptor, CXCR3; in addition, the ligand chemokine for this receptor, CXCL10, is overexpressed in the bronchiolar epithelium of smokers with COPD [29]. These data indicate that the CXCR3/CXCL10 interaction may lead to the recruitment of CD8+ T cells in the peripheral airways of smokers with COPD.

## Pathophysiological changes in COPD

With biochemical and cellular changes in the small airways and surrounding alveoli, structural damage leads to a loss of elastic lung recoil [30]. The lungs start to increase in size and forced vital capacity (FVC) increases. In early stages of COPD, the ratio of $FEV_1$ to FVC may decrease without any change in $FEV_1$. Both a loss of elastic lung recoil and an increase in lung resistance occur when alveoli become damaged or lost, with a reduction in the elastic supporting structure of the lung, since the airways are no longer tethered by the radial traction forces of the surrounding alveolar attachments [31]. Mural inflammation of the small airways and airways remodelling also reduce the airway lumen [32]. The site of airways obstruction in COPD is in the smaller conducting airways including bronchi and bronchioles of less than 2 mm in diameter [33]. Therefore, the causes of airflow obstruction in COPD are a combination of airways inflammation and remodelling, bronchospasm, mucus hypersecretion and loss of elastic lung recoil.

## Clinical presentation of COPD

The diagnosis of COPD is based on the detection of airflow limitation. Since the umbrella of COPD covers a range of overlapping conditions such as chronic bronchitis, bronchiolitis and emphysema, the clinical presentation can be varied. Many patients who have smoked for many years may be asymptomatic and the diagnosis may not be made because spirometry has not been performed. Otherwise, patients often present with shortness of breath on effort that is chronic; these patients also often present without cough. Other associated symptoms of COPD may include wheezing and chest tightness.

The association of current cigarette smoking with cough is well known [34,35], and the risk of cough is increased with the amount of tobacco smoked. Cough is frequently the first symptom reported by patients with COPD [36]. Some patients may have had a history of chronic bronchitis, with persistent cough and sputum production over a period of months during the winter, although this may or may not be associated with airflow obstruction. In fact, cough and sputum production may precede by many years the development of airflow limitation. Patients with COPD may have a persistent troublesome cough that is either productive or non-productive.

Given the enormous number of potential variables, which may play different roles at different stages of the COPD patient's clinical progress, it should be no surprise that simple questions about the frequency of cough and how troublesome it is often yield confusing results of uncertain value. In one selected series of patients 81% complained of cough but only 12% found this a very troublesome symptom and only half reported regular sputum production [37]. This illustrates how limited our knowledge of this important complaint really is in this group of patients. We urgently need a validated cough questionnaire that can be applied to sufficient numbers of patients for a reliable estimate of the severity, type and natural history of cough to be obtained. Only then will it be possible to relate some of the currently rather fragmentary mechanistic data to recognizable clinical settings.

A further useful development would be to agree a satisfactory acoustic definition of cough and apply it to COPD patients. Attempts to do this have been made [38], and studies of objectively recorded overnight cough suggest that most coughing in COPD occurs

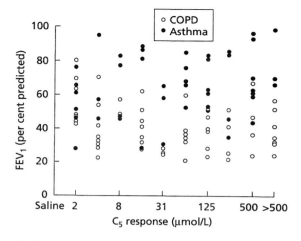

**Fig. 13.1** Relationship between $FEV_1$ as a percentage of predicted and directly measured capsaicin cough threshold in chronic obstructive pulmonary disease (COPD) (O) and chronic asthma (●). No significant relationship is present in either disease. Reproduced with permission from [37].

during periods of wakefulness rather than disturbing sleep, as occurs in other patients with chronic cough [39]. Measures of lung function like the $FEV_1$ are not well related to self-reported cough or to measures of capsaicin sensitivity (Fig. 13.1) [37]. This is another illustration of how one aspect of the COPD patient's disability, in this case expiratory airflow obstruction, does not capture the extent of their clinical problems with cough.

## Severity of COPD

The severity of COPD is usually categorized by spirometric measurements, as proposed by GOLD. Stage 0 is early disease usually presenting with persistent cough with sputum in the absence of airflow obstruction. It has been proposed that these individuals with persistent cough and sputum have inflammation of the large airways, as well as the small airways and alveoli, due to cigarette smoke. The presence of symptoms of cough and sputum may indicate the presence at sites of pathology which can lead later to airflow limitation. Unfortunately, many smokers consider their cough to be a 'normal' accompaniment of smoking, and this may be the reason why early diagnosis of COPD may be missed. In addition, the use of spirometry necessary for the diagnosis of COPD is not prevalent in most primary

care settings. The value of Stage 0 is unknown. One study has suggested that Stage 0 has no predictive value in detecting subsequent airflow obstruction [10].

The later established stages of COPD are described according to the degree of airflow obstruction:

*Stage I (mild):* Early development of airflow obstruction reflected by a reduction in the $FEV_1/FVC$ ratio <70%, with $FEV_1$ in the normal range (>80% predicted).

*Stage II (moderate):*

A: $FEV_1$ between 50 and 80% of predicted; $FEV_1/FVC$ ratio <70%; with or without symptoms.

B: $FEV_1$ between 30 and 50% of predicted; $FEV_1/FVC$ ratio <70%; with or without symptoms.

*Stage III (severe):* $FEV_1$ less than 30% of predicted, usually with evidence of current or previous respiratory failure or of right-sided heart failure. Cough and sputum production may be present at any stage of COPD.

### Exacerbations of COPD

Patients with severe COPD may deteriorate, with increased dyspnoea and productive cough associated with increased sputum volume or purulence [40], into an exacerbation. Cough is sometimes a very prominent symptom. Other symptoms may include wheeze, sore throat, nasal discharge or fever. Exacerbations of OPD that are more common in winter months are often due to viral or bacterial infections, and sometimes environmental pollutants, but the cold weather could be a predisposing trigger. Recurrent exacerbations are more usual in patients at a more severe stage of the disease.

## Cough reflex sensitivity

Data about the cough reflex in COPD have produced a somewhat contradictory picture reflecting differences in the method of selection of the subjects included and in the technique used to test the reflex (see Chapter 5). Even when the same stimulus is applied using the same protocol rather different results can emerge. Thus, a study of 11 patients with COPD with 'productive' cough demonstrated a normal sensitivity of the cough response to capsaicin [41], and this lends support to the concept that the cough of COPD was due to clearing of excessive secretions. However, in a larger cohort of

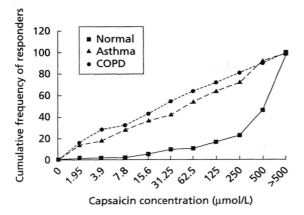

**Fig. 13.2** Cumulative frequency plot of the capsaicin concentration at which the $C_5$ threshold was reached in stable chronic obstructive pulmonary disease (COPD) patients (●), chronic asthma patients (▲) and normal individuals (■). Note that at any concentration more patients with airflow obstruction have a reduced threshold to coughing. Reproduced with permission from [37].

current or ex-smokers with COPD with a mean $FEV_1$ of 42% of predicted values, there was an increase in cough sensitivity [42]. The capsaicin cough sensitivity was related to the presence of cough, and to the patient's assessment of cough severity. In general the reduction in cough threshold was similar to that seen in a group of chronic asthmatics and significantly lower than that in a control population of somewhat younger subjects (Fig. 13.2). One strength of this study is that patients were not selected on the basis of having a clinically troublesome cough as in most other investigations. This may explain why they rated their cough as being of mild to moderate severity but also suggests that reductions in capsaicin cough threshold are not uncommon in established COPD. As yet there are no data regarding cough sensitivity during an exacerbation of COPD, but one presumes that it is further increased given the prominence of the cough and the triggering bacterial or viral infections which are known to increase cough sensitivity.

The increase in the cough reflex in COPD raises several interesting issues. First, the basis for the increased cough reflex is not known. Apart from possible mucus stimulation of cough, chronic smoking may increase airway sensitivity to capsaicin [43], and cough sensitivity to capsaicin in awake guinea-pigs [44].

Inflammatory mechanisms may sensitize afferent nerves in the airways through several mediators such as prostaglandins, or bradykinin may be implicated. Neurotrophins such as nerve growth factor and ciliary neurotrophic factor induce proliferation of airway sensory nerves and change their phenotype, with a reduced threshold of activation and increased expression of neuropeptides [45]. Substance P levels are elevated in induced sputum of patients with COPD [46], suggesting a role for neurogenic inflammation. Substance P may also be an important mechanism for augmentation and persistence of the cough reflex through 'peripheral' and 'central' mechanisms which integrate various inputs from sensory nerve subtypes in the central nervous system to initiate exaggerated reflexes and sensation [47]. The effect of products of activated neutrophils such as neutrophil myeloperoxidase or neutrophil elastase on the cough reflex is not known, but neutrophil elastase can cause goblet cell mucus secretion, epithelial damage and slowing of ciliary beat frequency [24,25].

## Mucus hypersecretion

As noted above, early epidemiological studies failed to find an association between mucus hypersecretion and rapid progression of COPD [3], but more recent population-based studies have now reported an association [48]. These latest epidemiological data support the concept that the development of cough and sputum in a smoker may be an early indicator of the development of COPD. It is also possible that the underlying cause of mucus hypersecretion and cough may also apply to the accelerated decline in lung function. Chronic bronchitis is associated with hyperplasia of both epithelial goblet cells and submucosal glands [20], and with submucosal gland hypertrophy [49]. Partial or complete occlusion of the airways of less than 2 mm in diameter with mucus plugs is commonly observed in COPD [33], with the clinical consequence of impairment of gas exchange, and morphometric measurements of distal airways of patients dying from COPD showed more mucus in the airway lumen when compared with controls without respiratory disease [49]. A positive correlation between the amount of submucosal glands and both the amount of mucus in the airway lumen and the daily sputum volume was reported. Many COPD patients also have areas of localized bronchiectasis identifiable on computed tomographic scans but not evident on the ordinary chest radiograph [50], which could also contribute to the total amount of sputum produced each day.

Increased mucus production could overwhelm the normal mucociliary clearance mechanisms and lead to the pooling of secretions and activation of the cough reflex. Alternatively the direct ciliotoxic effects of tobacco smoke coupled with delayed or ineffective epithelial healing following infective injury could impair the capacity of this system to clear more normal amounts of mucus produced physiologically in the airways. This would yield the same result but might explain why the amount of sputum produced by many patients is so meagre. Changes in the viscosity and physical properties of the sputum itself, as well as the production of this material in more distal airways than occurs in health due to goblet cell hyperplasia, could also make it harder to develop sufficiently high expiratory flows to clear mucus effectively. The residual material could act as a chronic irritant that repeatedly provokes relatively ineffective spells of coughing in the affected patient.

Whole-lung mucociliary clearance is reduced in COPD [51,52], and slowing of mucus clearance was observed to be greatest within the central airways [53]. In severe airflow obstruction, cough is usually an ineffective adjunct to mucociliary clearance. However, in asymptomatic smokers, normal values of mucus transport velocity were found in central airways with delays in clearance of mucus from peripheral airways [54]. This was reversed by β-agonist therapy.

Airway mucus is an aqueous solution of glycoconjugates, made predominantly of mucins, in addition to proteoglycans, enzymes and electrolytes. Mucins are important in determining the viscoelastic properties of airway mucus, and up to nine mucin genes have been identified so far [55]. MUC5AC is a predominant mucin in airway secretions from normal healthy children and in sputum samples from patients with chronic bronchitis [56]. In healthy smokers compared to non-smokers a fourfold increase in mucin-like material was detected in bronchoalveolar lavage fluid [57]. Mucus hypersecretion may also be induced by inflammation in the absence of substantial gland enlargement. For example, neutrophil elastase induces mucus secretion, together with epithelial damage and slowing of ciliary beat frequency [24,25]. Cigarette

smoke activates C fibres in airways and may result in mucus hypersecretion and goblet cell discharge [58], and tachykinins are potent stimuli of mucus secretion in human airways [59].

The differentiation of epithelial cells into goblet cells is another aspect underlying mucus hypersecretion and this is determined by the expression of mucin genes that encode the mucin glycoproteins in epithelial cells. Mucin genes can be up-regulated by exposure of epithelial cells to environmental factors including infections and pollutants, and to neutrophil elastase, while acrolein, a component of cigarette smoke, induces MUC5AC gene expression, and mucus metaplasia in rats [60, 61]. These effects may occur through the induction of oxidative stress [62], that leads to the ligand-independent transactivation of epidermal growth factor receptor (EGFR) and to airway mucin synthesis. Enhanced EGFR expression in the airway epithelium on exposure to cigarette smoke has been observed [63].

## Treatment of COPD

The treatment of COPD is mainly aimed towards the relief of symptoms. Although $FEV_1$ remains the basis for classification of severity, the change in $FEV_1$ with treatment is not used as a marker of response because such change may be small or within the error of the measurement, yet still be associated with significant symptomatic relief and improvement in well-being. Such symptomatic improvement can be obtained by the use of bronchodilators. The rate of decline in $FEV_1$ is used as an indication of disease progression, and there are no treatments that appear to be able to reverse the accelerated decline in lung function in these patients. Only cessation of cigarette smoking has been shown to lead to a normalization of the decline in $FEV_1$ [64]. Therefore, an important therapeutic approach is to get the patient to cease smoking. Nicotine replacement therapy with either gum, skin patches or inhaler is beneficial, and addition of buproprion provides additive effects [65].

In one study, cough markedly decreased in most patients following smoking cessation, with an improvement in the cough noticeable within 4 weeks in more than 50% of cases [66]. On the basis of this information, one would assume that the cough reflex would be reduced with smoking cessation.

## Bronchodilators

Bronchodilators, while not modifying the rate of decline in FEV$_1$, provide the most symptomatic relief in COPD. Although a small bronchodilator response is usually observed, they may relieve symptoms of effort dyspnoea probably through a reduction in dynamic hyperinflation. Short-acting β-agonists (e.g. salbutamol or terbutaline) and short-acting anticholinergic drugs (e.g. oxitropium or ipratropium) are often used, and may be used in combination, usually provided on a regular basis up to six times per day. Long-acting β-agonists for regular use are more conveniently used because of their 12-h duration of action, and beneficial effects on quality of life without significant effect on FEV$_1$ have been demonstrated [67,68]. Tiotropium bromide, a long-acting anticholinergic, is now available for the treatment of COPD. This drug is clearly superior to short-acting anticholinergic therapy in terms of improving FEV$_1$, reducing the number of exacerbations and improving health status [69]. β-Agonists or anticholinergics may be combined with theophylline. Although little emphasized in the reports of trials with all these agents, the self-reported cough score is little influenced in most cases, although occasional studies reporting some benefit can be found [70]. This may reflect the many different mechanisms underlying cough in COPD (see above) as well as the insensitive nature of these questionnaires. However, it is possible that specific mechanisms underlie cough in this disease and these are not as closely related to those producing airflow obstruction and hence do not change with treatment primarily directed at this endpoint.

There are data suggesting that patients who receive short-acting anticholinergic drugs have a lower cough threshold than those on other treatments, while this test is not influenced by inhaled corticosteroids [37]. However, it is not clear whether this is just a selection by severity or a true pharmacological effect.

## Corticosteroids

The role of anti-inflammatory agents in the treatment of COPD remains unclear. Several trials of inhaled corticosteroid therapy have shown that these agents do not slow the decline in lung function, although they do provide slightly more bronchodilator responses to short-acting β-agonists, and they may reduce the number of exacerbations in severe COPD [71–73]. One reason

put forward for the lack of clinical response to corticosteroid treatment is that the inflammation of COPD is not steroid responsive [74]. Therefore, other more specific anti-inflammatory approaches may be necessary, such as those targeted against neutrophils or macrophage activation.

It is not deemed necessary to use the response to a course of oral steroids to determine whether a patient with COPD should be given inhaled corticosteroid therapy [72]. More severe COPD patients are more likely to benefit, and a trial of 3–6 months is recommended. Inhaled corticosteroids should be considered in patients who do not experience benefit from bronchodilators.

## Combination of corticosteroids and bronchodilators

Recent studies using a combination of fluticasone and salmeterol have shown a better improvement in FEV$_1$ improvement of the order of 50–70 mL and in dyspnoeic index when compared to placebo or salmeterol alone; in addition, the combination therapy significantly improved quality of life [75]. These results provide some optimism for using such combination therapies in COPD. The combination of inhaled steroids and inhaled tiotropium will be of interest.

## Specific treatment for cough in COPD

If cough is an important part of COPD and contributes to deterioration in quality of life, it would make sense to control the symptom. There are two approaches, which are to suppress the amount of airway secretions and to reduce the enhanced cough reflex to a 'normal' range. Other potential causes of cough must be looked for such as rhinosinusitis, gastro-oesophageal reflux, or being on angiotensin-converting enzyme inhibitor therapy.

There is no specific treatment of airway mucus hypersecretion currently available. The currently available anticholinergics do not affect mucus secretion. Inhaled corticosteroid therapy does not have an inhibitory effect on goblet cells or on the expression of mucins in the airways [76–78]. Steroids do not inhibit the neutrophilic inflammation [74] which may be responsible for excessive mucus secretion. Leukotriene receptor antagonists may be tried because the cysteinyl leukotrienes are potent mucus secretagogues, but it is unlikely that these mediators are involved in COPD.

## Mucolytic therapy

There has been a trend in the past to use mucolytic agents such as N-acetylcysteine or sodium 2-mercaptoethane sulphonate, which break down disulphide bonds in mucins, to reduce the viscosity of mucus, and therefore improve mucus clearance. N-acetylcysteine has been shown to have some beneficial effects, particularly in reducing exacerbations [79], although this may result from its antioxidant effects. However, their efficacy is not good, and there is no general acceptance of their use in the treatment of COPD.

## Cough suppressants

It is not recommended that centrally acting antitussives such as opiates be used because of their potential suppressive effect on breathing (although in severe breathlessness opiates are sometimes used), and also because of the risk of retaining secretions and of infections. Whether the latter are serious risks is not known. To what degree the bronchodilators such as β-agonists or anticholinergics may influence cough in COPD is not known, although in asthma the reduction in airway tone achieved by bronchodilators may be a reason why cough can be controlled. The use of tachykinin receptor antagonists as antitussives has been proposed particularly for cough in COPD, and this action may result from suppression of the effects of tachykinin on airways and sputum production.

## References

1 Murray CJ, Lopez AD. Alternative projections of mortality and disability by cause 1990–2020: Global Burden of Disease Study. *Lancet* 1997; **349**: 1498–504.
2 Pauwels RA, Buist AS, Calverley PM, Jenkins CR, Hurd SS. Global strategy for the diagnosis, management, and prevention of chronic obstructive pulmonary disease. NHLBI/WHO Global Initiative for Chronic Obstructive Lung Disease (GOLD) Workshop summary. *Am J Respir Crit Care Med* 2001; **163**: 1256–76.
3 Fletcher C, Peto R. The natural history of chronic airflow obstruction. *Br Med J* 1977; **1**: 1645–8.
4 Peto R, Speizer FE, Cochrane AL, Moore F, Fletcher CM, Tinker CM et al. The relevance in adults of air-flow obstruction, but not of mucus hypersecretion, to mortality from chronic lung disease. Results from 20 years of prospective observation. *Am Rev Respir Dis* 1983; **128**: 491–500.
5 Prescott E, Lange P, Vestbo J. Chronic mucus hypersecretion in COPD and death from pulmonary infection. *Eur Respir J* 1995; **8**: 1333–8.
6 Seemungal TA, Donaldson GC, Paul EA, Bestall JC, Jeffries DJ, Wedzicha JA. Effect of exacerbation on quality of life in patients with chronic obstructive pulmonary disease. *Am J Respir Crit Care Med* 1998; **157**: 1418–22.
7 Kanner RE, Anthonisen NR, Connett JE. Lower respiratory illnesses promote FEV(1) decline in current smokers but not ex-smokers with mild chronic obstructive pulmonary disease: results from the lung health study. *Am J Respir Crit Care Med* 2001; **164**: 358–64.
8 Jones PW, Quirk FH, Baveystock CM, Littlejohns P. A self-complete measure of health status for chronic airflow limitation. The St. George's Respiratory Questionnaire. *Am Rev Respir Dis* 1992; **145**: 1321–7.
9 Mannino DM, Gagnon RC, Petty TL, Lydick E. Obstructive lung disease and low lung function in adults in the United States: data from the National Health and Nutrition Examination Survey, 1988–1994. *Arch Intern Med* 2000; **160**: 1683–9.
10 Vestbo J, Lange P. Can GOLD Stage 0 provide information of prognostic value in chronic obstructive pulmonary disease? *Am J Respir Crit Care Med* 2002; **166**: 329–32.
11 Eriksson S. A 30-year perspective on alpha 1-antitrypsin deficiency. *Chest* 1996; **110**: 237S–42S.
12 Sandford AJ, Weir TD, Spinelli JJ, Pare PD. Z and S mutations of the alpha$_1$-antitrypsin gene and the risk of chronic obstructive pulmonary disease. *Am J Respir Cell Mol Biol* 1999; **20**: 287–91.
13 Retamales I, Elliott WM, Meshi B, Coxson HO, Pare PD, Sciurba FC et al. Amplification of inflammation in emphysema and its association with latent adenoviral infection. *Am J Respir Crit Care Med* 2001; **164**: 469–73.
14 Pilette C, Godding V, Kiss R, Delos M, Verbeken E, Decaestecker C et al. Reduced epithelial expression of secretory component in small airways correlates with airflow obstruction in chronic obstructive pulmonary disease. *Am J Respir Crit Care Med* 2001; **163**: 185–94.
15 Wanner A. Clinical aspects of mucociliary transport. *Am Rev Respir Dis* 1977; **116**: 73–125.
16 Di SA, Capelli A, Lusuardi M, Balbo P, Vecchio C, Maestrelli P et al. Severity of airflow limitation is associated with severity of airway inflammation in smokers. *Am J Respir Crit Care Med* 1998; **158**: 1277–85.
17 Rutgers SR, Postma DS, ten Hacken NH, Kauffman HF, Der Mark TW, Koeter GH et al. Ongoing airway inflam-

mation in patients with COPD who do not currently smoke. *Thorax* 2000; **55**: 12–8.

18 Chung KF. Cytokines in chronic obstructive pulmonary disease. *Eur Resp J* 2001; **18** (Suppl. 34): 50s–59s.

19 Finkelstein R, Fraser RS, Ghezzo H, Cosio MG. Alveolar inflammation and its relation to emphysema in smokers. *Am J Respir Crit Care Med* 1995; **152**: 1666–72.

20 Saetta M, Turato G, Baraldo S, Zanin A, Braccioni F, Mapp CE *et al.* Goblet cell hyperplasia and epithelial inflammation in peripheral airways of smokers with both symptoms of chronic bronchitis and chronic airflow limitation. *Am J Respir Crit Care Med* 2000; **161**: 1016–21.

21 Confalonieri M, Mainardi E, Della PR, Bernorio S, Gandola L, Beghe B *et al.* Inhaled corticosteroids reduce neutrophilic bronchial inflammation in patients with chronic obstructive pulmonary disease [see comments]. *Thorax* 1998; **53**: 583–5.

22 Yoshioka A, Betsuyaku T, Nishimura M, Miyamoto K, Kondo T, Kawakami Y. Excessive neutrophil elastase in bronchoalveolar lavage fluid in subclinical emphysema. *Am J Respir Crit Care Med* 1995; **152**: 2127–32.

23 Abboud RT, Fera T, Johal S, Richter A, Gibson N. Effect of smoking on plasma neutrophil elastase levels. *J Lab Clin Med* 1986; **108**: 294–300.

24 Sommerhoff CP, Nadel JA, Basbaum CB, Caughey GH. Neutrophil elastase and cathepsin G stimulate secretion from cultured bovine airway gland serous cells. *J Clin Invest* 1990; **85**: 682–9.

25 Smallman LA, Hill SL, Stockley RA. Reduction of ciliary beat frequency in vitro by sputum from patients with bronchiectasis: a serine proteinase effect. *Thorax* 1984; **39**: 663–7.

26 Saetta M, Baraldo S, Corbino L, Turato G, Braccioni F, Rea F *et al.* CD8+ve cells in the lungs of smokers with chronic obstructive pulmonary disease. *Am J Respir Crit Care Med* 1999; **160**: 711–7.

27 Saetta M, Di Stefano A, Maestrelli P, Ferraresso A, Drigo R, Potena A *et al.* Activated T-lymphocytes and macrophages in bronchial mucosa of subjects with chronic bronchitis. *Am Rev Respir Dis* 1993; **147**: 301–6.

28 Turato G, Di Stefano A, Maestrelli P, Mapp CE, Ruggieri MP, Roggeri A *et al.* Effect of smoking cessation on airway inflammation in chronic bronchitis. *Am J Respir Crit Care Med* 1995; **152**: 1262–7.

29 Saetta M, Mariani M, Panina-Bordignon P, Turato G, Buonsanti C, Baraldo S *et al.* Increased expression of the chemokine receptor CXCR3 and its ligand CXCL10 in peripheral airways of smokers with chronic obstructive pulmonary disease. *Am J Respir Crit Care Med* 2002; **165**: 1404–9.

30 Petty TL, Silvers GW, Stanford RE. Mild emphysema is associated with reduced elastic recoil and increased lung size but not with air-flow limitation. *Am Rev Respir Dis* 1987; **136**: 867–71.

31 Mead J, Turner JM, Macklem PT, Little JB. Significance of the relationship between lung recoil and maximum expiratory flow. *J Appl Physiol* 1967; **22**: 95–108.

32 Matsuba K, Thurlbeck WM. The number and dimensions of small airways in emphysematous lungs. *Am J Pathol* 1972; **67**: 265–75.

33 Hogg JC, Macklem PT, Thurlbeck WM. Site and nature of airway obstruction in chronic obstructive lung disease. *N Engl J Med* 1968; **278**: 1355–60.

34 Barbee RA, Halonen M, Kaltenborn WT, Burrows B. A longitudinal study of respiratory symptoms in a community population sample. Correlations with smoking, allergen skin-test reactivity, and serum IgE. *Chest* 1991; **99**: 20–6.

35 Cullinan P. Persistent cough and sputum: prevalence and clinical characteristics in south east England. *Respir Med* 1992; **86**: 143–9.

36 Burrows B, Earle RH. Course and prognosis of chronic obstructive lung disease. A prospective study of 200 patients. *N Engl J Med* 1969; **280**: 397–404.

37 Doherty MJ, Mister R, Pearson MG, Calverley PM. Capsaicin responsiveness and cough in asthma and chronic obstructive pulmonary disease. *Thorax* 2000; **55**: 643–9.

38 Power JT, Stewart IC, Connaughton JJ, Brash HM, Shapiro CM, Flenley DC *et al.* Nocturnal cough in patients with chronic bronchitis and emphysema. *Am Rev Respir Dis* 1984; **130**: 999–1001.

39 Hsu J-Y, Stone RA, Logan-Sinclair R, Worsdell M, Busst C, Chung KF. Coughing frequency in patients with persistent cough using a 24-hour ambulatory recorder. *Eur Resp J* 1994; **7**: 1246–53.

40 Anthonisen NR, Manfreda J, Warren CP, Hershfield ES, Harding GK, Nelson NA. Antibiotic therapy in exacerbations of chronic obstructive pulmonary disease. *Ann Intern Med* 1987; **106**: 196–204.

41 Choudry NB, Fuller RW. Sensitivity of the cough reflex in patients with chronic cough. *Eur Respir J* 1992; **5**: 296–300.

42 Doherty MJ, Mister R, Pearson MG, Calverley PM. Capsaicin induced cough in cryptogenic fibrosing alveolitis. *Thorax* 2000; **55**: 1028–32.

43 Bergren DR. Enhanced lung C-fiber responsiveness in sensitized adult guinea pigs exposed to chronic tobacco smoke. *J Appl Physiol* 2001; **91**: 1645–54.

44 Bergren DR. Chronic tobacco smoke exposure increases cough to capsaicin in awake guinea pigs. *Respir Physiol* 2001; **126**: 127–40.

45 Carr MJ, Hunter DD, Undem BJ. Neurotrophins and asthma. *Curr Opin Pulm Med* 2001; **7**: 1–7.

46 Tomaki M, Ichinose M, Miura M, Hirayama Y, Yamauchi

H, Nakajima N *et al*. Elevated substance P content in induced sputum from patients with asthma and patients with chronic bronchitis. *Am J Respir Crit Care Med* 1995; 151: 613–7.

47 Canning BJ. Interactions between vagal afferent nerve subtypes mediating cough. *Pulm Pharmacol Ther* 2002; 15: 187–92.

48 Vestbo J, Prescott E, Lange P. Association of chronic mucus hypersecretion with FEV1 decline and chronic obstructive pulmonary disease morbidity. Copenhagen City Heart Study Group. *Am J Respir Crit Care Med* 1996; 153: 1530–5.

49 Aikawa T, Shimura S, Sasaki H, Takishima T, Yaegashi H, Takahashi T. Morphometric analysis of intraluminal mucus in airways in chronic obstructive pulmonary disease. *Am Rev Respir Dis* 1989; 140: 477–82.

50 O'Brien C, Guest PJ, Hill SL, Stockley RA. Physiological and radiological characterisation of patients diagnosed with chronic obstructive pulmonary disease in primary care. *Thorax* 2000; 55: 635–42.

51 Camner P, Mossberg B, Philipson K. Tracheobronchial clearance and chronic obstructive lung disease. *Scand J Respir Dis* 1973; 54: 272–81.

52 Wanner A. Clinical aspects of mucociliary transport. *Am Rev Respir Dis* 1977; 116: 73–125.

53 Smaldone GC, Foster WM, O'Riordan TG, Messina MS, Perry RJ, Langenback EG. Regional impairment of mucociliary clearance in chronic obstructive pulmonary disease. *Chest* 1993; 103: 1390–6.

54 Foster WM, Langenback EG, Bergofsky EH. Disassociation in the mucociliary function of central and peripheral airways of asymptomatic smokers. *Am Rev Respir Dis* 1985; 132: 633–9.

55 Rose MC, Gendler SJ. Airway mucin genes and gene products. In: Rogers DF, Lethem MI, eds. *Airway Mucus: Basic Mechanisms and Clinical Perspectives*. Boston, MA: Birkhauser-Verlag, 1997: 41–66.

56 Hovenberg HW, Davies JR, Carlstedt I. Different mucins are produced by the surface epithelium and the submucosa in human trachea: identification of MUC5AC as a major mucin from the goblet cells. *Biochem J* 1996; 318 (1): 319–24.

57 Steiger D, Fahy J, Boushey H, Finkbeiner WE, Basbaum C. Use of mucin antibodies and cDNA probes to quantify hypersecretion in vivo in human airways. *Am J Respir Cell Mol Biol* 1994; 10: 538–45.

58 Kuo HP, Rohde JAL, Barnes PJ, Rogers DF. Cigarette smoke-induced airway goblet cell secretion: dose dependent differential nerve activation. *Am J Physiol* 1992; L161–L167.

59 Rogers DF, Aursudkij B, Barnes PJ. Effect of tachykinins on mucus secretion on human bronchi in vitro. *Eur J Pharmacol* 1989; 174: 283–6.

60 Borchers MT, Wert SE, Leikauf GD. Acrolein-induced MUC5ac expression in rat airways. *Am J Physiol* 1998; 274: L573–L581.

61 Voynow JA, Young LR, Wang Y, Horger T, Rose MC, Fischer BM. Neutrophil elastase increases MUC5AC mRNA and protein expression in respiratory epithelial cells. *Am J Physiol* 1999; 276: L835–L843.

62 Takeyama K, Dabbagh K, Jeong SJ, Dao-Pick T, Ueki IF, Nadel JA. Oxidative stress causes mucin synthesis via transactivation of epidermal growth factor receptor: role of neutrophils. *J Immunol* 2000; 164: 1546–52.

63 Barsky SH, Roth MD, Kleerup EC, Simmons M, Tashkin DP. Histopathologic and molecular alterations in bronchial epithelium in habitual smokers of marijuana, cocaine, and/or tobacco. *J Natl Cancer Inst* 1998; 90: 1198–205.

64 Anthonisen NR, Connett JE, Kiley JP, Altose MD, Bailey WC, Buist AS *et al*. Effects of smoking intervention and the use of an inhaled anticholinergic bronchodilator on the rate of decline of FEV1. The Lung Health Study. *JAMA* 1994; 272: 1497–505.

65 Jorenby DE, Leischow SJ, Nides MA, Rennard SI, Johnston JA, Hughes AR *et al*. A controlled trial of sustained-release bupropion, a nicotine patch, or both for smoking cessation. *N Engl J Med* 1999; 340: 685–91.

66 Wynder EL, Kaufman PL, Lesser RL. A short-term follow-up study on ex-cigarette smokers. With special emphasis on persistent cough and weight gain. *Am Rev Respir Dis* 1967; 96: 645–55.

67 Jones PW, Bosh TK. Quality of life changes in COPD patients treated with salmeterol. *Am J Respir Crit Care Med* 1997; 155: 1283–9.

68 Dahl R, Greefhorst LA, Nowak D, Nonikov V, Byrne AM, Thomson MH *et al*. Inhaled formoterol dry powder versus ipratropium bromide in chronic obstructive pulmonary disease. *Am J Respir Crit Care Med* 2001; 164: 778–84.

69 Vincken W, van Noord JA, Greefhorst AP, Bantje TA, Kesten S, Korducki L *et al*. Improved health outcomes in patients with COPD during 1 year's treatment with tiotropium. *Eur Respir J* 2002; 19: 209–16.

70 Boyd G, Morice AH, Pounsford JC, Siebert M, Peslis N, Crawford C. An evaluation of salmeterol in the treatment of chronic obstructive pulmonary disease (COPD). *Eur Respir J* 1997; 10: 815–21.

71 Vestbo J, Sorensen T, Lange P, Brix A, Torre P, Viskum K. Long-term effect of inhaled budesonide in mild and moderate chronic obstructive pulmonary disease: a randomised controlled trial. *Lancet* 1999; 353: 1819–23.

72 Burge PS, Calverley PM, Jones PW, Spencer S, Anderson JA, Maslen TK. Randomised, double blind, placebo controlled study of fluticasone propionate in patients with moderate to severe chronic obstructive pulmonary

disease: the ISOLDE trial. *Br Med J* 2000; **320**: 1297–303.

73 Pauwels RA, Lofdahl CG, Laitinen LA, Schouten JP, Postma DS, Pride NB. Long-term treatment with inhaled budesonide in persons with mild chronic obstructive pulmonary disease who continue smoking. European Respiratory Society Study on Chronic Obstructive Pulmonary Disease. *N Engl J Med* 1999; **340**: 1948–53.

74 Culpitt SV, Maziak W, Loukidis S, Nightingale JA, Matthews JL, Barnes PJ. Effect of high dose inhaled steroid on cells, cytokines, and proteases in induced sputum in chronic obstructive pulmonary disease. *Am J Respir Crit Care Med* 1999; **160**: 1635–9.

75 Calverley PMA, Pauwels RA, Vestbo J, Jones PW, Pride NB, Gulsvik A, Anderson J, Maden C. Combined salmeterol and fluticasone in the treatment of chronic obstructive pulmonary disease: a randomised controlled trial. *Lancet* 2003; **361**: 449–56.

76 Laitinen LA, Laitinen A, Haahtela T. A comparative study of the effects of an inhaled corticosteroid, budesonide, and a beta 2-agonist, terbutaline, on airway inflammation in newly diagnosed asthma: a randomized, double-blind, parallel-group controlled trial. *J Allergy Clin Immunol* 1992; **90**: 32–42.

77 Fahy JV, Boushey HA. Effect of low-dose beclomethasone dipropionate on asthma control and airway inflammation. *Eur Respir J* 1998; **11**: 1240–7.

78 Groneberg DA, Eynott PR, Lim S, Oates T, Wu R, Carlstedt I *et al.* Expression of respiratory mucins in fatal status asthmaticus and mild asthma. *Histopathology* 2002; **40**: 367–73.

79 Boman G, Backer U, Larsson S, Melander B, Wahlander L. Oral acetylcysteine reduces exacerbation rate in chronic bronchitis: report of a trial organized by the Swedish Society for Pulmonary Diseases. *Eur J Respir Dis* 1983; **64**: 405–15.

# 14 Cough in suppurative airway diseases

*Robert Wilson*

## Introduction

Airway suppurative diseases are characterized by production of purulent sputum containing large numbers of bacteria and neutrophils. They usually occur because the local host defences are in some way deficient, permitting inhaled bacteria to persist and multiply. Neutrophils are attracted into the airway lumen by the products of bacteria themselves and also by mediators released from host cells, e.g. interleukin-8 (IL-8), C5a and leukotriene $B_4$ ($LTB_4$). Serum levels of the adhesion molecules E-selectin, ICAM-1 and VCAM-1 are elevated, suggesting that endothelial activation occurs, probably within the lung [1]. The failure of the inflammatory response to eradicate the infection once it is established is due partly to the impaired defences but also to the number of bacteria present and their pathogenic determinants [2]. Chronic neutrophilic inflammation has the potential to cause tissue damage via spillage of proteolytic enzymes such as elastase and reactive oxygen species. Immune complexes are formed between antibodies that are produced locally and those arriving via transudation, and bacterial antigens. These stimulate other inflammatory processes. Infection and inflammation may spread to involve adjacent areas of normal bystander lung. The lung defences are further weakened by the tissue damage caused by inflammation, and this in turn promotes continued infection, which perpetuates the inflammatory response. Epithelial cells, lymphocytes and macrophages release cytokines and other factors which orchestrate this sequence of events which has been termed 'a vicious circle' (Fig. 14.1).

Bronchiectasis results from loss of structural proteins such as elastin from the bronchial wall, and the muscle and cartilage layers also show signs of damage. These changes lead to abnormal chronic dilatation of the affected bronchi. Copious secretions produced by increased numbers of goblet cells and hypertrophic submucosal glands partially obstruct the airway lumen. Mucus is poorly cleared from the bronchiectatic airways for several reasons: there is pooling of excess secretions in the abnormal dilated airways; ciliated cells are lost when the epithelium is damaged; and the mucus is less elastic and more viscous making it difficult to clear by ciliary beat or cough. Side branches of the tortuous airways are frequently obliterated, and there may be complete fibrosis of small airways. There may be peribronchial pneumonic changes with evidence of parenchymal damage. Lymphocytes predominate in the bronchial wall, which contains lymphoid follicles and nodes, whereas neutrophils are abundant in the lumen. As well as B lymphocytes, plasma cells and CD4+ T lymphocytes in the follicles, there is a well-developed cell-mediated immune response, with increased numbers of activated T lymphocytes, mainly of the suppressor/cytotoxic CD8+ phenotype, antigen processing cells and mature macrophages [3].

What is often difficult to establish is the starting point of the pathological processes described above. Bronchiectasis can occur as a result of an acute insult which damages the bronchial wall, e.g. inhalation of a toxic gas, or following a serious infection, e.g. tuberculosis or whooping cough. In other cases, there may be a recognized deficiency in the local host defences, e.g. primary ciliary dyskinesia or cystic fibrosis; or there may be a deficiency of the systemic host defences, e.g.

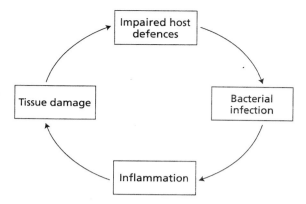

**Fig. 14.1** A vicious circle of events which begins because impaired host defences predispose the airway to bacterial infection. Persistent infection provokes chronic inflammation which damages lung tissue and further impairs host defences promoting continued infection.

hypogammaglobulinaemia, and in these cases damage is caused by repeated pneumonias. However, in many cases the origin of the bronchiectasis is much less clear. There may be a history of childhood pneumonia, but the significance of this when the patient presents in adult life with widespread bronchiectasis is uncertain. A history of wheezy bronchitis in childhood is also common. In some patients a particularly bad viral-like illness occurs at the onset of their problems, and the resultant cough and sputum never resolve. Persistent viral infection might in some way alter the host defences causing permissive conditions for what follows [4].

Patients with smoking-related chronic obstructive pulmonary disease (COPD) are prone to exacerbations caused by bacterial infection, sometimes preceded by a viral illness which impairs the airway defences by destroying ciliated cells and altering mucus rheology. A proportion of patients, about one-third in several studies, have lower airway bacterial colonization in the stable state which can be associated with chronic neutrophilic airway inflammation [5]. One community-based study has suggested that the prevalence of bronchiectasis in this population is much higher than had previously been recognized [6], and was present in 29% of patients. This is also suggested by the occurrence of *Pseudomonas aeruginosa* as a significant pathogen in COPD patients with severe airflow obstruction [7]. Therefore various aspects of the management of cough in suppurative airway diseases may have wider application in some COPD patients.

## Cough in bronchiectasis

Cough in bronchiectasis may be contributed by several factors, of which the continuous presence of sputum and airway secretions, often containing bacteria, is likely to be the most important. Excessive production of mucus and damage to mucociliary clearance mechanisms both contribute to mucus stasis in damaged airways of bronchiectasis. The induction of cough itself is a powerful additional mechanism for clearing mucus from the lungs. This cough clearance is independent of the action of cilia, but cough efficiency is dependent on the volume of liquid on the airway surface and the viscosity of the intraluminal material [8]. Although patients with primary ciliary dyskinesia have abnormalities in ciliary structure that leads to absent or slow ciliary beating and defective mucociliary clearance [9], their cough clearance is well preserved [10] and mucus clearance is entirely achieved by repetitive coughing. This illustrates the important therapeutic role of coughing (e.g. when performing physiotherapy) in conditions associated with bronchiectasis. The importance of cough as a clearing mechanism in bronchiectasis is also emphasized by a group of patients in whom cough suppression had an adverse effect on their clinical condition [11]. In cystic fibrosis, it has been hypothesized that the reduction of periciliary liquid surface is associated with both an inefficiency of mucociliary and of cough clearance, and perhaps results in a more severe disease phenotype when compared to primary ciliary dyskinesia [12]. One possibility is that this loss of periciliary liquid fluid may cause increased attachment between certain mucin components, to cause bonding between mucus and the epithelial surface.

## Capsaicin cough reflex

In a small group of bronchiectatic patients, the cough response to inhaled capsaicin was found to be comparable to that of normal subjects, but the severity of the bronchiectasis was not specified [13]. There may be several reasons why there could be an enhanced cough reflex in patients with more severe bronchiectasis. First, the presence of severe neutrophilic bronchial inflammation and damage may be expected to stimulate cough receptors. Second, the occurrence of concomitant diseases such a rhinosinusitis and gastrooesophageal reflux may contribute to or exacerbate cough. These associated conditions, of course, need to be treated specifically.

## Clinical features

The most common symptoms are cough and sputum production. Patients suffer from recurrent bronchial infections or may have chronic infection causing regular production of purulent sputum that can total several hundred millilitres in a day. Although most often an exacerbation is associated with increased purulent sputum production, sometimes the volume decreases because it becomes more sticky and difficult to expectorate. High temperature is unusual and may indicate an acute viral infection or pneumonia if it occurs. Chronic rhinosinusitis is very common. There is a positive correlation between the severity of airflow obstruction present and the severity of bronchiectasis [14]. There may be some reversibility indicating an asthmatic component, but most of the obstruction is usually fixed. Over half of patients have airway hyperresponsiveness to methacholine [15].

Chest pains and discomfort are common and increase during exacerbations. Joint pains also occur. Haemoptysis when present is usually small. Undue tiredness and difficulty concentrating usually reflects poorly controlled disease. Symptoms of anxiety and/or depression may be present as in any chronic illness. We have found that depression correlates with severity of disease, but the level of anxiety may be much higher than is appropriate. This is important to recognize, because it may not improve with treatment of the lung disease, and would therefore need to be dealt with separately [16]. Exercise tolerance, the frequency of exacerbations, requirement for hospital admission and the presence or absence of *P. aeruginosa* infection are the best predictors of quality of life in bronchiectasis [17,18].

There may be coarse inspiratory crackles heard over the site of bronchiectasis, but sometimes there are no signs in the lung to suggest the diagnosis. Wheezes and squeaks may be heard due to obstructed airways. Clubbing is quite unusual nowadays, because severe cases

with cystic bronchiectasis are seen infrequently. Weight should always be recorded because it often falls during a spell of poor control. Patients' description of their sputum colour and volume is often inaccurate and a 24-h sputum collection is very informative. Mucus plugs that form a cast of the airway may indicate allergic bronchopulmonary aspergillosis (ABPA).

The prevalence of severe cystic bronchiectasis has decreased because of the introduction of vaccination against childhood infections, improved socioeconomic conditions and the availability of antibiotics, but in parts of the world where social conditions are poor and health care less available bronchiectasis remains a much more common cause of morbidity and mortality. The availability of high-resolution computed tomography has increased the recognition of milder forms of disease. This cylindrical or tubular form has been termed 'modern' bronchiectasis [19]. The disease is usually bilateral and may be diffuse, although the lower lobes are usually worst affected. Progression of disease may be bimodal, with most patients stable or declining slowly, whereas a smaller number progress more rapidly for reasons that may not be clear. It is important to identify those patients that are deteriorating in order that treatment can be given in an attempt to halt the decline.

## Investigations

Suspicion of the presence of bronchiectasis should lead to investigation of possible causes (Table 14.1) and associated conditions (Table 14.2). The protocol of investigations performed in our unit is given in Table 14.3. In a study of 150 patients, Pasteur *et al.* [20] found that similar intensive investigation influenced management in 44 instances: 12 had immunological defects, 11 ABPA, 6 aspiration or reflux, 5 Young's syndrome, 4 cystic fibrosis, 3 primary ciliary dyskinesia, 2 ulcerative colitis and 1 diffuse panbronchiolitis. Younger patients, those with associated conditions, e.g. infertility, and those in whom respiratory function is deteriorating and/or infective exacerbations are becoming more frequent or prolonged should be seen by a respiratory physician with a special interest in bronchiectasis who has access to all of the investigations listed.

A chest radiograph is a relatively insensitive test for bronchiectasis. In one study less than 50% of patients who subsequently had positive bronchography

**Table 14.1** Causes of bronchiectasis.

---

*Congenital*, e.g. defective bronchial wall, pulmonary sequestration

*Postinfective*, e.g. tuberculosis, whooping cough, non-tuberculous mycobacteria especially *Mycobacterium avium* complex

*Mechanical obstruction* within lumen (e.g. tumour or foreign body) or external compression (e.g. lymph node), bronchial stenosis

*Deficient immune response*, e.g. common variable hypogammaglobulinaemia, disorders of phagocyte function, human immunodeficiency virus

*Inflammatory pneumonitis*, e.g. aspiration of gastric contents, inhalation of toxic gases

*Excessive immune response*, e.g. allergic bronchopulmonary aspergillosis, lung transplant rejection, chronic graft vs. host disease

*Abnormal mucociliary clearance*, e.g. primary ciliary dyskinesia, cystic fibrosis*, Young's syndrome

*Fibrosis*, e.g. cryptogenic fibrosing alveolitis, sarcoidosis, radiation pneumonitis

---

*Note: Delayed mucociliary clearance in cystic fibrosis may be part of the primary defect or could be secondary to infection. Other mechanisms are likely to cause bacterial infection in cystic fibrosis, e.g. altered bacterial adherence to airway epithelium or defective bacterial killing by defensins due to high sodium content of airway fluids.

**Table 14.2** Conditions associated with bronchiectasis.

---

*Infertility*, e.g. primary ciliary dyskinesia, cystic fibrosis, Young's syndrome

*Inflammatory bowel disease*, e.g. ulcerative colitis, Crohn's disease, coeliac disease

*Connective tissue disorders*, e.g. rheumatoid arthritis, systemic lupus erythematosus, Sjögren's syndrome

*Malignancy*, e.g. acute or chronic lymphatic leukaemia

*Diffuse panbronchiolitis*. Predominantly seen in Japanese

*Yellow nail syndrome*. Discoloured (usually yellow) nails, lymphoedema and pleural effusions

$\alpha_1$-*Antiproteinase deficiency*. More commonly causes emphysema

*Mercury poisoning*. May cause Young's syndrome (obstructive azospermia, sinusitis and bronchiectasis)

---

were detected [21]. High-resolution thin-section (1–2 mm) computed tomography scans, performed with a fast scan time (1 s or less) to reduce artefacts from respiratory motion and cardiac pulsation, have replaced bronchography in establishing the diagnosis and assessing the extent of the disease. The whole of the lung should be examined with 10 mm intersection spacing. Characteristic findings are illustrated in Fig. 14.2. Although certain features may suggest a cause of bronchiectasis, e.g. cystic fibrosis (upper lobe disease), ABPA (proximal disease), non-tuberculous mycobacteria (mild disease with peripheral nodules that may be cavitating) or diffuse panbronchiolitis (widespread small nodules), they do not usually allow a confident diagnosis [22].

Lung function tests provide a measure of functional impairment and an assessment of change with time. Airflow obstruction, which is largely fixed, and gas trapping are very common. Gas transfer values that

have been adjusted for alveolar volume are usually well preserved unless the disease is severe. Antibody deficiency is a relatively common cause of bronchiectasis. Immunoglobulin G subclass deficiency by itself is not a cause of susceptibility to infection. Specific antibody levels should be measured, and if these are low the ability to respond appropriately to vaccination with polysaccharide (pneumococcal and *Haemophilus influenzae* type b) and protein (tetanus) antigens should be tested. All cases of immune deficiency may be secondary to malignancy, particularly of the lymphoreticular system, so a high index of suspicion must be maintained.

Sputum should be examined by microscopy as well as culture for respiratory pathogens including fungi and mycobacteria, since eosinophils may cause purulence, and their presence may indicate asthma and/or ABPA. *H. influenzae*, *H. parainfluenzae* and *Pseudomonas aeruginosa* (which develops a mucoid

**Table 14.3** Investigation of bronchiectasis.

*All patients*
Chest radiograph (PA and lateral)
Sinus radiographs
High-resolution thin-section computed tomography scan
Respiratory function tests
Blood investigations*
Sputum microscopy including eosinophils
Sputum culture and sensitivities
Sputum smear and culture for acid-fast bacilli
Skin tests (atopy, *Aspergillus*)
Sweat test (nasal potential difference, genotyping)
Nasal mucociliary clearance and exhaled nasal nitric oxide
Proceed to cilia studies if these tests are abnormal

*Selected patients*
Fibreoptic bronchoscopy
Barium swallow (video fluoroscopy)
Respiratory muscle function
Semen analysis
Tests for associated conditions
Blood tests for rarer immune deficiencies

*To include: differential white cell count; erythrocyte sedimentation rate and C-reactive protein; total immunoglobulin (Ig) levels of IgG, IgM, IgA, IgE and IgG subclasses; specific antibodies; protein electrophoretic strip; *Aspergillus* radioallergosorbent test and precipitins; rheumatoid factor and antinuclear antibodies; $\alpha_1$-antiproteinase.

phenotype after chronic infection) are the species identified most frequently.

The saccharin test can be used as a simple screening test to determine if there is a mucociliary clearance problem [23]. We use exhaled nasal nitric oxide, which is very low in patients with primary ciliary dyskinesia, as another screening test. When a ciliary problem is suspected a sample of epithelium is taken from the inferior turbinate of the nostril using a cytology brush. The ciliary beat frequency and the pattern of ciliary beating are assessed under light microscopy, and the rest of the sample is processed for electron microscopy and study of ultrastructure [24].

## Specific causes of bronchiectasis

We remain ignorant of many of the underlying causes of bronchiectasis, and about half of cases are still con-

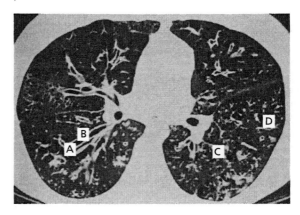

**Fig. 14.2** High-resolution thin-section computed tomography scan of a patient with bronchiectasis. Several characteristic features are demonstrated: a non-tapering bronchus (A); airway wall thickening (B); the signet ring sign in which the airway is larger than the accompanying pulmonary artery (C); mucus filled bronchi which appear as branching tubes or nodules (D).

sidered idiopathic. Some of the more important causes are briefly described in this section. Microorganisms causing severe lung infections that are particularly associated with subsequent bronchiectasis are *Mycobacterium tuberculosis*, *M. avium* complex, *Bordetella pertussis*, measles virus and adenovirus. A history of chronic cough and sputum production follows the severe illness. Localized bronchiectasis may occur due to infection occurring distal to a bronchial obstruction from any cause, and this can either be in the lumen or due to compression from outside. Acquired common variable hypogammaglobulinaemia is the most common immunological deficiency discovered in adults [25]. ABPA is caused by an immune reaction to *Aspergillus fumigatus* fungus colonizing the airway involving eosinophils. Atelectasis occurs due to obstruction by plugs of inspissated secretions containing fungal hyphae. Acute episodes of fever, wheeze, expectoration of viscid sputum plugs and pleuritic pain, sometimes associated with fleeting shadows on the chest radiograph, merge insidiously over time as bronchiectasis develops into chronic purulent sputum production where exacerbations of ABPA are difficult to distinguish from infective exacerbations of bronchiectasis.

Three different forms of impaired mucociliary clearance result in chronic bacterial infection and bronchiectasis. Cystic fibrosis is caused by a recessive mutation of a gene on the long arm of chromosome 7, which codes for CFTR (cystic fibrosis transmembrane conductance regulator), a cyclic AMP-dependent chloride channel, which has wide-ranging effects in addition to mucociliary clearance. Childhood infections with *Staphylococcus aureus* and non-typeable *H. influenzae* progress inexorably to severe bronchiectasis and chronic *P. aeruginosa* infection and death in early adult life due to respiratory failure. Primary ciliary dyskinesia is rare and is thought to be an autosomal recessive condition with incomplete penetrance. Ultrastructural abnormalities in the cilia cause them to be immotile or move in a slow disorganized fashion. About half of patients have dextrocardia, and a smaller percentage full situs inversus. They may present in the neonatal period with segmental collapse due to mucus impaction. Cough is incessant, as it is the only way the patient has to clear mucus. Diffuse bronchiectasis is associated with chronic sinusitis, middle ear disease and often, but not invariably, in men infertility due to immotile sperm. Young's syndrome is a combination of bronchiectasis, chronic sinusitis and azoospermia due to functional blockage of sperm in the caput epididymis. The condition has been linked to mercury positioning, the incidence of which has fallen since mercurous chloride was removed from teething powders and worm medication in the UK.

## Non-antibiotic treatment

Poor clearance of mucus from bronchiectatic airways is probably the fundamental reason that patients become infected. Therefore physiotherapy exercises to clear secretions are a critical aspect of management. Patients are advised to perform postural drainage at least once daily, and increase the frequency to twice or three times daily if they suffer an exacerbation. Patients should be taught by a trained physiotherapist to adopt the correct position to drain affected areas, and clear mucus by controlled breathing techniques, sometimes aided by chest clapping by the patient or partner. About 10 min in any one productive position is required. Understandably compliance with physiotherapy is poor, because of the nature of the process and the time involved, so medical staff should regularly remind the patient of its importance. Physical exercise should also be encouraged.

Any asthmatic component of bronchiectasis should be treated in the usual way. Systemic corticosteroids have unacceptable side-effects when used long-term to reduce airway inflammation, although they are used for short periods during severe exacerbations; however, in some patients systemic corticosteroids are required. Treatment of ABPA with high-dose inhaled corticosteroids may prevent exacerbations. The antifungal antibiotic itraconazole may act as a steroid sparing agent [26]. Inhaled corticosteroids are commonly given to bronchiectasis patients in an attempt to reduce airway inflammation and relieve airflow obstruction [27]. However, there is little evidence that this is beneficial, and an objective assessment of symptoms and lung function tests should be made after their introduction.

Acid reflux and rhinosinusitis should be treated if present. Influenza (annual) and pneumococcal vaccination should be encouraged. Nebulized saline may be given in an attempt to promote cough clearance by liquefying secretions. Nebulized recombinant human DNase gives some benefit to cystic fibrosis patients in this way, but not in other forms of bronchiectasis, and other mucolytic agents have no proven benefit. Patients with chronic respiratory failure due to bronchiectasis are managed in the usual way. Nasal intermittent positive pressure ventilation is often surprisingly well tolerated despite sinusitis and excess bronchial secretions [28].

The only curative treatment of bronchiectasis is surgical resection. Cylindrical bronchiectasis is usually bilateral and surgery is rarely considered for this reason. Palliative surgical resection may be considered if a localized area of severe bronchiectasis defies medical management and acts as a sump for infection, even if less severe bronchiectasis is present elsewhere. Emergency surgical resection may be necessary for life-threatening haemoptysis, but embolization of the appropriate bronchial artery is usually attempted first. Lung transplantation (usually two lungs or heart–lung otherwise infection in the remaining lung may spread to the new organ) has been used to treat end-stage respiratory failure due to bronchiectasis.

## Antibiotic management

When bronchiectasis is mild to moderate, antibiotics can reduce the bacterial numbers in the airway to low levels leading to resolution of the symptoms of the exacerbation. The lung defences are then able to control bacterial numbers at levels which do not attract an overt inflammatory response. The next exacerbation occurs either when a new bacterial infection occurs or when an event, such as a viral infection, impairs the host defences, so that bacterial numbers can increase. When lung damage is more severe, the bronchial tree is usually chronically infected and the patient's symptoms may return soon after stopping the antibiotic. In these different circumstances, antibiotics may be needed only during an infective exacerbation when there is a change in sputum production, breathlessness and malaise, or at the other end of the spectrum continuously if relapse following antibiotic treatment is rapid.

The choice of antibiotic is influenced by the high frequency of β-lactamase production by strains of *H. influenzae* and *Moraxella catarrhalis*, isolated from bronchiectasis patients who have taken frequent antibiotic courses in the past, and the presence or absence of *P. aeruginosa* which is resistant to most oral antibiotics. Co-amoxyclavulanate and ciprofloxacin are our first-line choices. If patients are severely unwell at presentation and/or are infected by resistant strains, intravenous antibiotics are used. Ceftriaxone (non-*Pseudomonas* patients) and ceftazidime plus an aminoglycoside (*Pseudomonas* patients) are our first-line antibiotics in these circumstances, with piperacillin-tazobactam and meropenem second line. Intravenous antibiotics should be commenced in hospital where supportive treatment such as physiotherapy can also be given, but increasingly patients are being taught to administer their own injections, so that when they are improving their hospital stay can be shortened by finishing the course at home.

Patients with frequent exacerbations who relapse quickly following intravenous treatment may be considered for long-term prophylactic antibiotics. This decision should only be taken after careful consideration, and only after other aspects of management have been optimized. There are several concerns about this approach: development of antibiotic resistance in the strains already present, promotion of infection by more antibiotic-resistant species, e.g. *P. aeruginosa*, and side-effects of antibiotics, e.g. *Clostridium difficile* infection. Three different approaches to antibiotic prophylaxis have been used: oral antibiotics, which can either be with a single antibiotic, or a rotation of several antibiotics from different classes [29]; inhaled

antibiotics given as an isotonic solution via a nebulizer [30]; and regular pulsed courses of intravenous antibiotics [31]. Each approach has been shown to reduce exacerbation frequency, as well as having other benefits. In broad terms we use oral prophylaxis in patients not infected with *Pseudomonas*, nebulized antibiotics for patients with chronic *Pseudomonas* infection, and pulsed intravenous antibiotics for patients with the most severe disease in whom other forms of prophylaxis have failed.

Continuous treatment with macrolide antibiotics has been used effectively to treat diffuse panbronchiolitis, even when there is chronic bronchial infection involving *P. aeruginosa*. This condition was first described in Japan, where it seems to be much more common. There are unique radiological and histological features, but it bears some resemblance clinically to idiopathic bronchiectasis. The benefit of macrolides is unlikely to involve bacterial killing, although macrolides do influence *P. aeruginosa* virulence determinants; it is more likely that the anti-inflammatory properties of the macrolide class are responsible [32]. A recent study has shown promising results in cystic fibrosis, and further studies in bronchiectasis are under way [33].

## Treatment of cough in bronchiectasis

Because cough clearance is important in bronchiectasis, antitussive therapy is relatively contraindicated. If cough appears to be a debilitating symptom for the patient, then various treatment approaches directed at the airway may well reduce the burden of cough. This is illustrated by treatments for the infective exacerbations of bronchiectasis. Corticosteroid therapy may reduce cough by inhibiting the inflammatory process in bronchiectatic airways, and inhaled β-agonist bronchodilator therapy by reversing airway smooth muscle tone and by improving mucociliary clearance. However, evidence is lacking that either of these two approaches is beneficial in non-asthmatic patients [34]. Macrolide antibiotics have been shown to reduce sputum volume and to normalize mucus rheology in two small studies [35,36], to suppress secretion of respiratory glycoconjugates from human airway cells [37], and to reduce neutrophil accumulation and activation [38]. In the future, demonstration of sensitization of the cough reflex may be a justification to intensify anti-inflammatory and mucus inhibitory approaches.

## References

1 Zheng L, Tipoe G, Lam WK *et al.* Up-regulation of circulating adhesion molecules in bronchiectasis. *Eur Respir J* 2000; **16**: 691–6.

2 Wilson R, Dowling R, Jackson AD. The biology of bacterial colonization and invasion of the respiratory mucosa. *Eur Respir J* 1996; **9**: 1523–30.

3 Lapa e Silva JR, Jones JAH, Cole PJ, Poulter LW. The immunological component of the cellular inflammatory infiltrate in bronchiectasis. *Thorax* 1989; **44**: 668–73.

4 Elliot WM, Hayashi S, Hogg JC. Immunodetection of adenoviral EIA proteins in human tissue. *Am J Respir Cell Mol Biol* 1995; **12**: 642–8.

5 Wilson R. Bacterial infection and chronic obstructive pulmonary disease. *Eur Respir J* 1999; **13**: 233–5.

6 O'Brien C, Guest PJ, Hill SL *et al.* Physiological and radiological characterisation of patients diagnosed with chronic obstructive pulmonary disease in primary care. *Thorax* 2000; **55**: 635–42.

7 Miravitlles M, Espinosa C, Ferandez-Laso E *et al.* Relationship between bacterial flora in sputum and functional impairment in patients with acute exacerbations of COPD. *Chest* 1999; **116**: 40–6.

8 King M, Zahm JM, Pierrot D, Vaquez-Girod S, Puchelle E. The role of mucus gel viscosity, spinnability, and adhesive properties in clearance by simulated cough. *Biorheology* 1989; **26**: 737–45.

9 Camner P, Mossberg B, Afzelius BA. Measurements of tracheobronchial clearance in patients with immotile-cilia syndrome and its value in differential diagnosis. *Eur J Respir Dis Suppl* 1983; **127**: 57–63.

10 Noone PG, Bennett WD, Regnis JA, Zeman KL, Carson JL, King M *et al.* Effect of aerosolized uridine-5'-triphosphate on airway clearance with cough in patients with primary ciliary dyskinesia. *Am J Respir Crit Care Med* 1999; **160**: 144–9.

11 Wells A, Rahman A, Woodhead M, Pfeiffer J, Wilson R, Cole PJ. Voluntary cough suppression associated with chronic pulmonary suppuration: a new syndrome. *Eur Respir J* 1992; **5** (Suppl. 15): 141S.

12 Knowles MR, Boucher RC. Mucus clearance as a primary innate defense mechanism for mammalian airways. *J Clin Invest* 2002; **109**: 571–7.

13 Choudry NB, Fuller RW. Sensitivity of the cough reflex in patients with chronic cough. *Eur Respir J* 1992; **5**: 296–300.

14 Hansell DM. Imaging of obstructive pulmonary disease. Bronchiectasis. *Radiol Clin N Am* 1998; **36**: 107–28.

15 Bahous J, Cortier A, Pineau L *et al.* Pulmonary function tests and airway responsiveness to metacholine in chronic bronchiectasis of the adult. *Bull Eur Physiopathol Respir* 1984; **20**: 375–80.

16 O'Leary CJ, Wilson CB, Hansell DM, Cole PJ, Wilson R, Jones PW. Relationship between psychological well-being and lung health status in patients with bronchiectasis. *Respir Med* 2002; **96**: 686–92.

17 Wilson CB, Jones PW, O'Leary CJ *et al.* Health status assessment in bronchiectasis using the St George's Respiratory Questionnaire. *Am J Respir Crit Care Med* 1997; **156**: 536–41.

18 Wilson CB, Jones PW, O'Leary CJ *et al.* Effect of sputum bacteriology on the quality of life of patients with bronchiectasis. *Eur Respir J* 1998; **12**: 820–4.

19 Cole PJ. Bronchiectasis. In: Brewis RAL, Corrin B, Geddes DM, Gibson GJ, eds. *Respiratory Medicine*, 2nd edn. London: W.B. Saunders, 1995: 1286–317.

20 Pasteur MC, Helliwell SM, Houghton SJ *et al.* An investigation into causative factors in patients with bronchiectasis. *Am J Respir Crit Care Med* 2000; **162**: 1277–84.

21 Currie DC, Cooke JC, Morgan AD *et al.* Interpretation of bronchograms and chest radiographs in patients with chronic sputum production. *Thorax* 1987; **42**: 278.

22 Reiff DB, Wells AU, Carr DH *et al.* CT findings in bronchiectasis: limited value in distinguishing between idiopathic and specific types. *Am J Roentgenol* 1995; **165**: 261–7.

23 Stanley P, MacWilliam L, Greenstone M *et al.* Efficacy of a saccharin test for screening to detect abnormal mucociliary clearance. *Br J Dis Chest* 1984; **78**: 62–5.

24 Rutland J, Dewar A, Cox T, Cole PJ. Nasal brushing for the study of ultrastructure. *J Clin Pathol* 1982; **35**: 357–9.

25 Watts WJ, Watts MB, Dai W *et al.* Respiratory dysfunction in patients with common variable hypogammaglobulinaemia. *Am Rev Respir Dis* 1986; **134**: 699–703.

26 Stevens DA, Schwartz HJ, Lee JY *et al.* A randomised trial of itraconazole in allergic bronchopulmonary aspergillosis. *N Engl J Med* 2000; **342**: 756–62.

27 Tsang KWT, Ho PL, Lam WK *et al.* Inhaled fluticasone reduces sputum inflammatory indices in severe bronchiectasis. *Am J Respir Crit Care Med* 1998; **158**: 723–7.

28 Gacouin A, Desrues B, Lena H *et al.* Long-term nasal intermittent positive pressure ventilation (NIPPV) in sixteen consecutive patients with bronchiectasis: a retrospective study. *Eur Respir J* 1996; **9**: 1246–50.

29 Rayner CFJ, Tillotson G, Cole PJ, Wilson R. Efficacy and safety of long term ciprofloxacin in the management of severe bronchiectasis. *J Antimicrob Chemother* 1994; **34**: 149–56.

30 Mukopadhyay S, Singh M, Cater JL *et al.* Nebulised antipseudomonal antibiotic therapy in cystic fibrosis: a meta-analysis of benefits and risks. *Thorax* 1996; **51**: 364–8.

31 Szaff M, Holby N, Flensborg FW. Frequent antibiotic therapy improves survival of cystic fibrosis patients with chronic *Pseudomonas aeruginosa* infection. *Acta Paediatr Scand* 1983; **72**: 651–7.

32 Kudoh S, Uetake T, Hagiwara K *et al.* Clinical effects of low dose long-term erythromycin chemotherapy on diffuse panbronchiolitis. *Jpn J Thorac Dis* 1987; **25**: 632–42.

33 Wolter J, Seeney S, Bell S, Bowler S, Masel P, McCormack J. Effect of long term treatment with azithromycin on disease parameters in cystic fibrosis: a randomised trial. *Thorax* 2002; **57**: 212–6.

34 Elborn JS, Johnston B, Allen F, Clarke J, McGarry J, Varghese G. Inhaled steroids in patients with bronchiectasis. *Respir Med* 1992; **86**: 121–4.

35 Tamaoki J, Takeyama K, Tagaya E, Konno K. Effect of clarithromycin on sputum production and its rheological properties in chronic respiratory tract infections. *Antimicrob Agents Chemother* 1995; **39**: 1688–90.

36 Rubin BK, Druce H, Ramirez OE, Palmer R. Effect of clarithromycin on nasal mucus properties in healthy subjects and in patients with purulent rhinitis. *Am J Respir Crit Care Med* 1997; **155**: 2018–23.

37 Goswami SK, Kivity S, Marom Z. Erythromycin inhibits respiratory glycoconjugate secretion from human airways in vitro. *Am Rev Respir Dis* 1990; **141**: 72–8.

38 Culic O, Erakovic V, Parnham MJ. Anti-inflammatory effects of macrolide antibiotics. *Eur J Pharmacol* 2001; **429**: 209–29.

# 15 Cough in cancer patients

*Sam H. Ahmedzai & Nisar Ahmed*

## Prevalence and epidemiology

Cough is a normal basic mechanism for self-preservation, and is experienced by all people frequently and often subconsciously. In respiratory diseases, cough is sometimes necessary to expectorate excess mucus, but its frequency and severity may increase to the point that it impinges on normal daily activities. In the cancer patient, who is usually already burdened by several physical and psychological symptoms, cough can become a major source of distress.

The cancers that are most commonly associated with cough and other respiratory symptoms such as dyspnoea and haemoptysis are, naturally, those arising from the airways, lungs, pleura and other mediastinal structures. However, cancers from many other primary sites can metastasize to the thorax and produce the same symptoms. As discussed below, the various anticancer treatments given for all types of malignancy can themselves be a potent cause of cough, amongst many other side-effects. For these reasons, it is difficult to state the exact prevalence of cough in cancer patients, as this varies between different primary types, their stage and therapies used.

At presentation, cough is one of the commonest symptoms of lung cancer. Cumulative experience of 650 patients entering the UK Medical Research Centre's multicentre lung cancer trials shows that, overall, cough was the fourth commonest symptom reported at presentation [1]. The actual frequency of cough was 80% in small cell lung cancer (SCLC) and in 70% of non-small cell lung cancer (NSCLC). Male patients reported 7% more cough, and 12% more coughing up of blood (haemoptysis), than females. A survey of patients with a variety of other cancers attending a large US cancer hospital found that cough was a troublesome symptom for 22% of patients with colon cancer, 26% with prostate cancer, 28% with ovarian cancer and 37% with breast cancer [2]. The overall prevalence of cough was 29%.

Much of the literature on the palliation of cough in lung and other primary cancers focuses on the 'advanced' stages of disease. Usually this means that the cancer has failed to respond to first-line curative treatment and has progressed either locally or metastatically. The reporting of cough in these patients is therefore subject to bias from the impact of prior anticancer therapies as well as intercurrent respiratory infections that are increasingly common in patients with increasing frailty and reduced immunity. Another cause for lack of precision in stating the frequency of cough—as well as most other symptoms in cancer patients—is that standardized and validated measures, ideally rated by patients themselves, are not directly comparable. Indeed, in much of the older oncological literature, symptoms were evaluated by attending clinicians rather than the patients.

A standard quality of life (QoL) questionnaire commonly used in lung cancer studies is the European Organization for Research and Treatment of Cancer (EORTC) Lung Cancer 13-item Module (LC-13). Two international studies, conducted for the validation of this patient-rated instrument, which included 883 patients with inoperable NSCLC who were about to start palliative radiotherapy or chemotherapy, found that the prevalence of cough which was scored as 'quite a bit' or 'very much' was altogether 39% [3]. In contrast, combined data on a total of 673 patients from two US studies in advanced (stage III and IV) NSCLC which used another self-rated tool, the Lung Cancer Symptom Scale (LCSS), showed the baseline prevalence of cough overall to be much higher (86%) [4]. The difference probably arises because the EORTC study only reported those who reported the more severe grades of cough. This assumption is backed up by a later study using the LCSS, which confirmed that cough was the least severe of the self-reported symptoms [5].

Several surveys of patients referred to palliative care services have measured symptom prevalence on admission. One US teaching hospital study found cough to be present in 52% of 100 consecutively admitted patients [6]. Of this series, 59 had cancer, 22 AIDS and the rest a variety of terminal conditions. In contrast, a UK palliative care team investigating the problems presented by heart failure and cancer patients at referral found the former were more likely to report cough as a troublesome symptom (44% compared with 26%, respectively) [7].

Table 15.1 summarizes the evidence on the prevalence of cough in cancer and palliative care patients.

The prevalence of cough in children with cancer was assessed in an Australian study which used another self-rated instrument, the Memorial Symptom Assessment Scale [8]. In 160 children aged 10–18, cough fell into the group of symptoms experienced by >35% of the sample. However, it was not amongst the symptoms that the patients identified as causing severe distress.

Does the presence of cough have prognostic significance in cancer patients? A multivariate analysis of several factors concerning 260 patients with surgically resected stage I and II NSCLC did indeed show that median survival in patients with cough was 39 months, compared with 57 months for patients without cough ($P=0.04$) [9]. In a further analysis of this series, using the Cox proportional hazards model, cough was a significant predictor of shorter survival (present vs. absent, $P=0.01$) [10]. Furthermore, the presence of cough was a significant ($P=0.02$) predictor of disease-free survival. A Japanese study has also revealed that during the course of hospice care, cough frequency rose from 29% on admission to 48% nearer to death [11]. However, many other symptoms also deteriorated during the hospice stay, and the analysis did not reveal whether cough was an independent prognostic factor.

When is cough in cancer patients a new symptom of that disease? This is a relevant question, as most patients who present with lung cancer are smokers who may already have a chronic cough. A case-control study of Czech women with newly diagnosed lung cancer (140 cases, 280 matched controls) investigated this issue. It found that chronic cough and sputum (defined as occurring at least 3 months per year) was associated with an excess risk of lung cancer (odds ratio=6.07), but only if the cough was of less than 2 years in duration [12]. Thus it was argued that the cough associated with lung cancer patients, at least, was a new symptom resulting from preclinical changes arising from the malignancy. A further epidemiological study from Sweden which investigated 364 new cases of lung cancer supports this interpretation [13]. Only 7% of the patients

Table 15.1 Prevalence of cough in cancer and palliative care patients.

| Source | Primary site | Stage of disease | n | Cough (%) | Haemoptysis (%) | Dyspnoea (%) |
|---|---|---|---|---|---|---|
| [1] | SCLC | Advanced | 232 | 81 | 26 | 87 |
| [1] | NSCLC | Advanced | 423 | 87 | 36 | 86 |
| [3] | NSCLC | Inoperable | 833 | – | – | – |
| [4] | NSCLC | Advanced | 673 | 86 | 41 | 87 |
| [2] | Breast | Mixed | 70 | 37 | nr | 26 |
| [2] | Colon | Mixed | 60 | 22 | nr | 29 |
| [2] | Prostate | Mixed | 63 | 26 | nr | 25 |
| [2] | Ovary | Mixed | 50 | 29 | nr | 25 |
| [11] | Mixed | Terminal | 350 | 29–48* | nr | 33–66* |
| [7] | Mixed | Terminal | 213 | 26 | nr | 49 |

* First figure is at admission; second figure is near death.
SCLC, small cell lung cancer; NSCLC, non-small cell lung cancer; nr, not recorded.

were asymptomatic at diagnosis, and cough was the most common *first* symptom to be reported.

It is not altogether clear why cough should be such a sensitive indicator of a new lung cancer and may also signify a poorer outcome. One possible explanation comes from a study of the rheological properties of mucus taken by bilateral paired sampling in patients being bronchoscoped for a unilateral radiological abnormality [14]. Eight of the 20 patients studied were found to have lung cancer. Mucus from the side with the radiological abnormality had a lower value for the loss tangent tan d100 ($P=0.004$), indicating greater mucus recoil. This would be consistent with poor mucus clearability on the affected side. All of the eight cancer patients had a low tan d100 value ($P=0.007$), and two of those who were initially negative from bronchoscopy but had abnormal mucus values were later diagnosed with cancer on follow-up. These interesting findings need to be confirmed, but may have implications for therapeutic management as well as their diagnostic value.

## Causes and consequences of cough in cancer patients

The study by Zayas *et al.* [14] described above sheds light on one of the possible causes of cough as a troublesome symptom in cancer patients. If the presence of malignant change in the bronchial tree can induce changes which lead to mucus that is more difficult to clear and expectorate, then it is evident that the patient could complain of difficulty in coughing.

Several other causative and associated factors also need to be considered [15,16]. Table 15.2 gives a summary of the conditions which may initiate or provoke cough in cancer patients. Infection of the respiratory tract is naturally a major suspect, as is chronic obstructive pulmonary disease, since most patients with lung cancer, at least, have a longstanding smoking history. It is important to consider unusual pathogens, especially in immunocompromised patients. In one series of such patients, invasive pulmonary aspergillosis was accompanied by cough in 54% of cases, fever in 54%, haemoptysis in 30% and dyspnoea in 8% [17]. Since cancer in adults is a disease that is commoner in the middle-aged and elderly, it is important to consider comorbidity as a causative factor. Heart failure, the use of angiotensin-converting enzyme (ACE) inhibiting drugs

for cardiac disease, systemic inflammatory diseases and pulmonary thromboembolism should be excluded. The latter is particularly relevant in view of the increased blood coaguability associated with some cancers, and the insidious nature of recurrent thromboembolic episodes which may be individually subclinical.

Complications of lung cancer and sometimes other malignancies which give rise to increased coughing include pleural or pericardial effusion, superior vena cava obstruction, bronchopleural fistula and lymphangitis carcinomatosa. These are usually evident clinically or on routine chest radiographs or computed tomography (CT) scan, although lymphangitis may be difficult to diagnose in a patient with pre-existing pulmonary disease or heart failure.

Unfortunately, cough is a common consequence of many of the treatments which are used against cancer itself. Studies of long-term survivors of cancer have reported cough as one of the symptoms which both children and adults suffer long after the disease has been treated. The Childhood Cancer Survivor Study which investigated 12 390 ex-patients in the USA 5 years or more after their illness found that, compared with siblings, survivors had significantly increased relative risk of chronic cough as well as recurrent pneumonia, lung fibrosis, pleurisy and exercise-induced breathlessness [18]. Specifically, the study identified the association of chronic cough with prior chest radiation therapy ($RR = 2.0$, $P<0.001$); with bleomycin exposure ($RR=1.9$, $P<0.001$); and with cyclophosphamide therapy ($RR=1.3$, $P=0.004$). The propensity for these anticancer therapies to cause pulmonary damage has been known for a long time, although cyclophosphamide-induced lung damage is relatively rare [19].

A recent study in Sweden has investigated the relatively new approach of allogeneic haematopoietic stem cell transplantation (HSCT) in adult cancer patients [20]. Twenty-five patients who had received HSCT 2–4 years previously were surveyed using a variety of symptom and health-related QoL measures. More than half the patients reported cough, dry mouth and eye problems, as well as tiredness, sexual difficulties and anxiety. It should be noted that, in spite of these reported problems, 80% of the cancer survivors estimated their general health as 'quite good' or 'excellent'. In contrast, another Swedish follow-up study of 277 men who had been cured of testicular teratoma, compared with 392 controls, revealed that they reported significantly *less*

**Table 15.2** Conditions that may initiate or provoke cough in cancer patients.

| System | Site | Pathology/mechanism |
|---|---|---|
| Respiratory | Upper airways | Laryngeal tumour |
| | | Tracheal tumour |
| | | Iatrogenic, e.g. radiation tracheitis |
| | Bronchi | Lung cancer |
| | | Metastatic cancer |
| | | Infection |
| | | Chronic obstructive pulmonary disease |
| | Lung parenchyma | Infection |
| | | Lymphangitis carcinomatosa |
| | | Iatrogenic, e.g. pneumonitis and/or fibrosis after radiation, chemotherapy, biological therapies |
| | Pleura | Mesothelioma |
| | | Pleural effusion |
| Cardiovascular | Heart | Pericardial effusion |
| | | Pulmonary congestion |
| | | Pulmonary thromboembolism |
| | | Iatrogenic, e.g. angiotensin-converting enzyme inhibitor |
| Gastrointestinal | Oesophagus | Tracheo-oesophageal fistula |
| | | Reflux |

cough, as well as less backache, leg pains and eye problems than the controls [21].

Autologous peripheral blood stem cell transplantation which uses busulphan chemotherapy can also cause an acute or subacute idiopathic pneumonia syndrome (IPS) characterized by cough, hypoxaemia and pulmonary infiltrates, sometimes with pleural effusions. Although IPS only arose in 10 out of a series of 271 patients, it was fatal in eight of these [22]. A more insidious form of this condition has also been described as delayed pulmonary toxicity syndrome (DPTS), following the use of high-dose chemotherapy with cyclophosphamide/cisplatin/BCNU and autologous bone marrow transplantation [23].

Table 15.3 gives a summary of the common treatments used for cancer that have been shown to be associated with pulmonary damage, cough and dyspnoea. Many 'traditional' anticancer drugs can cause interstitial pneumonia, leading to pulmonary fibrosis. Among the newer agents that are being used for cancers of the breast and thorax are the taxanes. Six out of 30 NSCLC and mesothelioma patients who received paclitaxel with concurrent chest radiotherapy developed significant lung injury manifested by a persistent cough [24].

**Table 15.3** Common treatments used for cancer that have been shown to be associated with pulmonary damage, cough and dyspnoea.

| Type of therapy | Pathology |
|---|---|
| Radiation | Acute lymphocytic alveolitis |
| | Acute pneumonitis |
| | Bronchiolitis obliterans organizing pneumonia (BOOP) |
| | Late pulmonary fibrosis |
| Anticancer chemotherapy | Acute idiopathic pneumonia syndrome (IPS) |
| | Delayed pulmonary toxicity syndrome (DTPS) |
| | Interstitial pneumonitis |
| | Late pulmonary fibrosis |
| Biological therapies | Idiopathic cough — herceptin; interleukin |

Irinotecan is another new antineoplastic agent which is increasingly being used in the management of colorectal cancer. Cumulative evidence from clinical trials in Japan and the US suggests that up to 20% of patients may develop pulmonary toxicity, causing dyspnoea and cough. The drug initiates an interstitial pneumonitis that may not respond to corticosteroids and can be fatal [25]. It is claimed that patients with pre-existing lung disease may be at a higher risk of irinotecan pulmonary toxicity.

Amplification of the human epidermal growth factor receptor 2 protein (HER2) correlates with poor prognosis in breast cancer, and herceptin is a recombinant humanized monoclonal immunoglobulin antibody that binds to the HER2 receptor. It is being increasingly used in breast cancer trials. One of its commoner side-effects is cough, along with fever and chills, pain and tiredness [26]. Interleukin-2 (IL-2) is used as an anticancer agent for metastatic melanoma. One of its many dose-dependent side-effects is cough [27].

Radiation therapy may causes an acute lymphocytic alveolitis or hypersensitivity pneumonitis, which is associated with dyspnoea and cough within weeks or a few months of the dose [28]. In a study of 256 lung cancer patients receiving radical doses of radiotherapy, 49% developed acute radiation pneumonitis although it was severe in only 13% [29]. Late radiation damage is evident as pulmonary fibrosis, and may take several months or years to develop. The fibrosis results from the effects of tissue repair mechanisms following pneumonitis within the irradiated area, which involve the activation of fibroblasts by transforming growth factor-$\beta$, fibronectin and platelet-derived growth factor [28]. For longer-term survivors of cancer, radiation fibrosis is a sinister development as it can lead to severe symptoms and terminal respiratory failure. There is evidence that a smoking history can protect patients from developing radiation-induced pneumonitis [30].

Apart from lung cancer, breast cancer is another malignancy that often involves thoracic radiation. The syndrome of bronchiolitis obliterans organizing pneumonia (BOOP) has been described as a rare (2.5%) complication of postoperative radiotherapy following breast-conserving surgery [31]. These patients develop fever, non-productive cough and patchy unilateral or bilateral pulmonary infiltrates 5–6 months after radiotherapy. Postradiation BOOP is a serious condition which tends to recur even after long-term corticosteroid therapy. Modern radiation planning techniques, which limit the total dose to normal lung, have minimized the risk of BOOP and IPS, but they may still be a risk for patients requiring radiation therapy, who have pre-existing chronic pulmonary disease.

There are some other less common but interesting iatrogenic causes of disordered or diminished cough in cancer patients. For example, with concurrent radiotherapy and chemotherapy for head and neck cancer, 14% of patients in one study exhibited aspiration prior to treatment, 65% soon after therapy and 62% in the late post-therapy stage (aspiration rates pre-therapy vs. post-therapy $P = 0.0002$) [32]. This typically silent aspiration was a result of disordered epiglottal and pharyngeal muscle coordination, leading to a diminished cough reflex or cough which was delayed or ineffective in expectorating the aspirated material. Reduced cough effectiveness is also seen after unilateral vocal cord paralysis, which is often the result of mediastinal encroachment of a bronchial cancer, but may also result iatrogenically during thoracic surgery for the disease [33].

## Assessment of cough in cancer patients

The formal methods of assessing cough are covered elsewhere in this volume. Specific symptom measurement tools devised for cancer patients, which could be useful for evaluating the impact of cough on functioning and QoL include the EORTC LC-13; the Lung Cancer Symptom scale; and the Functional Assessment of Cancer Treatment (FACT) lung cancer module.

Investigations used in determining the source of cough in cancer patients are the same as for other disease groups. Thus, the most useful tests will include thoracic imaging by X-ray or CT scan; ultrasound in the case of suspected pleural or pericardial effusion; and ventilation/perfusion scanning for suspected pulmonary thromboembolism. Bronchoscopy is rarely necessary once a diagnosis of cancer is made, unless an endobronchial metastasis from a remote primary site is being considered.

## Management of cough in cancer patients

This topic will be approached under the following sections—specific anticancer therapies; laser and photodynamic therapy; palliative drug therapies; and management in terminal care. Table 15.4 summarizes these methods of managing cough. One of the difficulties of presenting and comparing different methods of cough palliation is that most studies have used a variety of outcome measures, timescales and definitions of 'successful' palliation. The UK Medical Research Council has also found that success depends on the starting point: whereas 90% of patients with lung cancer who had severe or moderate grades of cough at baseline reported improvement after treatment, only 53% who started with mild cough did so [34].

### Anticancer therapies

#### *Radiation therapy*
Radiotherapy may be offered to the cancer patient for two reasons—with the primary aim of curing disease or extending survival (radical treatment), or with the primary aim of palliating symptoms (palliative treatment). Table 15.5 gives a summary of the results of radiotherapy for palliation of respiratory symptoms. Most of the radiation studies have concentrated on the former, until recent years. Unfortunately, symptom relief was often considered of less importance compared with survival and tumour response in the case of radical treatment, and so the earlier research shed little light on subjective response. Thus, a US review of 156 patients with clinical stage I NSCLC, who were medically inoperable and therefore treated with radical intent (median dose 64 Gy) between 1980 and 1995, states that before

treatment 23% of patients had cough [35]. However, the paper does not reveal to what extent radiotherapy relieved the cough. The analysis did show that the presence of cough prior to treatment was associated with a higher local failure rate.

A European EORTC study, however, did investigate respiratory symptoms as well as QoL changes in 164 patients with NSCLC receiving a radical (60 Gy) dose of radiotherapy [36]. This study showed that there was a significant association between objective tumour response and the palliation of pain and physical functioning. During radiation treatment, many general symptoms and QoL deteriorated. However, after treat-

Table 15.4 Methods used to manage cough in cancer patients.

| Type of therapy | Examples |
| --- | --- |
| Anticancer chemotherapy | Single agents, e.g. gemcitabine<br>Combination regimens |
| Radiotherapy | Hypofractionated regimens |
| Laser therapy | Nd-YAG laser<br>Photodynamic therapy |
| Palliative drugs | Anti-inflammatory, e.g. corticosteroid<br>Suppressant, e.g. opioid<br>Antimuscarinic, e.g. hyoscine, glycopyrrolate |

Table 15.5 Summary of the results of radiotherapy for palliation of respiratory symptoms in non-small cell lung cancer (figures quoted are response rates for each symptom).

| Dose | Study | Cough (%) | Haemoptysis (%) | Dyspnoea (%) |
| --- | --- | --- | --- | --- |
| Radical (curative) 60 Gy | [36] | 31 | 83 | 37 |
| Conventional palliation | [39] | 49 | 79 | 3 |
| Hypofractionated 17 Gy | [37] | 48 | 95 | 46 |
| Hypofractionated 17 Gy | [42] | 24 | 60 | 55 |
| Hypofractionated 20 Gy | [41] | 68 | 77 | 42 |

Gy, Gray.

ment, cough improved in 31% of patients, haemoptysis in 83% and dyspnoea in 37%. Global QoL improved in 36%.

In order to improve tumour response to radical radiotherapy, there has been a move towards increasing the number of doses given daily (hyperfractionation). Continuous hyperfractionated radiotherapy (CHART) is being used in potentially curable cancer patients who are unable to have surgical resection. Studies of CHART have focused, not surprisingly, on long-term objective outcomes. However, short-term monitoring of patients with head and neck cancer having CHART has revealed that cough and hoarseness were improved, compared with conventional dose radiotherapy, at 6 weeks [38].

Studies of palliative regimens for radiotherapy have naturally focused on symptom control as a key endpoint. The same EORTC group just mentioned above also reported on palliative responses in patients with locally advanced and metastatic NSCLC [39]. In comparison with their radical treatment study, cough was relieved in 49% of patients, haemoptysis in 79% and dyspnoea in 39%. Once again, global QoL improved in 37% of patients after completion of radiotherapy and there was a tendency for patients who had an objective tumour response to have a symptomatic benefit.

A Cochrane systematic review examined 10 published randomized trials of palliative radiotherapy for lung cancer. Meta-analysis of the results was not possible because of great heterogeneity in the doses, patient characteristics and outcome measures used. There was no convincing evidence that any particular regime gave a better symptom resolution. The conclusion from this review was that most patients should be treated with minimum doses delivered in one or two fractions (hypofractionation) [40]. This approach would be specially useful for patients who are ill, cannot be admitted to hospital or cannot attend for long outpatient courses. In India a study examined the effect of giving four small weekly doses to a total of 20 Gy to 47 inoperable patients with NSCLC [41]. Not only was the regime well tolerated and convenient for patients who had long distances to travel, but it also gave relief of cough in 68%, of haemoptysis in 77% and of dyspnoea in 42%. Hypofractionation was also used in a Greek study of 48 NSCLC patients who had two doses of 8.5 Gy 1 week apart [42]. Cough was palliated in 24% with a median palliation duration of 70 days; haemoptysis in 60% over 133 days; and dyspnoea in 55% over 74 days.

Should palliative radiotherapy be offered routinely at the time of diagnosis, or only as needed when symptoms develop? This question was tackled by the UK Medical Research Council in an international study involving 230 patients with advanced inoperable NSCLC, who had no immediate reasons for radiotherapy [43]. The results showed that there was no difference between the immediate or deferred treatment approaches in terms of symptom relief, psychological distress or survival. Adverse effects were more likely after immediate radiotherapy.

When lung cancer recurs after a course of radiotherapy, it is unusual but it may be feasible to offer a second course of treatment. A retrospective study evaluating the outcome of reirradiation showed that 60% of patients achieved improvement in cough, 73% in dyspnoea, and all patients with haemoptysis had a reduction or complete resolution [44]. In recent years, the preferred approach in specialist centres for such patients is to offer endobronchially delivered intraluminal irradiation (brachytherapy). This involves subjecting the patient to a bronchoscopy and placing a catheter in the airway down to the level of the tumour. An after-loading device then sends a radioactive source via the catheter to the tumour site for a short time before withdrawal [45]. Several recent small studies have documented good palliative benefit after brachytherapy—relief of cough, haemoptysis and dyspnoea occurring in 54%, 74% and 54%, respectively [46]; 65%, 86% and 64%, respectively [47]; and 43%, 95% and 80%, respectively [48]. One problem with brachytherapy is that it is only available in a few centres with the necessary radioisotope equipment; another is that it has been associated with dose-dependent late toxicities, especially massive haemoptysis. Tauelle et al. [46] reported severe or fatal haemoptysis occurring in 7% of their patients; Hatlevoll et al. [47] in 27% (22% within 6 months); and Anacak et al. [48] in 11%.

## Chemotherapy

As with radiation therapy, in the past the emphasis in research was on achieving 'cure', so that the end-points were usually survival and objective tumour response rather than symptom relief. In SCLC, chemotherapy has long been the preferred option as the disease is often disseminated and, unlike NCSLC, is very sensitive to antimitotic drugs. It is well established that objective tumour response in SCLC is associated with symptom improvement. In various trials of standard combina-

Table 15.6 Summary of the results of chemotherapy for palliation of respiratory symptoms in non-small cell lung cancer (figures quoted are response rates for each symptom).

| Regimen | Study | Cough (%) | Haemoptysis (%) | Dyspnoea (%) |
|---|---|---|---|---|
| Cisplatin/vindesine+ mitomycin or ifosfamide | [51] | 45 | 91 | 78 |
| Mitomycin/ifosfamide/ cisplatin | [52] | 70 | 92 | 46 |
| Gemcitabine alone | [53] | 44 | 63 | 26 |
| Gemcitabine/cisplatin | [50] | 44 | 75 | 36 |

tion chemotherapy regimens, relief of cough has been reported in between 45% and 70% of patients; of haemoptysis in up to 92%; and of dyspnoea in between 46% and 78% [45]. A recent study in poor prognosis SCLC patients comparing combination chemotherapy vs. single-agent carboplatin showed that even in this very sick population, good symptom palliation could be achieved [49]. The combination regime (CAV) gave 21% relief of cough compared with 7% after carboplatin; dyspnoea improved in 66% and 41%, respectively. In terms of toxicity and objective tumour response, there were few differences.

Gemcitabine is a new anticancer drug which is given singly or in combination with others. As a single agent for inoperable NSCLC it has given relief of cough in 44%, of haemoptysis in 63% and of dyspnoea in 26% [45]. In combination with cisplatin these response rates were 44%, 75% and 36%, respectively [50]. It is likely that other new agents such as the taxanes will be used increasingly for symptom palliation in NSCLC. Single-agent chemotherapy (as well as talc and tetracycline) is also used to prevent the recurrence of pleural and pericardial effusions [54]. Table 15.6 summarizes the results of recent studies of palliating respiratory symptoms in NSCLC.

## Laser and photodynamic therapy

Laser therapy for the palliation of cough is delivered intraluminally via a bronchoscope. Unlike brachytherapy which was described above, laser therapy works by macroscopically heating and destroying tissues. Photodynamic therapy (PDT) is a refinement of the laser process by premedicating patients with tissue sensitiz-

ers which allow greater killing of tumour as compared with normal cells [15]. Both of these techniques are much less commonly available than radiotherapy (either external or endobronchial) or chemotherapy. Studies of their effectiveness have been relatively small and mostly uncontrolled. However, a recent randomized controlled trial was performed in 31 patients with tracheobronchial obstruction due to inoperable NSCLC [55]. The study directly compared laser resection using an Nd-YAG laser with dihaematoporphyrin ether and argon dye laser photoradiation. There was no difference between the two techniques in terms of symptom relief, but PDT gave a longer time till recurrence of symptoms and a longer median survival.

## Drug therapies

The drug management of cough is described in detail elsewhere in this volume, as well as in palliative medicine texts [15,16], so only a few points specific to cancer patients will be highlighted. Most palliative care units use codeine-based drugs for relieving cough. For patients who are resistant to codeine, other drugs which have been recommended include hydrocodone [56], benzonatate [57] and levodropropizine [58]. There are no published trials comparing the relative benefits or side-effects of these agents in cancer patients. A potential problem arises when a cancer patient is already receiving a potent opioid (morphine, hydromorphone, fentanyl, etc.) for pain, and then complains of a cough. It does not make sense pharmacologically to add a second opioid drug, as there is no evidence that incomplete cross-tolerance exists between opioids for cough (unlike the situation with pain modulation).

In this situation, it would be appropriate to use another class of drug or another approach entirely, such as radiotherapy.

In palliative care centres, nebulized lidocaine or bupivacaine have sometimes been advocated for the relief of intractable unproductive cough [16]. This method is thought to work by anaesthesizing sensory nerve endings in the hypopharynx, larynx and upper airways that are involved in generating the cough reflex. Other drugs which have theoretical actions on cough and may be tried in refractory cases include baclofen and mexilitine [16].

As discussed above, cough can arise as a symptom of pulmonary toxicity after some anticancer drugs. Recently there have been attempts to prevent or reverse the pulmonary damage using novel drug approaches. In an open uncontrolled US study, 63 patients with breast cancer who were starting high-dose chemotherapy prior to autologous bone marrow transplantation were given an inhaled corticosteroid — fluticasone propionate [59]. After 12 weeks of taking this drug twice daily, the study found that, compared with the centre's historical controls, $DL_{CO}$ (the diffusing capacity of the lungs) declined by a smaller amount (21% fluticasone vs. 33% historical controls). Delayed pulmonary toxicity syndrome developed in 35% of fluticasone patients compared to 73% of historical controls. Because of the grave significance of such pulmonary toxicity, further randomized trials of this and similar regimens are required.

## Management in terminal care

In the care of cancer patients, cough may become very distressing in the terminal stage. The act of coughing may cause or aggravate pain, it may disturb precious sleep and it can impede communication between patients and carers. If the cough is productive, it is helpful to position the patient so that expectoration is assisted, and gentle chest physiotherapy may be used [15]. It may be appropriate to offer an antibiotic for a respiratory tract infection, if the symptoms of cough and dyspnoea are very distressing. Patients with cancer are often prescribed drugs which can cause dry mouth and reduction of tracheobronchial mucus (opioids, anticholinergics, antihistamines) and this can cause difficulty in expectoration. It may be helpful in such situations to humidify the air or oxygen, if the patient needs the latter for hypoxaemia.

Some patients develop noisy breathing as they slip into unconsciousness (so-called death rattle). The cause of this is thick mucus lying in the major airways or hypopharynx, which partly obstructs the airflow, but which the patient is unable to cough up. The patient is usually unaware of the noise, but it can be very upsetting to family carers or others nearby. Suction may help if there is mucus in or above the larynx. Often the most practical management is to prevent further mucus production by giving an antimuscarinic agent, preferably by subcutaneous injections or by continuous infusions. The best agents for this purpose are hysoscine butylbromide or glycopyrrolate [60].

## References

1 Hopwood P, Stephens RJ on behalf of the Medical Research Council (MRC) Lung Cancer Working Party. Symptoms at presentation for treatment in patients with lung cancer: implications for the evaluation of palliative treatment. *Br J Cancer* 1995; **71**: 633–6.
2 Portenoy RK, Thaler HT, Kornblith AB *et al*. Symptom prevalence, characteristics and distress in a cancer population. *Qual Life Res* 1994; **3**: 183–9.
3 Bergmann B, Aaronson NK, Ahmedzai S *et al*. The EORTC QLC-LC13: a modular supplement to the EORTC Core Quality of Life Questionnaire (QLC-C30) for use in lung cancer clinical trials. *Eur J Cancer* 1994; **30A**: 635–42.
4 Hollen PJ, Gralla RJ, Kris MG *et al*. Normative data and trends in quality of life from the Lung Cancer Symptom Scale (LCSS). *Support Care Cancer* 1999; **7**: 140–8.
5 Lutz S, Norrell R, Bertucio C *et al*. Symptom frequency and severity in patients with metastatic or locally recurrent lung cancer: a prospective study using the Lung Cancer Symptom Scale in a community hospital. *Palliat Med* 2001; **4**: 157–65.
6 Ng K, von Gunten CF. Symptoms and attitudes of 100 consecutive patients admitted to an acute hospice/palliative care unit. *J Pain Symptom Manage* 1998; **16**: 307–16.
7 Anderson H, Ward C, Eardley A *et al*. The concerns of patients under palliative care and a heart failure clinic are not being met. *Palliat Med* 2001; **15**: 279–86.
8 Collins JJ, Byrns ME, Dunkel IJ *et al*. The measurement of symptoms in children with cancer. *J Pain Symptom Manage* 2000; **19**: 363–77.
9 Mehdi SA, Etxell JE, Newman NB *et al*. Prognostic significance of Ki-67 immunostaining and symptoms in resected stage I and II non-small cell lung cancer. *Lung Cancer* 1998; **20**: 99–108.

**155**

10 Mehdi SA, Tatum AH, Newman NB *et al*. Prognostic markers in resected stage I and II non-small-cell lung cancer: an analysis of 260 patients with 5 year follow-up. *Clin Lung Cancer* 1999; 1: 59–67.

11 Morita T, Tsunoda J, Inoue S *et al*. Contributing factors to physical symptoms in terminally-ill cancer patients. *J Pain Symptom Manage* 1999; 18: 338–46.

12 Kubik A, Zatloukal P, Boyle P *et al*. A case-control study of lung cancer among Czech women. *Lung Cancer* 2001; 31: 111–22.

13 Koyi H, Hillerdal G, Branden E. A prospective study of a total material of lung cancer from a county in Sweden 1997–1999; gender, symptoms, type, stage and smoking habits. *Lung Cancer* 2002; 36: 9–14.

14 Zayas JG, Rubin BK, York EL *et al*. Bronchial mucus properties in lung cancer: relationship with site of lesion. *Can Respir J* 1999; 6: 246–52.

15 Ahmedzai SH. Palliation of respiratory symptoms. In: Doyle D, Hanks GWC, McDonald N, eds. *Oxford Textbook of Palliative Medicine*, 2nd edn. Oxford: Oxford University Press, 1998: 583–616.

16 Twycross R, Wilcock A. Respiratory symptoms. In: Twycross R, Wilcock A, eds. *Symptom Management in Advanced Cancer*, 2nd edn. Oxford: Radcliffe Press, 1997: 141–79.

17 Pidhorecky I, Urschel J, Anderson T. Resection of invasive pulmonary aspergillosis in immunocompromised patients. *Ann Surg Oncol* 2000; 7: 312–7.

18 Mertens AC, Yasui Y, Liu Y *et al*. Pulmonary complications in survivors of childhood and adolescent cancer. A report from the Childhood Cancer Survivor Study. *Cancer* 2002; 95: 2431–41.

19 Segura A, Yuste A, Cercos A *et al*. Pulmonary fibrosis induced by cyclophosphamide. *Ann Pharmacother* 2001; 35: 894–7.

20 Edman L, Larsen J, Hagglund H *et al*. Health-related quality of life, symptom distress and sense of coherence in adult survivors of allogeneic stem-cell transplantation. *Eur J Cancer Care (Engl)* 2001; 10: 124–30.

21 Rudberg L, Carlsson M, Nilsson S *et al*. Self-perceived physical, psychologic, and general symptoms in survivors of testicular cancer 3–13 years after treatment. *Cancer Nurs* 2002; 25: 187–95.

22 Bilgrami SF, Metersky ML, McNally D *et al*. Idiopathic pneumonia syndrome following myeloablative chemotherapy and autologous transplantation. *Ann Pharmacother* 2001; 35: 196–201.

23 Wilczynski SW, Erasmus JJ, Petros WP *et al*. Delayed pulmonary toxicity syndrome following high-dose chemotherapy and bone marrow transplantation for breast cancer. *Am J Respir Crit Care Med* 1998; 157: 565–73.

24 Herscher LL, Hahn SM, Kroog G *et al*. Phase I study of pa-clitaxel as a radiation sensitizer in the treatment of mesothelioma and non-small-cell lung cancer. *J Clin Oncol* 1998; 16: 635–41.

25 Madarnas Y, Webster P, Shorter AM *et al*. Irinotecan-associated pulmonary toxicity. *Anticancer Drugs* 2000; 11: 709–13.

26 Goldenberg MM. Trastuzumab, a recombinant DNA-derived humanized monoclonal antibody, a novel agent for the treatment of metastatic breast cancer. *Clin Ther* 1999; 21: 309–18.

27 Eton O, Rosenblum MG, Legha SS *et al*. Phase I trial of subcutaneous recombinant human interleukin-2 in patients with metastatic melanoma. *Cancer* 2002; 95: 127–34.

28 Abratt RP, Morgan GW. Lung toxicity following chest irradiation in patients with lung cancer. *Lung Cancer* 2002; 35: 103–9.

29 Inoue A, Kunitoh H, Sekine I *et al*. Radiation pneumonitis in lung cancer patients: a retrospective study of risk factors and the long-term prognosis. *Int J Radiat Oncol Biol Phys* 2001; 49: 649–55.

30 Johansson S, Bjermer L, Franzen L *et al*. Effects of ongoing smoking on the development of radiation-induced pneumonitis in breast cancer and oesophagus cancer patients. *Radiother Oncol* 1998; 49: 41–7.

31 Takigawa N, Segawa Y, Saeki T *et al*. Bronchiolitis obliterans organizing pneumonia syndrome in breast-conserving therapy for early breast cancer: radiation-induced lung toxicity. *Int J Radiat Oncol Biol Phys* 2000; 48: 751–5.

32 Eisbruch A, Lyden T, Bradford CR *et al*. Objective assessment of swallowing dysfunction and aspiration after radiation concurrent with chemotherapy for head-and-neck cancer. *Int J Radiat Oncol Biol Phys* 2002; 53: 23–8.

33 Abraham MT, Bains MS, Downey RJ *et al*. Type I thyroplasty for acute unilateral vocal fold paralysis following intrathoracic surgery. *Ann Otol Rhinol Laryngol* 2002; 111: 667–71.

34 Stephens RJ, Hopwood P, Girling DJ. Defining and analysing symptom palliation in cancer clinical trials: a deceptively difficult exercise. *Br J Cancer* 1999; 79: 538–44.

35 Sibley GS, Jamieson TA, Marks LB *et al*. Radiotherapy alone for medically inoperable stage I non-small-cell lung cancer: the Duke experience. *Int J Radiat Oncol Biol Phys* 1998; 40: 149–54.

36 Langendijk JA, Aaronson NK, de Jong JM *et al*. Prospective study on quality of life before and after radical radiotherapy in non-small-cell lung cancer. *J Clin Oncol* 2001; 19: 2123–33.

37 Medical Research Council Lung Cancer Working Party. Randomized trial of palliative two-fraction versus more intensive 13 fraction radiotherapy for patients with inop-

erable non-small cell lung cancer and good performance status. *Clin Oncol* 1996; **8**: 167–75.

38 Griffiths GO, Parmar MK, Bailey AJ. Physical and psychological symptoms of quality of life in the CHART randomized trial in head and neck cancer: short-term and long-term patient reported symptoms. CHART Steering Committee. Continuous hyperfractionated accelerated radiotherapy. *Br J Cancer* 1999; **81**: 1196–205.

39 Langendijk JA, ten Velde GP, Aaronson NK *et al.* Quality of life after palliative radiotherapy in non-small cell lung cancer: a prospective study. *Int J Radiat Oncol Biol Phys* 2000; **47**: 149–55.

40 Macbeth F, Toy E, Coles B *et al.* Palliative radiotherapy regimens for non-small cell lung cancer. [Update of *Cochrane Database Syst Rev* 2001; **2**: CD002143; PMID: 11406035.] *Cochrane Database Syst Rev* Issue 4, 2002.

41 Bhatt ML, Mohani BK, Kumar L *et al.* Palliative treatment of advanced non small cell lung cancer with weekly fraction radiotherapy. *Indian J Cancer* 2000; **37**: 148–52.

42 Plataniotis GA, Kouvaris JR, Dardoufas C *et al.* A short radiotherapy course for locally advanced non-small cell lung cancer (NSCLC): effective palliation and patients' convenience. *Lung Cancer* 2002; **35**: 203–7.

43 Falk SJ, Girling DJ, White RJ *et al.* Immediate versus delayed palliative thoracic radiotherapy in patients with unresectable locally advanced non-small cell lung cancer and minimal thoracic symptoms: randomised controlled trial. *Br Med J* 2002; **325**: 465.

44 Gressen EL, Werner-Wasik M, Cohn J *et al.* Thoracic reirradiation for symptomatic relief after prior radiotherapeutic management for lung cancer. *Am J Clin Oncol* 2000; **23**: 160–3.

45 Hoskin P, Ahmedzai SH. Assessment and management of respiratory symptoms of malignant disease. In: Ahmedzai SH, Muers M, eds. *Supportive Care of the Respiratory Disease Patient.* Oxford: Oxford University Press, 2003 (in press).

46 Taulelle M, Chauvet B, Vincent P *et al.* High dose rate endobronchial brachytherapy: results and complications in 189 patients. *Eur Respir J* 1998; **11**: 162–8.

47 Hatlevoll R, Karlsen KO, Skovlund E. Endobronchial radiotherapy for malignant bronchial obstruction or recurrence. *Acta Oncol* 1999; **38**: 999–1004.

48 Anacak Y, Mogulkoc N, Ozkok S *et al.* High dose rate endobronchial brachytherapy in combination with external beam radiotherapy for stage III non-small cell lung cancer. *Lung Cancer* 2001; **34**: 253–9.

49 White SC, Cheeseman S, Thatcher N *et al.* Phase II study of oral topotecan in advanced non-small cell lung cancer. *Clin Cancer Res* 2000; **6**: 868–73.

50 Jassem J, Krzakowski M, Roszkowski K *et al.* A phase II study of gemcitabine plus cisplatin in patients with advanced non-small cell lung cancer: clinical outcomes and quality of life. *Lung Cancer* 2002; **35**: 73–9.

51 Fernandez C, Rosell R, Abad-Esteve A *et al.* Quality of life during chemotherapy in non-small cell lung cancer. *Acta Oncol* 1989; **28**: 29–33.

52 Cullen MH. The MIC regimen in non-small cell lung cancer. *Lung Cancer Suppl* 1993; **2**: 81–98.

53 Thatcher N, Anderson H, Betticher DC *et al.* Symptomatic benefit from gemcitabine and other chemotherapy in advanced non-small cell lung cancer: changes in performance status and tumour-related symptoms. *Anticancer Drugs* 1995; **6** (Suppl.): 39–48.

54 Paz-Ares L, Garcia-Carbonera R. Medical emergencies. In: Cavalli F, Hansen HE, Kaye SB, eds. *Textbook of Medical Oncology*, 2nd edn. Martin Dunitz, 2000: 619–49.

55 Diaz-Jimenez JP, Martinez-Ballarin JE, Llunell A *et al.* Efficacy and safety of photodynamic therapy versus Nd-YAG laser resection in NSCLC with airway obstruction. *Eur Respir J* 1999; **14**: 800–5.

56 Homsi J, Walsh D, Nelson KA *et al.* Pain and symptom management. Hydrocodone for cough in advanced cancer. *Am J Hospice Palliative Care* 2000; **17**: 342–6.

57 Doona M, Walsh D. Benzonatate for opioid-resistant cough in advanced cancer. *Palliat Med* 1998; **12**: 55–8.

58 Luporini G, Barni S, Marchi E *et al.* Efficacy and safety of levodropropizine and dihydrocodeine on nonproductive cough in primary and metastatic lung cancer. *Eur Respir J* 1998; **12**: 97–101.

59 McGaughey DS, Nikcevich DA, Long GD *et al.* Inhaled steroids as prophylaxis for delayed pulmonary toxicity syndrome in breast cancer patients undergoing high-dose chemotherapy and autologous stem cell transplantation. *Biol Blood Marrow Transplant* 2001; **7**: 274–8.

60 Bennett M, Lucas V, Brennan M *et al.* Using antimuscarinic drugs in the management of death-rattle: evidence-based guidelines for palliative care. *Palliat Med* 2002; **16**: 369–74.

# Pathophysiology

# 16 Sensory pathways for the cough reflex

*Stuart B. Mazzone, Brendan J. Canning & John G. Widdicombe*

## Introduction

The cough reflex is one of several defensive reflexes that serve to protect the airways from the potentially damaging effects of inhaled particulate matter, aeroallergens, pathogens, aspirate and accumulated secretions. In some airways diseases, cough may become excessive and non-productive, and is potentially harmful to the airway mucosa. An understanding of the neural pathways involved in the cough reflex may facilitate the development of therapeutic strategies that prevent excessive and non-productive cough, whilst preserving the important innate defensive role of this respiratory reflex.

Much of our current understanding of the neural pathways involved in the cough reflex is derived from studies in animals. In cats, dogs, rabbits, guinea-pigs and monkeys it is clear that vagal afferent nerves are responsible for initiating the cough reflex [1–6]. Although poorly described, afferent nerves innervating other viscera as well as somatosensory nerves innervating the chest wall, diaphragm and abdominal musculature also likely play an integral role in regulating cough. In this chapter the broad classes of vagal afferent nerves innervating the airways and their role in regulating the cough reflex will be defined.

## Defining airway afferent nerve subtypes

Airway afferent nerve subtypes can be distinguished based on their physicochemical sensitivity, adaptation to sustained lung inflation, neurochemistry, origin, myelination, conduction velocity and sites of termination in the airways. The utility of each of these approaches for defining airway afferent nerve subtypes is limited in large part by the lack of specificity of the various characteristics studied. When used in combination, however, these physiological and morphological attributes can be used to identify at least three broad classes of airway afferent nerves: rapidly adapting mechanoreceptors (RARs), slowly adapting mechanoreceptors (SARs) and unmyelinated C-fibres (Fig. 16.1).

The value of this now widely accepted classification scheme used to define airway afferent nerve subtypes is confirmed by its established utility in all species thus far studied. Most airway afferent nerves found in any of these species are described reasonably well as either RAR, SAR or C-fibre. The observations that stereotypical reflexes are initiated by stimuli selective (even if not specific) for these afferent nerve subtypes and that these reflexes are modulated by interventions that preferentially alter the activity or actions of the afferent nerve subtypes studied is further evidence for the utility of this classification scheme. Studies of central nervous system (CNS) termination sites of the various afferent nerve subtypes identified also confirm the utility of the classification scheme [7]. Such analyses reveal the necessary divergence of afferent nerve terminals within the CNS, divergence that is required to differentially and specifically control homeostatic and defensive reflexes initiated from the airways.

The characteristics of the afferent nerve subtypes innervating the airways are described briefly in Table 16.1 and in detail below.

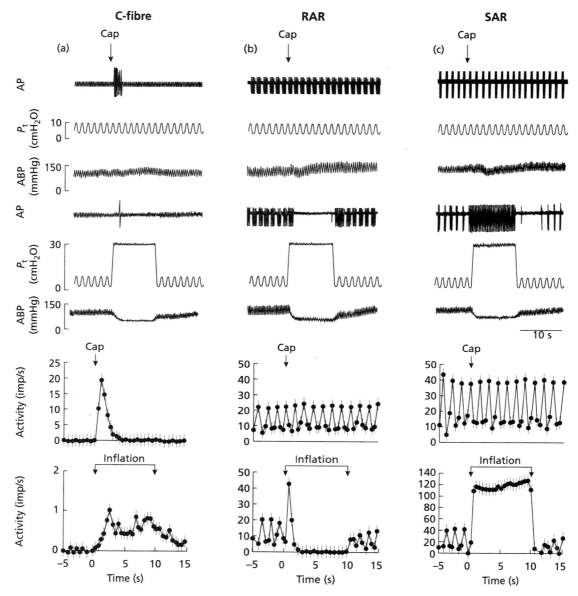

**Fig. 16.1** Afferent nerve subtypes innervating the mammalian airways. Representative traces (upper panels) and mean data (lower panels) obtained from single-fibre recordings of afferent nerve activity in the vagus nerve of anaesthetized rats. (a) Airway C-fibres are generally quiescent during tidal breathing and relatively unresponsive to lung inflation (peak activity ~ 1 impulse/s). C-fibres, however, respond vigorously to intravenous injections of the vanilloid capsaicin (peak activity ~ 20 impulses/s). Rapidly adapting receptors (RARs) (b) and slowly adapting receptors (SARs) (c) are sporadically active during the respiratory cycle (10–40 impulses/s). Neither subtype of mechanoreceptor responds to capsaicin (Cap), but both fire intensely when the lungs are inflated (peak activity ~ 40–120 impulses/s). Note that RARs are easily differentiated from SARs since they rapidly adapt during sustained lung inflation. Modified with permission from [10].

**Table 16.1** *In vivo* properties of vagal afferent nerve subtypes innervating the mammalian airways.

| | Rapidly adapting receptor | Slowly adapting receptor | C-fibre |
|---|---|---|---|
| *Electrophysiological properties* | | | |
| Conduction velocity (m/s) | 14–23 | 15–32 | 1.3–1.5 |
| Fibre type | Myelinated | Myelinated | Unmyelinated |
| Eupnoeic activity (impulses/s) | 0–20 | 10–40 | 0.3–1.5 |
| *Physical sensitivity* | | | |
| Lung deflation | Increased | Decreased | No effect |
| Oedema | Increased | No effect | Increased |
| *Chemical sensitivity* | | | |
| $CO_2$ | No effect | Decreased | Increased |
| $H^+$ | Increased | No effect | Increased |
| Capsaicin | Increased* | No effect | Increased† |
| Bradykinin | Increased* | No effect | Increased† |
| *Reflex effects* | | | |
| Parasympathetic | Excitatory | Inhibitory | Excitatory |
| Respiratory | Hyperpnoea | Inhibit inspiration | Apnoea |
| Oedema formation | Promote | No effect | Promote |
| *Neurokinin positive* | No | No | Yes |

* Increased RAR activity is prevented by bronchodilator pretreatment, suggesting that activation occurs secondary to obstruction in the lung.
† Increased C-fibre activity is enhanced by bronchodilator pretreatment, suggesting that bradykinin and capsaicin directly stimulate C-fibres in the airways. See text for further details and references.

## Afferent nerve subtypes innervating the airways and their role in regulating cough

### Rapidly adapting receptors

Although relatively little is known about the anatomical arrangement of RAR terminations in the airway wall, functional studies suggest that RARs terminate within or beneath the epithelium and are localized to both intra- and extrapulmonary airways [8–11]. RARs are typically differentiated from other airway afferent nerves by their rapid (1–2 s) adaptation to sustained lung inflations (Fig. 16.1) [10–14]. Other distinguishing properties of RARs include their sensitivity to lung collapse and/or lung deflation, their responsiveness to alterations in dynamic lung compliance (and thus their sensitivity to bronchospasm), and their conduction velocity (4–18 m/s, suggestive of small, myelinated axons) [8–11,15]. Careful analysis of the responsive-

ness of RARs to mechanical stimulation reveals that their adaptation to sustained lung inflation is not attributable to an electrophysiological adaptation, as with sustained, dynamic mechanical stimulation, RARs are continually activated [16,17]. RARs may also adapt comparatively slow to lung deflation [10]. Perhaps RARs are thus better defined as dynamic receptors that respond to changes in airway mechanical properties (e.g. diameter, length, interstitial pressures).

RARs are sporadically active throughout the respiratory cycle, activated by the dynamic mechanical forces accompanying lung inflation and deflation and becoming more active as the rate and volume of lung inflation increases [10,16,17]. It follows therefore that RAR activity during respiration correlates to respiratory rate and is higher in guinea-pigs and rats (16–27 impulses/s) and almost unmeasurable in larger animals such as dogs (<1 impulse/s). It also follows that, at least in smaller animals, RAR-dependent reflexes require a heightened activity in the already active RARs. This

**163**

CHAPTER 16

sensitivity to the dynamic forces associated with lung inflation and deflation suggests a mechanism by which stimuli activate RARs. RARs may be insensitive to many 'direct' chemical stimuli (Fig. 16.1). However, RAR activity can be increased by stimuli that evoke bronchospasm or obstruction resulting from mucus secretion or oedema [11,18–23]. Not surprisingly, then, the ability of substances such as histamine, capsaicin, substance P and bradykinin to activate RARs can be markedly inhibited or abolished by preventing the local end-organ effects that these stimuli evoke (e.g. mucus secretion, bronchospasm).

Activation of RARs increases parasympathetic nerve activity in the airways [13,21]. RARs also respond to stimuli that evoke cough in many species including humans (see below), and fulfil all of the accepted criteria for mediating cough [1,4,13,24]. Further evidence for their role in the cough reflex comes from studies of vagal cooling, which blocks cough at temperatures that selectively abolish activity in myelinated fibres (including RARs) whilst preserving unmyelinated C-fibre activity [25].

Slowly adapting mechanoreceptors

SARs, like RARs, are active during the respiratory cycle, their activity increasing sharply during the inspiratory phase and peaking just prior to the initiation of expiration (Fig. 16.1) [10,26]. SARs are thus believed to be the primary afferent fibres involved in the Hering–Breuer reflex, which terminates inspiration and initiates expiration when the lungs are adequately inflated [26]. SARs, however, can be differentiated from RARs in some species based on action potential conduction velocity, and in most species by their lack of adaptation during sustained lung inflations. SARs may also be differentially distributed throughout the airways [26]. In cats, guinea-pigs and rats, few if any SARs but many RARs and C-fibres can be found in the extrapulmonary airways. Rather, SARs appear to be associated with the smooth muscle of the intrapulmonary airways (in dogs, SARs may also be localized to extrapulmonary airways). SARs also differ from RARs with respect to the reflexes they precipitate. SAR activation results in central inhibition of respiration and inhibition of cholinergic drive to the airways, leading to decreased phrenic nerve activity and decreased airway smooth muscle tone (due to a withdrawal of cholinergic nerve activity) [22,26].

The role of SARs in the cough reflex is poorly understood. Single-unit recordings from the vagus nerve in rabbits suggest that SAR activity does not increase prior to or during ammonia-induced coughing [5]. Although this suggests that SARs are unlikely to play a primary role in the cough reflex, their profound influence over respiratory pattern makes it likely that they, in some way, play a role in cough and other airway defensive reflexes. It has been proposed, for example, that enhancing baseline SAR activity with the loop diuretic frusemide (furosemide) may account for the reported antitussive effects of this agent in animals and in human subjects [27]. In contrast, preloading, which will likely increase baseline SAR activity, has been reported to increase expiratory efforts during cough [28,29]. Consistent with this latter assertion, experiments performed on rabbits in which inhaled sulphur dioxide has been used in an attempt to selectively block SAR activity show that the cough reflex is coincidentally attenuated [4,30]. However, it must be noted that the selectivity of sulphur dioxide for airway SARs is questionable since several reports indicate an excitatory action of sulphur dioxide on airway C-fibres [31,32]. C-fibre activation may be inhibitory to cough (see below).

Studies of CNS processing also suggest that SARs may facilitate coughing. Shannon and colleagues have proposed a central cough network in which SARs facilitate cough via activation of brainstem second-order neurones (termed pump cells) of the SAR reflex pathway [2]. In this model, SARs, through activation of pump cells, open an as yet unidentified 'gate' in the brainstem that is thought to promote cough. An excitatory role of pump cells in cough, however, is difficult to reconcile with studies showing that SARs (via pump cells) inhibit other RAR-mediated reflex pathways [20,33].

C-fibres

Unmyelinated afferent C-fibres are physiologically and morphologically similar to the unmyelinated nociceptors of the somatic nervous system and comprise the majority of afferent nerves innervating the airways [11,14,34,35]. In addition to their conduction velocity, afferent C-fibres are distinguished from RARs and SARs by their relative insensitivity to mechanical stimulation and lung inflation and their responsiveness to bradykinin and capsaicin (Fig. 16.1) [9–12,21,34]. C-fibre afferent nerves are further distinguished from

RARs by the observation that bradykinin and capsaicin-evoked activation of their endings in the airways is not inhibited by pretreatment with bronchodilators. On the contrary, bronchodilators such as prostaglandin $E_2$ ($PGE_2$), adrenaline (epinephrine) and adenosine may enhance excitability of airway afferent C-fibres [34,36]. This indicates that unlike RARs, C-fibres are directly activated by substances such as bradykinin and capsaicin.

Morphological studies in rats and in guinea-pigs indicate that C-fibre afferent nerves innervate the airway epithelium as well as other effector structures within the airway wall [9,37–39]. C-fibres may synthesize neuropeptides that are subsequently transported to their central and peripheral nerve terminals [9,37,39,40]. This unique neurochemical property of bronchopulmonary C-fibres has been exploited to describe the distribution and peripheral nerve terminals of these unmyelinated airway afferent nerve endings. Although the expression of neuropeptides in their peripheral afferent nerve terminals may be species dependent, it seems likely that C-fibres innervating the airways of other species are morphologically (if not neurochemically) similar to those well characterized in guinea-pigs and rats [38,41].

In dogs, airway afferent C-fibres may be further subdivided into bronchial and pulmonary C-fibres, a distinction based both on sites of termination but also on responsiveness to chemical and mechanical stimuli [14]. Notably, pulmonary C-fibres in dogs may be unresponsive to histamine, whilst bronchial C-fibres (in dogs at least) are activated by histamine. Whether similar physiological distinctions between bronchial and pulmonary afferent C-fibres can be defined in other species is unknown.

C-fibre afferent nerves play a key role in airway defensive reflexes. Although C-fibre afferent endings are polymodal and thus respond to both chemical and mechanical stimulation, their threshold for mechanical activation is substantially higher than that of RARs and SARs [9,10]. Accordingly, C-fibres are generally quiescent throughout the respiratory cycle but are readily activated by chemical stimuli such as capsaicin, bradykinin, citric acid, hypertonic saline and sulphur dioxide [9–11,34]. Reflex responses evoked by C-fibre activation include increased airway parasympathetic nerve activity and the chemoreflex, characterized by apnoea (followed by rapid shallow breathing), bradycardia and hypotension [11,14,21,34]. In some species

(particularly rats and guinea-pigs) C-fibre activation evokes peripheral release of neuropeptides (via an axon reflex) leading to bronchospasm and neurogenic inflammation [34,42].

The role of bronchopulmonary C-fibres in the cough reflex is controversial. Several lines of evidence support the hypothesis that activation of airway C-fibres precipitates cough. For example, putatively selective stimulants of airway C-fibres such as capsaicin, bradykinin and citric acid evoke cough in conscious animals and in humans [3,14,18,43–45]. Furthermore, capsaicin pretreatment, a technique that is used to selectively deplete C-fibres of neuropeptides, abolishes cough in guinea-pigs induced by citric acid, but has no effect on cough evoked by mechanical probing of the airway mucosa in these same animals [43]. Finally, pharmacological studies which take advantage of the somewhat unique expression of neurokinins by airway C-fibres have shown that citric acid- and capsaicin-induced cough in cats and guinea-pigs is attenuated if not abolished by prior treatment with selective neurokinin receptor antagonists [46].

Although the evidence summarized above supports a role for C-fibres in the cough reflex, there is also considerable evidence to indicate that airway C-fibres do not evoke cough and may actually inhibit cough evoked by RAR stimulation. In anaesthetized animals, for example, C-fibre stimulation has consistently failed to evoke coughing, even though cough can be readily induced in these animals by mechanically probing mucosal sites along the airways [6,24,25,47]. Indeed, systemic administration of C-fibre stimulants has been shown to inhibit cough evoked by RAR stimulation in various species [24,25,47]. Given that vagal cooling abolishes cough and yet preserves C-fibre-dependent reflexes provides further evidence against a role for C-fibres in cough [25].

It is unclear why so much conflicting evidence about C-fibres in cough exists. It is possible that general anaesthesia in animals selectively disrupts the ability of C-fibres to evoke cough without adversely affecting cough induced by RAR stimulation. Consistent with this notion, general anaesthesia can also inhibit the cough reflex in human subjects [48]. It is unlikely that anaesthesia prevents C-fibre activation and C-fibre-mediated reflex effects entirely. C-fibres are readily activated in anaesthetized animals and can precipitate profound cardiorespiratory reflexes [14,21,49–52]. Rather, anaesthesia must selectively inhibit cough-related neural pathways, or may act by accentuating the inhibitory effects of C-fibre activation on cough. Alternatively, general anaesthesia may interfere with the conscious perception of airway irritation and the resulting urge to cough. In this context, it is interesting that capsaicin-evoked cough can be consciously suppressed in human subjects [53]. Yet an equally viable hypothesis is that C-fibre stimulation alone is simply insufficient to evoke cough but depends upon airway afferent nerve interactions both in the periphery and at the level of the central nervous system (see below).

### Other airway afferent nerve subtypes

Not all airway afferent nerves fit into the three classes of airway afferent nerves described above. In guinea-pigs (commonly used to study cough), a second type of nociceptor-like afferent nerve has been described *in vitro* [9,16,24,39,40]. Extracellular recording in the vagal sensory ganglia of guinea-pigs indicates that about half of the tracheal afferent nerves responsive to both bradykinin and capsaicin are small, myelinated, A$\delta$-fibres [9]. Physiologically, these myelinated airway nociceptors resemble the myelinated nociceptors described in somatic tissues [54]. The guinea-pig tracheal A$\delta$-nociceptors have their cell bodies in the jugular ganglia (superior vagal ganglia, which also contains the perikarya of bronchopulmonary C-fibres) and are readily distinguished from RAR-like A$\delta$-fibres innervating the guinea-pig trachea, which have their cell bodies in the nodose ganglia (inferior vagal ganglia). Unlike the jugular A$\delta$-fibres, nodose-derived RARs are utterly unresponsive to direct stimulation by either capsaicin or bradykinin *in vitro* and are 15-fold more sensitive to mechanical stimulation than the jugular A$\delta$-fibres. The adaptation index (a measurement of afferent responsiveness to sustained mechanical stimulation) of these fibres also differs considerably. McAlexander *et al.* [16] reported that the nodose-derived RARs had an adaptation index that averaged $95\pm2$, whereas the adaptation index of the jugular A$\delta$-fibres was comparable to the adaptation index of tracheal/bronchial C-fibres in the preparation, averaging $46\pm8$. Histological analyses reveal that like C-fibres, A$\delta$-nociceptors innervating the guinea-pig trachea express the capsaicin receptor VR1, but unlike airway C-fibres, do not synthesize neuropeptides [9,39,40].

The role of A$\delta$-nociceptors in airway homeostatic and defensive reflexes, and whether these afferent nerve subtypes are unique to the guinea-pig trachea, is unknown. No such fibres have been described in rats or dogs. Whether this is reflective of their peculiarity to the guinea-pig or of the fact that myelinated, nociceptor-like fibres innervating the airways of other species have been excluded from published analyses is also unknown. It is interesting, however, that only about half of the RARs studied in other species are responsive to capsaicin [12,18].

Subtypes of RARs and SARs have also been proposed [10,11,14,26,55,56]. Differences in the airway segments innervated and not differences in the physiological properties of the SARs and RARs likely account in part for some of the subtypes described. In other instances, it could be argued that the evidence for SAR and RAR subtypes is more an argument of semantics than physiology. For example, Bergren and Peterson [56] and Ho and colleagues [10] both described a population of myelinated afferent nerves innervating the airways of rats that were activated vigorously by lung deflation yet adapted rapidly to sustained lung inflation. These afferent nerves, which were active throughout the respiratory cycle, appeared to be physiologically identical in every way and yet Bergren and Peterson classified these fibres as SARs while Ho and colleagues called them RARs [10,56]. Such divergent interpretations of essentially identical data by experienced investigators highlight the importance of establishing universal criteria for identifying airway afferent nerve subtypes.

## Interactions between afferent nerve subtypes evoking cough

### Peripheral interactions

Activation of airway C-fibres, particularly by capsaicin, evokes axon reflex-dependent peripheral release of the neuropeptides substance P, neurokinin A and calcitonin gene-related peptide [42]. There are many consequences of axonal reflexes, including bronchospasm, vasodilatation, oedema, leucocyte recruitment, mucus secretion, altered parasympathetic nerve activity and stimulation of endothelial and epithelial cells [57–63]. This peripheral neuropeptide release from C-fibre endings in the lung is prominent in rats and in guinea-pigs, and can be problematic when studying mechanisms of airway defensive reflexes in these species.

Peripheral neuropeptide release in the airways may also activate RARs. Studies in rabbits and in guinea-pigs have shown that endogenously released or exogenously administered substance P increases RAR activity [22,23,64]. The neuropeptide-evoked RAR activation is unlikely to be a direct action on the afferent nerve ending. Rather, it probably occurs secondary to actions on structural cells in the airway wall that in turn indirectly activate RARs [13,19,20]. Consistent with this notion, capsaicin- and bradykinin-induced stimulation of RARs in anaesthetized guinea-pigs correlates with the increases in pulmonary insufflation pressure evoked by these agents. The associated increases in RAR activity can be substantially reduced or abolished by pretreating animals with isoproterenol,

thereby preventing the bronchospastic activity of these agents [19].

Given the ability of C-fibre stimulants to activate RARs secondary to axonal reflex-mediated effects, it is predictable that preventing the axon reflex would be effective at preventing cough (Fig. 16.2). Indeed, cough evoked by capsaicin, cigarette smoke, bronchospasm or the neutral endopeptidase inhibitor phosphoramidon is markedly inhibited in guinea-pigs pretreated with β-agonists, inhaled neurokinin receptor antagonists or inhaled neutral endopeptidase (which enzymatically inactivates neurokinins and bradykinin) [65–69].

Although it is clear that C-fibre stimulants readily evoke cough, it is unclear whether axon reflexes or any peripheral interactions between C-fibres and RARs play any role in defensive reflex responses in the

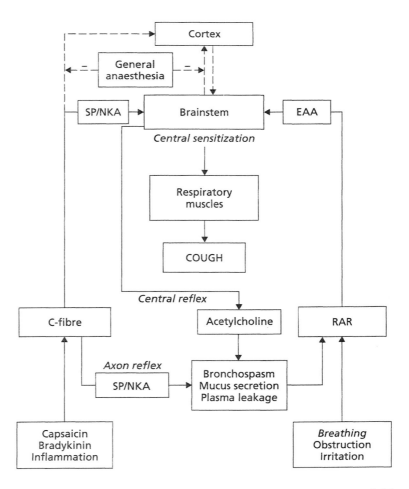

**Fig. 16.2** Highly schematic diagram showing the potential roles of airway C-fibres and rapidly adapting receptors (RARs) in the cough reflex. *In vivo*, the brainstem continuously receives input from RARs as a result of the mechanical effects of breathing. Additional obstruction or mechanical irritation likely evokes a distinct activity pattern in RARs which directly promotes coughing. C-fibres may also contribute to cough by (a) further activating RARs secondary to either central or axon reflex mediated airways obstruction; (b) facilitating ongoing RAR activity in the brainstem via central sensitization; or (c) directly activating cough pathways in the brainstem possibly by promoting the urge to cough through the perception of airway irritation. EAA, excitatory amino acids; NKA, neurokinin A; SP, substance P.

CHAPTER 16

airways of humans or in the airways of any species other than guinea-pigs. In cats and dogs, for example, bradykinin and capsaicin evoke bronchospasm, bronchial vasodilatation and mucus secretion, but these responses can be prevented entirely with atropine or by vagotomy. Unlike those seen in rats and guinea-pigs, therefore, parasympathetic reflexes account for the end-organ effects mediated by airway C-fibre activation in the airways of dogs and cats [14,70,71]. Similar findings have been reported in humans [72]. Morphological studies also call into question the importance of the axon reflex in humans, as there are few substance P-containing nerve fibres in human airways, and there is no evidence that these nerves correspond to the terminals of capsaicin-sensitive afferent C-fibres [38]. Although studies *in vitro* suggest that capsaicin can evoke contractions of the airway smooth muscle and enhance mucus secretion in human tissue preparations, these effects are not mediated by neurokinins [73–75].

The apparent lack of the axon reflex in humans (and other species) has to be reconciled with data showing that C-fibre stimulants are extremely effective at evoking cough. This would indicate that other mechanisms must underlie any potential involvement of C-fibres in coughing. It is possible that peripheral interactions between C-fibres and RARs may also proceed independent of axon reflexes (Fig. 16.2). For example, C-fibre activation evokes CNS-dependent parasympathetic reflex-induced alterations in airway and vascular tone and also induces mucus secretion [14,21,34,71,72]. These end-organ effects are mediated in large part by acetylcholine released from airway parasympathetic nerves and may be sufficient to activate RARs in the airway wall. This may account in part for the observation that inhaled anticholinergics have some antitussive properties in animals and in human subjects [76,77].

Central interactions

Our understanding of central integration of airway afferent fibres is somewhat limited. Insights into how C-fibres and RARs might interact in the brainstem may be obtained from studies in other systems, particularly the somatosensory system. C-fibres and mechanoreceptors arising from somatic tissues interact in the spinal cord in a process known as central sensitization [35,78]. The consequence of this central interaction

manifests as a heightened reflex responsiveness and exaggerated sensations of pain following cutaneous stimulation. Studies of central sensitization in the spinal cord have revealed two features of the somatosensory system that facilitate this hyperreflexia. Firstly, C-fibre and mechanoreceptor nerve terminals appear to converge onto common integrative neurones in the spinal cord. Secondly, this convergence allows for central amplification of afferent signalling (i.e. synergy) following the coincident activation of both afferent nerve subtypes. In many systems, this synergy and resulting hyperreflexia is precipitated by neurokinins released from the central terminals of somatosensory C-fibres. This results in a long-lasting hyperexcitability of spinal integrative neurones [35,78].

Several lines of evidence suggest that a process similar to central sensitization may play a role in airway defensive reflexes. The morphological, electrophysiological and pharmacological properties of airway C-fibres and mechanoreceptors are similar to those in the somatic nervous system [9,10,14,35,78]. In addition, anatomical and functional studies have shown considerable convergence of vagal afferents in brainstem integration sites such as the nucleus of the solitary tract (nTS) [7,79,80]. In many species, lung mechanoreceptors are sporadically active throughout the respiratory cycle, whereas C-fibres are typically quiescent, even during large lung inflations [10–14]. The central processing of C-fibre afferent nerve activity must therefore be integrated into a reflex pathway that is continuously receiving input from airway mechanoreceptors. C-fibre activation, via central interactions with RARs, may promote coughing by facilitating synaptic transmission at RAR relay neurones in the brainstem (Fig. 16.2). In support of this notion, substance P can facilitate synaptic transmission between lung afferents and nTS neurones in guinea-pigs [81].

Direct evidence for central interactions between airway C-fibres and RARs in the regulation of airway parasympathetic tone has been documented [80]. Activation of C-fibre afferent nerves in the lung evokes profound increases in cholinergic tone in the airways by facilitating airway mechanoreceptor activity in the brainstem. In the absence of airway mechanoreceptor activity, C-fibres are ineffective at evoking reflex responses. The facilitating effects of C-fibres on RAR reflex pathways in the brainstem appear to be mediated by neurokinins since the central synergistic interactions are prevented entirely by neurokinin receptor antagonists administered intracerebroventricularly. The sensitizing effect of nociceptor stimulation can also be mimicked, in the absence of C-fibre stimulation, by administering substance P to the brainstem [80]. Given that neurokinin receptor antagonists also inhibit cough, at least in part, via central mechanisms [47], it is tempting to speculate that they are acting to prevent the central sensitizing effects of C-fibre activation on RAR pathways.

## Concluding remarks

Studies that have delineated the afferent neural pathways regulating cough indicate that RARs subserve a primary role in the cough reflex. There remains some uncertainty about the role of other afferent nerve subtypes (particularly C-fibres) in this defensive reflex. The failure to clearly define the role of C-fibres in cough relates in part to the ability of general anaesthesia to selectively prevent cough mediated by C-fibre stimulants. The effects of general anaesthesia appear to be unique to the cough reflex, since C-fibres readily evoke other defensive reflexes under these same conditions. Anaesthesia must therefore selectively disrupt an as yet unidentified C-fibre-specific cough pathway in the brain. Further studies are required to identify the afferent pathways responsible for initiating cough, and the interactions between these pathways and other modulatory afferent nerves regulating this important defensive reflex.

## References

1 Widdicombe JG. Afferent receptors in the airways and cough. *Respir Physiol* 1998; **114**: 5–15.
2 Shannon R, Baekey DM, Morris KF, Lindsey BG. Ventrolateral medullary respiratory network and a model of cough motor pattern generation. *J Appl Physiol* 1998; **84**: 2020–35.
3 Karlsson JA. The role of capsaicin-sensitive C-fibre afferent nerves in the cough reflex. *Pulm Pharmacol* 1996; **9**: 315–21.
4 Sant'Ambrogio G, Sant'Ambrogio FB, Davies A. Airway receptors in cough. *Bull Eur Physiopathol Respir* 1984; **20**: 43–7.
5 Matsumoto S. The activities of lung stretch and irritant receptors during cough. *Neurosci Lett* 1988; **90**: 125–9.
6 Deep V, Singh M, Ravi K. Role of vagal afferents in the re-

7 Kubin L, Davies RO. Central pathways of pulmonary and airway vagal afferents. In: Hornbein TF, ed. *Regulation of Breathing*, Vol. 79. New York: Marcel Dekker, 1995: 219–84.
8 Bergren DR, Sampson SR. Characterization of intrapulmonary, rapidly adapting receptors of guinea-pigs. *Respir Physiol* 1982; **47**: 83–95.
9 Riccio MM, Kummer W, Biglari B, Myers AC, Undem BJ. Interganglionic segregation of distinct vagal afferent fibre phenotypes in guinea-pig airways. *J Physiol* 1996; **496**: 521–30.
10 Ho CY, Gu Q, Lin YS, Lee LY. Sensitivity of vagal afferent endings to chemical irritants in the rat lung. *Respir Physiol* 2001; **127**: 113–24.
11 Widdicombe J. Airway receptors. *Respir Physiol* 2001; **125**: 3–15.
12 Armstrong DJ, Luck JC. A comparative study of irritant and type J receptors in the cat. *Respir Physiol* 1974; **21**: 47–60.
13 Sant'Ambrogio G, Widdicombe J. Reflexes from airway rapidly adapting receptors. *Respir Physiol* 2001; **125**: 33–45.
14 Coleridge JC, Coleridge HM. Afferent vagal C fibre innervation of the lungs and airways and its functional significance. *Rev Physiol Biochem Pharmacol* 1984; **99**: 1–110.
15 Jonzon A, Pisarri TE, Coleridge JC, Coleridge HM. Rapidly adapting receptor activity in dogs is inversely related to lung compliance. *J Appl Physiol* 1986; **61**: 1980–7.
16 McAlexander MA, Myers AC, Undem BJ. Adaptation of guinea-pig vagal airway afferent neurones to mechanical stimulation. *J Physiol* 1999; **521**: 239–47.
17 Pack AI, DeLaney RG. Response of pulmonary rapidly adapting receptors during lung inflation. *J Appl Physiol* 1983; **55** (3): 955–63.
18 Mohammed SP, Higenbottam TW, Adcock JJ. Effects of aerosol-applied capsaicin, histamine and prostaglandin E2 on airway sensory receptors of anaesthetized cats. *J Physiol* 1993; **469**: 51–66.
19 Bergren DR. Sensory receptor activation by mediators of defense reflexes in guinea-pig lungs. *Respir Physiol* 1997; **108**: 195–204.
20 Morikawa T, Gallico L, Widdicombe J. Actions of moguisteine on cough and pulmonary rapidly adapting receptor activity in the guinea-pig. *Pharmacol Res* 1997; **35**: 113–8.
21 Canning BJ, Reynolds SM, Mazzone SB. Multiple mechanisms of reflex bronchospasm in guinea-pigs. *J Appl Physiol* 2001; **91**: 2642–53.
22 Joad JP, Kott KS, Bonham AC. Nitric oxide contributes to substance P-induced increases in lung rapidly adapting

flex effects of capsaicin and lobeline in monkeys. *Respir Physiol* 2001; **125**: 155–68.

receptor activity in guinea-pigs. *J Physiol* 1997; **503**: 635–43.

23 Bonham AC, Kott KS, Ravi K, Kappagoda CT, Joad JP. Substance P contributes to rapidly adapting receptor responses to pulmonary venous congestion in rabbits. *J Physiol* 1996; **493**: 229–38.

24 Canning BJ, Reynolds SM, Meeker S, Undem BJ. Electrophysiological identification of tracheal (T) and laryngeal (LX) vagal afferents mediating cough in guinea-pigs (GP). *Am J Respir Crit Care Med* 2000; **161**: A434.

25 Tatar M, Sant'Ambrogio G, Sant'Ambrogio FB. Laryngeal and tracheobronchial cough in anesthetized dogs. *J Appl Physiol* 1994; **76**: 2672–9.

26 Schelegle ES, Green JF. An overview of the anatomy and physiology of slowly adapting pulmonary stretch receptors. *Respir Physiol* 2001; **125**: 17–31.

27 Sudo T, Hayashi F, Nishino T. Responses of tracheobronchial receptors to inhaled furosemide in anesthetized rats. *Am J Respir Crit Care Med* 2000; **162**: 971–5.

28 Hanacek J, Korpas J. Modification of the intensity of the expiration reflex during short-term inflation of the lungs in rabbits. *Physiol Bohemoslov* 1982; **31**: 169–74.

29 Nishino T, Sugimori K, Hiraga K, Hond Y. Influence of CPAP on reflex responses to tracheal irritation in anesthetized humans. *J Appl Physiol* 1989; **67**: 954–8.

30 Hanacek J, Davies A, Widdicombe JG. Influence of lung stretch receptors on the cough reflex in rabbits. *Respiration* 1984; **45**: 161–8.

31 Atzori L, Bannenberg G, Corriga AM, Lou YP, Lundberg JM, Ryrfeldt A, Moldeus P. Sulfur dioxide-induced bronchoconstriction via ruthenium red-sensitive activation of sensory nerves. *Respiration* 1992; **59**: 272–8.

32 Wang AL, Blackford TL, Lee LY. Vagal bronchopulmonary C-fibers and acute ventilatory response to inhaled irritants. *Respir Physiol* 1996; **104**: 231–9.

33 Ezure K, Tanaka I. Lung inflation inhibits rapidly adapting receptor relay neurons in the rat. *Neuroreport* 2000; **11**: 1709–12.

34 Lee LY, Pisarri TE. Afferent properties and reflex functions of bronchopulmonary C-fibers. *Respir Physiol* 2001; **125**: 47–65.

35 Ma QP, Woolf CJ. Involvement of neurokinin receptors in the induction but not the maintenance of mechanical allodynia in rat flexor motoneurones. *J Physiol* 1995; **486**: 769–77.

36 Ho CY, Gu Q, Hong JL, Lee LY. Prostaglandin E(2) enhances chemical and mechanical sensitivities of pulmonary C fibers in the rat. *Am J Respir Crit Care Med* 2000; **162**: 528–33.

37 Baluk P, Nadel JA, McDonald DM. Substance P-immunoreactive sensory axons in the rat respiratory tract: a quantitative study of their distribution and role in neurogenic inflammation. *J Comp Neurol* 1992; **319**: 586–98.

38 Lundberg JM, Hokfelt T, Martling CR, Saria A, Cuello C. Substance P-immunoreactive sensory nerves in the lower respiratory tract of various mammals including man. *Cell Tissue Res* 1984; **235**: 251–61.

39 Hunter DD, Undem BJ. Identification and substance P content of vagal afferent neurons innervating the epithelium of the guinea-pig trachea. *Am J Respir Crit Care Med* 1999; **159**: 1943–8.

40 Myers AC, Kajekar R, Undem BJ. Allergic inflammation-induced neuropeptide production in rapidly adapting afferent nerves in guinea-pig airways. *Am J Physiol Lung Cell Mol Physiol* 2002; **282**: L775–81.

41 Dey RD, Altemus JB, Zervos I, Hoffpauir J. Origin and colocalization of CGRP- and SP-reactive nerves in cat airway epithelium. *J Appl Physiol* 1990; **68**: 770–8.

42 Barnes PJ. Neurogenic inflammation in the airways. *Respir Physiol* 2001; **125**: 145–54.

43 Forsberg K, Karlsson JA. Cough induced by stimulation of capsaicin-sensitive sensory neurons in conscious guinea-pigs. *Acta Physiol Scand* 1986; **128**: 319–20.

44 Choudry NB, Fuller RW, Pride NB. Sensitivity of the human cough reflex: effect of inflammatory mediators prostaglandin E2, bradykinin, and histamine. *Am Rev Respir Dis* 1989; **140**: 137–41.

45 Mazzone SB, Mori N, Canning BJ. Bradykinin-induced cough in conscious guinea-pigs. *Am J Respir Crit Care Med* 2002; **165**: A773.

46 Bolser DC, DeGennaro FC, O'Reilly S, McLeod RL, Hey JA. Central antitussive activity of the NK1 and NK2 tachykinin receptor antagonists, CP-99,994 and SR 48968, in the guinea-pig and cat. *Br J Pharmacol* 1997; **121**: 165–70.

47 Tatar M, Webber SE, Widdicombe JG. Lung C-fibre receptor activation and defensive reflexes in anaesthetized cats. *J Physiol* 1988; **402**: 411–20.

48 Nishino T, Tagaito Y, Isono S. Cough and other reflexes on irritation of airway mucosa in man. *Pulm Pharmacol* 1996; **9**: 285–92.

49 Roberts AM, Kaufman MP, Baker DG, Brown JK, Coleridge HM, Coleridge JC. Reflex tracheal contraction induced by stimulation of bronchial C-fibers in dogs. *J Appl Physiol* 1981; **51**: 485–93.

50 Davis B, Roberts AM, Coleridge HM, Coleridge JC. Reflex tracheal gland secretion evoked by stimulation of bronchial C-fibers in dogs. *J Appl Physiol* 1982; **53**: 985–91.

51 Pisarri TE, Coleridge JC, Coleridge HM. Capsaicin-induced bronchial vasodilation in dogs: central and peripheral neural mechanisms. *J Appl Physiol* 1993; **74**: 259–66.

52 Bergren DR. Enhanced lung C-fiber responsiveness in sensitized adult guinea-pigs exposed to chronic tobacco smoke. *J Appl Physiol* 2001; **91**: 1645–54.

53 Hutchings HA, Morris S, Eccles R, Jawad MS. Voluntary suppression of cough induced by inhalation of capsaicin in healthy volunteers. *Respir Med* 1993; **87**: 379–82.

54 Szolcsányi J. Actions of capsaicin on sensory receptors. In: Wood JN, ed. *Capsaicin in the Study of Pain*. London: Academic Press, 1993: 1–27.

55 Yu J. Spectrum of myelinated pulmonary afferents. *Am J Physiol Regul Integr Comp Physiol* 2000; **279**: R2142–8.

56 Bergren DR, Peterson DF. Identification of vagal sensory receptors in the rat lung: are there subtypes of slowly adapting receptors? *J Physiol* 1993; **464**: 681–98.

57 Lundberg JM, Saria A, Brodin E, Rosell S, Folkers K. A substance P antagonist inhibits vagally induced increase in vascular permeability and bronchial smooth muscle contraction in the guinea-pig. *Proc Natl Acad Sci USA* 1983; **80**: 1120–4.

58 Kuo HP, Rohde JA, Tokuyama K, Barnes PJ, Rogers DF. Capsaicin and sensory neuropeptide stimulation of goblet cell secretion in guinea-pig trachea. *J Physiol* 1990; **431**: 629–41.

59 Manzini S. Bronchodilatation by tachykinins and capsaicin in the mouse main bronchus. *Br J Pharmacol* 1992; **105**: 968–72.

60 Piedimonte G, Hoffman JI, Husseini WK, Snider RM, Desai MC, Nadel JA. NK1 receptors mediate neurogenic inflammatory increase in blood flow in rat airways. *J Appl Physiol* 1993; **74**: 2462–8.

61 Baluk P, Bertrand C, Geppetti P, McDonald DM, Nadel JA. NK1 receptors mediate leukocyte adhesion in neurogenic inflammation in the rat trachea. *Am J Physiol* 1995; **268**: L263–L269.

62 Ricciardolo FL, Rado V, Fabbri LM, Sterk PJ, Di Maria GU, Geppetti P. Bronchoconstriction induced by citric acid inhalation in guinea-pigs: role of tachykinins, bradykinin, and nitric oxide. *Am J Respir Crit Care Med* 1999; **159**: 557–62.

63 Canning BJ, Reynolds SM, Anukwu LU, Kajekar R, Myers AC. Endogenous neurokinins facilitate synaptic neurotransmission in guinea-pig airway parasympathetic ganglia *Am J Physiol Regul Integr Comp Physiol* 2002; **283**: R320–30.

64 Matsumoto S, Takeda M, Saiki C, Takahashi T, Ojima K. Effects of tachykinins on rapidly adapting pulmonary stretch receptors and total lung resistance in anesthetized, artificially ventilated rabbits. *J Pharmacol Exp Ther* 1997; **283**: 1026–31.

65 Ujiie Y, Sekizawa K, Aikawa T, Sasaki H. Evidence for substance P as an endogenous substance causing cough in guinea-pigs. *Am Rev Respir Dis* 1993; **148**: 1628–32.

66 Bolser DC, DeGennaro FC, O'Reilly S, Hey JA, Chapman RW. Pharmacological studies of allergic cough in the guinea-pig. *Eur J Pharmacol* 1995; **277**: 159–64.

67 Sekizawa K, Ebihara T, Sasaki H. Role of substance P in cough during bronchoconstriction in awake guinea-pigs. *Am J Respir Crit Care Med* 1995; **151**: 815–21.

68 Yasumitsu R, Hirayama Y, Imai T, Miyayasu K, Hiroi J. Effects of specific tachykinin receptor antagonists on citric acid-induced cough and bronchoconstriction in unanesthetized guinea-pigs. *Eur J Pharmacol* 1996; **300**: 215–9.

69 Kohrogi H, Nadel JA, Malfroy B, Gorman C, Bridenbaugh R, Patton JS, Borson DB. Recombinant human enkephalinase (neutral endopeptidase) prevents cough induced by tachykinins in awake guinea-pigs. *J Clin Invest* 1989; **84**: 781–6.

70 Russell JA, Lai-Fook SJ. Reflex bronchoconstriction induced by capsaicin in the dog. *J Appl Physiol* 1979; **47**: 961–7.

71 Ichinose M, Inoue H, Miura M, Yafuso N, Nogami H, Takishima T. Possible sensory receptor of nonadrenergic inhibitory nervous system. *J Appl Physiol* 1987; **63**: 923–9.

72 Fuller RW, Dixon CM, Barnes PJ. Bronchoconstrictor response to inhaled capsaicin in humans. *J Appl Physiol* 1985; **58**: 1080–4.

73 Baker B, Peatfield AC, Richardson PS. Nervous control of mucin secretion into human bronchi. *J Physiol* 1985; **365**: 297–305.

74 Rogers DF, Barnes PJ. Opioid inhibition of neurally mediated mucus secretion in human bronchi. *Lancet* 1989; **1**: 930–2.

75 Ellis JL, Sham JS, Undem BJ. Tachykinin-independent effects of capsaicin on smooth muscle in human isolated bronchi. *Am J Respir Crit Care Med* 1997; **155**: 751–5.

76 Jia YX, Sekizawa K, Sasaki H. Cholinergic influence on the sensitivity of cough reflex in awake guinea-pigs. *J Auton Pharmacol* 1998; **18**: 257–61.

77 Lowry R, Wood A, Johnson T, Higenbottam T. Antitussive properties of inhaled bronchodilators on induced cough. *Chest* 1988; **93**: 1186–9.

78 Woolf CJ, Salter MW. Neuronal plasticity: increasing the gain in pain. *Science* 2000; **288**: 1765–9.

79 Jordan D. Central nervous pathways and control of the airways. *Respir Physiol* 2001; **125**: 67–81.

80 Mazzone SB, Canning BJ. Synergistic interactions between airway afferent nerve subtypes mediating reflex bronchospasm in guinea-pigs. *Am J Physiol Regul Integr Comp Physiol* 2002; **283**: R86–98.

81 Mutoh T, Bonham AC, Joad JP. Substance P in the nucleus of the solitary tract augments bronchopulmonary C fiber reflex output. *Am J Physiol* 2000; **279**: R1215–23.

## Other modulatory influences on the cough motor pattern

Respiratory neurones of the ventrolateral medulla (BÖT/rVRG) mutually interact with other respiratory and non-respiratory modulated neurones in the medulla, pons and cerebellum to form a larger dynamic network. Results from neuronal recordings and lesioning studies are consistent with a modulatory role of neurones in the medullary midline (i.e. raphe nuclei and adjoining reticular formation) and lateral tegmental field, pontine respiratory group and cerebellum on generation of the cough pattern by BÖT/rVRG [7,21–25]. Additional studies are needed to elucidate pathways and connections between these regions and their specific modulatory roles.

## Cough is a gated process

The work of Bolser et al. [5] involved perturbation of the cough motor pattern and provided evidence for a gating mechanism in the tracheobronchial cough pattern generator. The location and identity of the gate are unknown. The gating mechanism is postulated to regulate the behaviour of the cough network by raising its excitability above a threshold (analogous to apnoeic threshold for breathing). Single coughs result from transient excitation of the gating mechanism, whereas repetitive coughing can occur as long as the cough threshold is exceeded. Furthermore, this gating mechanism regulates the magnitude of expiratory motor activation during cough.

## Evidence supporting the gating mechanism

Antitussive drugs do not inhibit tracheobronchial cough by suppression of the entire central cough generation mechanism, rather they have very specific effects on various components of this system. For example, low doses of antitussive drugs (administered via the vertebral artery) specifically decreased the number of coughs elicited per stimulus trial and the expiratory muscle electromyogram burst amplitude during tracheobronchial cough [5]. Inspiratory or expiratory phase durations and inspiratory burst amplitude were unchanged by these low doses of antitussive drugs.

Therefore, antitussive drugs must inhibit tracheobronchial cough number by an action 'upstream' from the components of the pattern generator that regulate cough cycle duration (Fig. 17.3a,b). This aspect of the model accounts for the fact that antitussive drugs do not decrease breathing frequency at doses that inhibit cough [5,26].

We propose that afferent input to the pattern generator is transmitted by cough receptor relay interneurones and pump cells through the gating mechanism (Fig. 17.3a). Direct suppression of pump cell activity by antitussive drugs is unlikely because in our study these drugs had no effect on eupnoeic respiratory phase durations or integrated diaphragm EMG amplitude [5]. These drugs can also selectively decrease expiratory motor activation during cough without reducing inspiratory motor activation. These findings do not support an action of antitussive drugs on cough receptor interneurones in the NTS. A caveat to this argument is that the population of NTS cough relay neurones may be composed of subsets that separately regulate the behaviour of inspiratory and expiratory motor pathways. The expiratory subset could have a high relative sensitivity to codeine. To our knowledge, no evidence exists supporting the existence of functional subsets of this population of NTS neurones. As such, we have depicted in Fig. 17.3(a) what we believe to be the simplest hypothesis. In this model, pump cells, NTS cough receptor neurones and the core of the cough network that controls cough phase durations do not participate in the gating mechanism (Fig. 17.3a).

## Proposed interaction of the gating mechanism with elements of the cough network

The model in Fig. 17.1 is specific to tracheobronchial cough and does not address any differences between this type of cough and that elicited from stimulation of the larynx. Furthermore, the model is based on the results of experiments in which single coughs were generated in each stimulus trial, whereas the gating mechanism (Fig. 17.3) is based largely on experiments in which repetitive coughing was produced during each stimulus. The differences in how elements participating in this network may interact during single and repetitive coughs are currently unknown.

Reconciliation of the gating mechanism with the

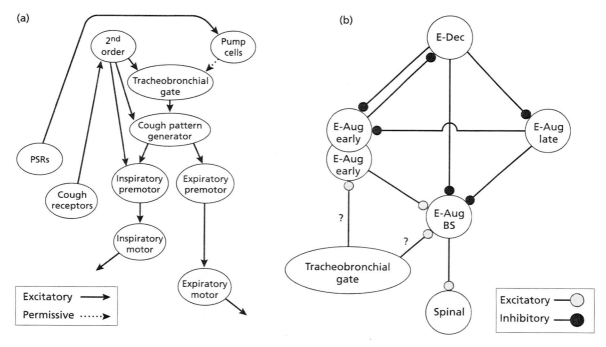

**Fig. 17.3** Proposed relationship of the tracheobronchial gate with elements of the cough pattern generator. (a) A generalized representation of the relationship of the gate to the cough pattern generator. (b) Potential synaptic relationships of the gate with elements of the cough network that control expiratory motor drive. Abbreviations as in Table 17.1.

detailed model of the cough network is challenging because the gate is a functional entity of unknown anatomical location. In essence, it is difficult to connect functional elements with specifically identified components of a model in the absence of specific knowledge of synaptic relationships between them. This problem in unifying a functional model with a specific network model highlights an important concept: namely, that it is at least as important to determine how the gating mechanism interacts with known elements of the cough pattern generator as it is to identify the neuronal groups that make up the gate itself. Our recent work has been aimed at determining how the gating mechanism interacts with neurones that control expiratory motor drive during cough [27]. We have not proposed a model of the specific synaptic mechanisms by which the gate is proposed to control the number of coughs per stimulus trial; more information is needed regarding the identity and activity patterns of neurones participating in the gate mechanism before this will become possible.

According to the model in Fig. 17.3(a,b), suppression of expiratory motor activity by antitussive drugs is

accomplished by inhibition of elements of the tracheobronchial gating system, preventing the excitatory effects of cough receptors from reaching bulbospinal premotor expiratory neurones. There currently is no evidence in the literature indicating the mechanism by which antitussive drugs suppress medullary or spinal expiratory motor activity during cough. Jakus *et al.* [28] have shown that the tracheobronchial cough-related discharge of caudal VRG expiratory neurones is reduced after systemic administration of codeine. These findings could be explained either by an inhibitory action of codeine on medullary expiratory neurones or by an action of this drug on neurones presynaptic to medullary expiratory neurones.

The determination of the mechanism by which antitussive drugs decrease the activity of expiratory motor pathways during cough represents a critical piece of information in determining how the gating mechanism interacts with specific elements of the cough network. We have obtained evidence that the responsiveness of expiratory motor pathways to other inputs is relatively unchanged after doses of codeine sufficient to almost completely eliminate cough [27]. In anaesthetized cats, we determined the response of abdominal expiratory EMG to cough and expiratory threshold loading (ETL). Expiratory loading results in increased activity of caudal ventral respiratory group expiratory premotor neurones and expiratory spinal motoneurones [29]. Central (intravertebral arterial) administration of codeine significantly suppressed expiratory muscle activation during tracheobronchial cough, but had no effect on the response to ETL [27]. This selective effect of codeine supports the concept that expiratory motor pathways activated by both stimuli are not directly inhibited by the drug. These data are consistent with the hypothesis that codeine inhibits one or more elements presynaptic to expiratory premotor and motoneurones. In the cough network (Fig. 17.1), a subset of 'core' expiratory augmenting neurones (E-Aug early), caudal medullary expiratory premotor neurones (E-Aug), and spinal expiratory motoneurones all contribute to increased expiratory muscle activity during cough, as well as the temporal regulation of the expulsive phase. Based on our evidence, we propose that the tracheobronchial gate mechanism is presynaptic to the 'core' early E-Aug and caudal VRG premotor neurones (Fig. 17.3b). We also hypothesize that there are, at least, two subpopulations of early E-Aug neurones. One subpopulation is involved in the regulation of expiratory phase durations during cough and the other group receives excitatory input from the tracheobronchial gate and in turn excites E-Aug bulbospinal (BS) neurones. This hypothesis is supported by evidence that the expiratory phase duration and magnitude of expulsive motor drive during cough are regulated independently [30].

The proposed interaction between the gate and the cough network shown in Fig. 17.3(b) is subject to several caveats. The model must be further tested by direct determination of the excitability of selected elements of the expiratory network during codeine administration. A presynaptic action of codeine would be supported by an unchanged excitability of E Aug BS neurones in the presence of this drug. However, if the excitability of E-Aug BS neurones were decreased by codeine, the model would have to be revised to incorporate these neurones in the gating mechanism.

## Identity of the gate elements

The gate could represent single or multiple groups of interneurones interposed between NTS cough receptor relay neurones and the cough network. Alternatively, suppression of selected presynaptic terminals of NTS cough receptor relay neurones by antitussive drugs could account for some of our observations. Candidate populations of neurones may exist in the raphe nuclei [24], pons [23], interposed nucleus of the cerebellum [25], reticular formation [31] and/or tegmental field [22]. We propose that some elements of the gating mechanism participate in excitation of expiratory premotor neurones during cough. Whether this excitation occurs by monosynaptic or multisynaptic interactions is currently unknown. The excitability of neurones participating in the gating mechanism should be decreased by antitussive drugs, leading to disfacilitation of elements of the cough network with which they interact. Of the candidate locations listed above, the most information is available on the effect of the cerebellum on the cough motor pattern [25]. Cerebellectomy or lesion of the interposed nucleus can elicit relative suppression of expiratory motor discharge during cough as well as a decrease in cough number [25]. However, cerebellectomy does not completely eliminate cough as is commonly observed after administration of antitussive drugs [32]. The role of the cerebellum in mediating proposed functions of the gate should be clarified by further investigation.

*Acknowledgements*
Work presented in this review was supported by National Heart, Lung, and Blood Institute grant HL-49813 and State of Florida Department of Health Biomedical Research grant BM-040.

## References

1 Shannon R, Bolser DC, Lindsey BG. Neural control of coughing and sneezing. In: Miller AD, Bianchi AL, Bishop BP, eds. *Neural Control of Breathing*. Boca Raton: CRC Press, 1996: 215–24.
2 Shannon R, Baekey DM, Morris KF, Lindsey BG. Brainstem respiratory networks and cough. *Pulm Pharmacol* 1997; 9: 343–7.
3 Shannon R, Morris KF, Lindsey BG. Ventrolateral medullary respiratory network and a model of cough

motor pattern generation. *J Appl Physiol* 1998; **84**: 2020–35.

4 Shannon R, Baekey DM, Morris KF, Li Z, Lindsey BG. Functional connectivity among ventrolateral medullary respiratory neurons and responses during fictive cough in the cat. *J Physiol* 2000; **525**: 207–24.

5 Bolser DC, Hey JA, Chapman RW. Influence of central antitussive drugs on the cough motor pattern. *J Appl Physiol* 1999; **86**: 1017–24.

6 Engelhorn R, Weller E. Zentrale representation hustenwirksamer Afferenzen in der Medulla oblongata der Katze. *Pflug Arch* 1965; **284**: 224–39.

7 Jakus J, Tomori Z, Boselova L, Nagyova B, Kubinec V. Respiration and airway reflexes after transversal brain stem lesions in cats. *Physiol Bohemoslov* 1987; **36**: 329–40.

8 Dawid-Milner MS, Lara JP, Milan A, Gonzalez-Baron S. Activity of inspiratory neurons of the ambiguous complex during cough in the spontaneously breathing decerebrate cat. *Exp Physiol* 1993; **78**: 835–8.

9 Oku Y, Tanaka I, Ezure K. Activity of bulbar respiratory neurons during fictive coughing and swallowing in the decerebrate cat. *J Physiol* 1994; **480**: 309–84.

10 Gestreau C, Milano S, Bianchi AL, Grelot L. Activity of dorsal respiratory group inspiratory neurons during laryngeal-induced fictive coughing and swallowing in decerebrate cats. *Exp Brain Res* 1996; **108**: 247–56.

11 Bongianni F, Mutolo D, Fontana GA, Pantaleo T. Discharge patterns of Botzinger complex neurons during cough in the cat. *Am J Physiol* 1998; **274**: R1015–24.

12 Baekey DM, Morris KF, Gestreau C, Lindsey BG, Shannon R. Medullary respiratory neurones and control of laryngeal motoneurones during fictive eupnoea and cough in the cat. *J Physiol* 2001; **534**: 565–81.

13 Tomori Z, Widdicombe JG. Muscular, bronchomotor, and cardiovascular reflexes elicited by mechanical stimulation of the respiratory tract. *J Physiol* 1969; **200**: 25–49.

14 Widdicombe JG. Afferent receptors in the airways and cough. *Respir Physiol* 1998; **114**: 5–15.

15 Balis UJ, Morris KF, Koleski J, Lindsey BG. Simulations of ventrolateral medullary neural network for respiratory rhythmogenesis inferred from spike train cross-correlation. *Biol Cybern* 1994; **70**: 311–27.

16 Hayashi F, Coles SK, McCrimmon DR. Respiratory neurons mediating the Breuer–Hering reflex prolongation of expiration in rat. *J Neurosci* 1996; **16**: 6526–36.

17 Ezure K, Tanaka I. Pump neurons of the nucleus of the solitary tract project widely to the medulla. *Neurosci Lett* 1996; **215**: 123–6.

18 Bolser DC, Davenport PW. Volume–timing relationships

19 Hanecek J, Davies A, Widdicombe JG. Influence of lung stretch receptors on the cough reflex in rabbits. *Respiration* 1984; **45**: 161–8.

20 Sant'Ambrogio G, Sant'Ambrogio FB, Davies A. Airway receptors in cough. *Bull Eur Physiopathol Respir* 1984; **20**: 43–7.

21 Jakus A, Stransky A, Poliacek I, Barani H, Boselova L. Effects of medullary midline lesions on cough and other airway reflexes in anaesthetized cats. *Physiol Res* 1998; **47**: 203–13.

22 Jakus J, Stransky A, Poliacek I, Barani H, Boselova L. Kainic acid lesions to the lateral tegmental field of medulla: effects on cough, expiration and aspiration reflexes in anesthetized cats. *Physiol Res* 2000; **49**: 387–98.

23 Baekey DM, Morris KF, Li Z, Nuding SC, Lindsey BG, Shannon R. Concurrent changes in pontine respiratory group neuron activities during fictive coughing. *FASEB J* 1999; **13**: A824.

24 Baekey DM, Morris KF, Nuding SC, Segers LS, Lindsey BG, Shannon R. Raphe neuron activity during fictive coughing. *FASEB J* 2002; **16**: 628.

25 Xu F, Frazier DT, Zhang Z, Shannon R. Influence of the cerebellum on the cough motor pattern. *J Appl Physiol* 1997; **83**: 391–7.

26 May AJ, Widdicombe JG. Depression of the cough reflex by pentobarbitone and some opium derivatives. *Br J Pharmacol* 1954; **9**: 335–40.

27 Bolser DC, Pampo CA, Ruble MA, Golder FJ. Evidence for disfacilitation of expiratory premotor pathways by antitussive drugs. *Am J Respir Crit Care Med* 2001; **163**: A629.

28 Jakus J, Tomori Z, Stransky A, Boselova L. Bulbar respiratory activity during defensive airways reflexes in cats. *Acta Physiol Hung* 1987; **70**: 245–54.

29 Baker JP, Frazier DT. Response of abdominal muscle to graded mechanical loads. *J Neurosci Res* 1985; **13**: 581–9.

30 Bolser DC, Davenport PW. Determinants of cough cycle duration in the cat. *FASEB J* 2001; **13**: 798.

31 Billig I, Foris JM, Enquist LW, Card JP, Yates BJ. Definition of neuronal circuitry controlling the activity of phrenic and abdominal motoneurons in the ferret using recombinant strains of pseudorabies virus. *J Neurosci* 2000; **20**: 7446–54.

32 Bolser DC, DeGennaro FC, O'Reilly S, McLeod RL, Hey JA. Central antitussive activity of the tachykinin receptor antagonists CP 99,994 and SR 48968 in the guinea pig and cat. *Br J Pharmacol* 1997; **121**: 165–70.

# 18 Plasticity of vagal afferent fibres mediating cough

*Marian Kollarik & Bradley J. Undem*

## Introduction

The coughing associated with acute respiratory tract infections and chronic airway diseases including bronchitis, asthma and chronic obstructive pulmonary disease (COPD) likely arises as a result of production of various tussigenic agonists in the airway wall. In addition, in these disorders as well as in cough related to gastro-oesophageal reflux (GOR), angiotensin-converting enzyme inhibitor treatment and idiopathic cough, the *sensitivity* of cough reflex pathways may be increased (Fig. 18.1). That is to say, cough is evoked by stimuli that are normally subthreshold for initiating the cough reflex. The increase in cough reflex sensitivity has been experimentally demonstrated in numerous studies. However, the molecular mechanisms by which this sensitization occurs and the structures involved remain unknown. One likely structure affected by processes resulting in increased sensitivity is the vagal afferent nerve.

Afferent nerves are not static entities, but rather are constantly changing in structure and activity. In general terms the change in structure and function of nerves is referred to as neuroplasticity [1]. In this chapter we use the term 'plasticity' rather liberally to denote changes in neuronal excitability, receptor expression, transmitter chemistry and the structure of the nerve. Regrettably, little is known about vagal nerve plasticity in human diseases associated with cough reflex hypersensitivity. Knowledge in this area has been obtained only by inference from studies on the somatosensory system, and from functional and electrophysiological studies of vagal afferent nerves using various cellular, tissue and animal models. With respect to the somatosensory system, the general concept of cough reflex hypersensitivity finds its analogy in the heightened sensitivity of pain pathways, i.e. hyperalgesia and allodynia associated, for example, with inflammation. A mechanistic understanding of the cough reflex plasticity may ultimately suggest novel therapeutic strategies aimed at normalizing the heightened reflex associated with chronic cough. In this chapter we focus on those aspects of neuroplasticity that are likely to contribute to the increases in cough sensitivity. Although not discussed in this chapter, it should be noted that increases in cough sensitivity may also occur independently of changes in nerve structure and function. This is exemplified by the convergent interactions among different types of airway afferent nerves, and is discussed elsewhere in this volume (Chapter 16).

## Clinical studies on cough reflex sensitivity

Cough reflex sensitivity can be quantified by several methods [2,3]. In general, these methods are based on the determination of the amount of tussigenic agent required to evoke a predetermined cough response. The most common tussive agents used are capsaicin and citric acid. The use of either of these agents has revealed that some diseases are associated with an appreciable increase in cough reflex sensitivity (i.e. a decrease in the amount of tussigenic agent required to evoke cough). Table 18.1 summarizes some studies on cough sensitivity [4–11].

Cough sensitivity studies need to be cautiously interpreted, because cough reflex hypersensitivity may be

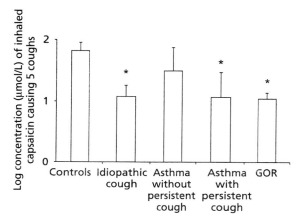

**Fig. 18.1** Cough reflex sensitivity to inhaled capsaicin in normal subjects and in patients with diseases presenting with cough. Cough threshold was determined as the concentration of capsaicin causing at least 5 coughs ($C_5$). Note that cough threshold is decreased in the asthma associated with persistent cough but not in the asthma without persistent cough (see also Table 18.1). *$P < 0.05$ compared with control. Data from [2].

stimulus specific. It is possible that more than one subtype of vagal afferents, each with its own stimulus specificity, are involved in the initiating of cough. Although capsaicin is a useful tool to evaluate an increase in cough reflexes mediated by nociceptive-type nerves, it is probably much less useful for the study of cough reflexes initiated by mechanical stimulation of nerve fibres with the rapidly adapting receptor (RAR) phenotype. As discussed below, the mechanisms of afferent nerve plasticity depend on the nerve phenotype. It would not be surprising, therefore, to find a clinical setting in which the cough response to mechanical stimuli is altered whereas the capsaicin-induced cough is unaltered (or vice versa). It will be important in the future to design protocols such that the sensitivity of cough to disparate stimuli can be quantitatively evaluated. This will be necessary to address the hypothesis of specificity in the changes of cough sensitivity associated with various pathologies.

## Afferent nerve fibres associated with the cough reflex

Detailed information on the characteristics of the subtypes of afferent nerve fibres involved in cough can be found elsewhere in this volume (Chapter 16). In

**Table 18.1** Studies showing increase in cough reflex sensitivity in the disorders presenting with cough.

| Disorder | Tussive agent | Cough reflex sensitivity | Reference |
|---|---|---|---|
| Asthma with persistent cough | Capsaicin | Increased | [2] |
| | | Increased | [4] |
| Asthma without persistent cough | Capsaicin | Unaffected | [2] |
| Asthma (unselected populations) | Capsaicin | Unaffected | [5] |
| | | Increased | [6] |
| | Tartaric acid | Unaffected | [7] |
| Gastro-oesophageal reflux | Capsaicin | Increased | [2] |
| | | Increased | [8] |
| Chronic obstructive pulmonary disease | Capsaicin | Increased | [6] |
| | Citric acid | Increased | [9] |
| Acute respiratory infections | Capsaicin | Increased | [10] |
| | Citric acid | Increased | [11] |

the context of the present chapter, however, we would like to stress the idea that activation of at least two fundamentally distinct types of afferent fibres can lead to cough in animal models. The 'cough fibre' described by the classical studies of Widdicombe and colleagues is a myelinated fibre that conducts action potentials in the Aδ range [12]. These fibres are very sensitive to mechanical perturbation. A defining characteristic of these fibres is the rapid adaptation of their action potential discharge to a prolonged suprathreshold mechanical stimulus. Accordingly, these fibres are commonly referred to as rapidly adapting receptors or RARs. The other fibre type involved in certain types of cough is the nociceptive fibre (nociceptor). These fibres are relatively insensitive to mechanical stimulation, but can be activated by inflammatory mediators, acid, changes in osmolarity, and chemicals such as capsaicin and bradykinin [13,14]. Nociceptors are typically characterized by non-myelinated axons (i.e. C-fibres); however, nociceptors also comprise a large number of Aδ-fibres [13]. It is worth emphasizing that in guinea-pig airways, nociceptive Aδ-fibres differ from RAR Aδ-fibres in that the latter are exquisitely mechanically sensitive and do not respond directly to capsaicin [13].

The RAR fibres and nociceptors are not only activated by different types of stimuli, but also appear to be situated in different compartments within the extrathoracic airway. In guinea-pig airways, circumstantial evidence supports the hypothesis that the nociceptive population of nerves appears to be the primary nerve type that extends into the epithelium, whereas the RAR type of fibres are situated in the submucosa just beneath the epithelium [15]. These two types of afferent nerves may also have different embryological origins. This speculation is based on the observation that, in guinea-pig airways, the RAR-type fibres arise from cell bodies situated in the nodose ganglia, whereas the nociceptive C and Aδ-fibres are derived from cell bodies in the jugular (supranodose) ganglia [13]. Embryologically, neurones within the nodose ganglia are thought to be derived from the epibranchial placodes, whereas the jugular ganglion neurones are derived from the neural crest as are the dorsal root ganglia neurones [16]. Thus, based on the nature of the activating stimuli, location within the airways and perhaps embryological origin, the RAR fibres and nociceptive fibres represent quite distinct subpopulations of airway afferent nerves in guinea-pig trachea/bronchus.

The characteristics and mechanisms of plasticity will likely therefore differ between these two general types of fibre.

## Plasticity

We use the term plasticity here to denote change in the neuronal excitability, receptor expression, neurotransmitter chemistry and nerve structure. As such, plasticity *per se* denotes change, and may lead to either increases or decreases in overall responsiveness of the afferent nerves. We have chosen to focus our discussion on those aspects of plasticity that would most likely lead to an increase in afferent nerve activity and the sensitivity of cough reflex.

### Excitability

*General principles of excitability*
Activators of afferent nerves (mechanical displacement, certain chemicals, changes in osmolarity, etc.) interact with the nerve terminals in a manner that leads to a membrane depolarization. This initial terminal membrane depolarization is referred to as the generator potential. The generator potential is electrotonically conducted along the axon until it reaches the so-called active zone characterized by a high concentration of voltage-gated sodium channels. If in the active zone the magnitude of membrane depolarization is sufficient (i.e. the threshold for action potential formation is reached), action potential discharge is evoked. The greater the amplitude of generator potential, the higher is the frequency of action potential discharge. These are theoretical considerations inasmuch as neither the structure nor location of the generator region and active zones has been described in vagal afferent nerve terminals. However, these mechanisms have been worked out in considerable detail in somatosensory systems and are likely to be shared with vagal afferent nerves [17].

Many chemical mediators affect the electrophysiological properties of the afferent nerve membrane without causing a generator potential and activating the nerve. One might say that these are not activators of the nerve, but rather are better characterized as modulators of nerve excitability. It is possible that a given stimulus may act both as an activator (causing a generator potential) and as a modulator of neuronal excitability. As discussed below, this is exemplified by some G-protein-coupled receptor agonists such as bradykinin. An obvious case of nerve modulation by prostaglandin $E_2$ ($PGE_2$) is illustrated in Fig. 18.2. In this nociceptive A$\delta$-fibre, bradykinin causes only modest discharge of ac-

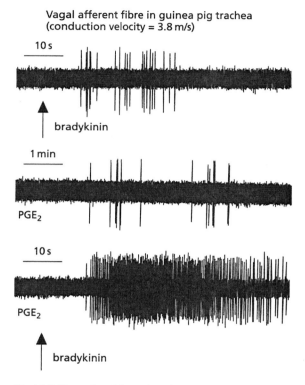

**Fig. 18.2** Examples of the action of activator and modulator of nerve excitability. Activation of airway nociceptive afferent nerve fibre by bradykinin (activator) and the sensitizing effect of prostaglandin $E_2$ ($PGE_2$) (modulator). Extracellular recording was made from the nociceptive A$\delta$-fibre projecting to the trachea in guinea-pig isolated perfused airway/nerve preparation. The tissue was pretreated with indomethacin (3 μmol/L) to suppress endogenous $PGE_2$ production. Upper trace: Transient (~3 s) administration of bradykinin (0.3 μmol/L, 500 μL) directly over the receptive field evoked a short delayed burst of action potential discharge. The delay in the onset of bradykinin-induced response is a consistent phenomenon. Middle trace: The tissue was incubated with $PGE_2$ (10 μmol/L, 10 min) that caused by itself no activation. Note the change in time scale. Lower trace: $PGE_2$-enhanced response to subsequent challenge with bradykinin.

tion potentials. Upon application of $PGE_2$, the nerve is not activated, but the activation by bradykinin is dramatically enhanced.

Mechanisms potentially leading to increased excitablity of afferent nerves are schematically illustrated in Fig. 18.3. The excitability of a cough fibre may be increased by processes that lead to an increase in the amplitude of the generator potential, an increase in the efficiency of electronic conduction, and/or a decrease in the membrane potential change required for action potential formation. The amplitude of the generator potential can be increased by increasing the probability of a stimulus opening the ion channels responsible for the generator potential and/or by increasing the average time the channel stays open. Both of these characteristics can be affected by a modulator acting through various intracellular signalling pathways. The amplitude of generator potential can also be increased by an increase in the membrane resistance, as the voltage change is a product of the current and membrane resistance (Ohm's law).

Decremental electrotonic conduction of generator potential to the active zone is governed by the time constant and the space constant. The time constant is a product of membrane resistance and capacitance, and characterizes the rate of membrane potential decay with time. The space constant depends on membrane resistance and resistance of the axoplasm, and characterizes the rate of membrane potential decay with distance. A modulator can affect these properties by, for example, increasing the membrane resistance. Such an increase in membrane resistance increases the excitability by the increased efficacy of generator potential conduction to the active zone. The extent to which these mechanisms participate in excitability changes will depend on the distance between the generator and active zones in the afferent nerve.

The membrane potential change required for action potential formation could be decreased by an increase in resting membrane potential and/or a decrease of the threshold for action potential discharge. Resting membrane potential largely depends on the potassium channels. The threshold for action potential formation is regulated by the number and activity of voltage-gated sodium channels in the active zone. In addition, neuronal excitability can be modulated by processes that affect the active (action potential) properties of the nerve. For example, a modulator may affect membrane repolarization in such a fashion that the refractory

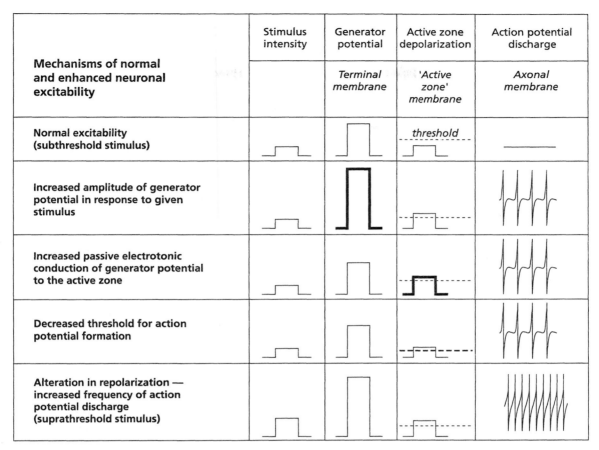

| Mechanisms of normal and enhanced neuronal excitability | Stimulus intensity | Generator potential | Active zone depolarization | Action potential discharge |
|---|---|---|---|---|
| | | *Terminal membrane* | *'Active zone' membrane* | *Axonal membrane* |
| **Normal excitability (subthreshold stimulus)** | | | *threshold* | |
| **Increased amplitude of generator potential in response to given stimulus** | | | | |
| **Increased passive electrotonic conduction of generator potential to the active zone** | | | | |
| **Decreased threshold for action potential formation** | | | | |
| **Alteration in repolarization — increased frequency of action potential discharge (suprathreshold stimulus)** | | | | |

Fig. 18.3 Theoretical mechanisms of normal and enhanced neuronal excitability. Stimulus interaction with the receptive field membrane results in membrane depolarization (generator potential). This depolarization propagates passively to the active zone which is responsible for initiation of action potentials. If the membrane depolarization at the active zone is of sufficient magnitude action potential discharge follows. Excitability of the nerve terminal could be enhanced by several mechanisms: (i) increase in the amplitude of the generator potential in response to the stimulus of given intensity by modification of transducer channels (for example by protein kinase A-mediated phosphorylation of the capsaicin receptor TRPV1); (ii) enhancement of passive propagation of the generator potential (for example by increasing membrane resistance through the inhibition of certain potassium channels); (iii) reduction of threshold for action potential formation (for example by modification of voltage-gated sodium channels); or (iv) increase in the frequency of action potential discharge due to change in repolarization (for example by modification of voltage-gated potassium channels involved in the membrane repolarization or hyperpolarization). The bars in 'generator potential' and 'active zone depolarization' columns denote the amplitude of membrane depolarization. The horizontal dashed lines in the 'active zone depolarization' column denote the threshold for action potential formation.

period is decreased and consequently the frequency of action potential discharge is increased.

It is important to realize that a single inflammatory mediator may affect multiple factors regulating neuronal excitability by signalling through divergent intracellular pathways. Moreover, inflammatory disorders lead to accumulation of numerous mediators at the site of nerve terminal. Therefore, within the complexity of airway disease, rather than an isolated change in a particular mechanism, multiple effects on excitability

**185**

could summate and result in greatly increased responsiveness of airway afferent nerves.

*Molecular mechanisms of increased excitability*

At a phenomenological level, allergic inflammation or various inflammatory mediators have been shown to increase cough reflex sensitivity as well as excitability of airway afferent nerves. Inhalation of $PGE_2$, for example, enhances capsaicin-induced cough in humans [18]. In addition to these types of studies, as discussed above, a large number of clinical studies have demonstrated that certain pathological conditions are accompanied by a substantial increase in cough reflex sensitivity in humans (Table 18.1). This can also be observed in animal models. For example, in guinea-pigs allergic inflammation or inhalation of bradykinin potentiated cough evoked by capsaicin and citric acid, respectively [19,20]. An increase in the excitability of the afferent nerve endings in the airways is likely to contribute to this phenomenon.

Inhalation of inflammatory mediators including $PGE_2$ and eosinophil major basic protein results in potentiation of capsaicin-induced action potential discharge in pulmonary nociceptive fibres in rats [21,22]. Some of these mediators also decrease the amount of mechanical force required to activate nociceptive C-fibres in the lungs [21]. Excitability of RAR fibres is also enhanced by inflammatory conditions. For example, exposing the trachea isolated from sensitized guinea-pigs to the antigen causes a substantial increase in the mechanosensitivity of RAR fibres [23]. Beyond these types of descriptive studies, there has been relatively little published relating to the mechanisms underlying increases in airway afferent excitability.

The vast majority of studies on the mechanistic basis of afferent nerve excitability and plasticity have been carried out on nociceptive-type somatosensory neurones isolated from the dorsal root ganglia [1]. Somatosensory nociceptors share many properties with airway nociceptive fibres, and thus may provide important clues to the mechanism of airway nociceptor excitability. On the other hand, the RAR phenotype fibre is not readily paralleled by any type of somatosensory afferent. Consequently relatively little has been published on the mechanisms by which airway RAR excitability is modulated. It nevertheless should be kept in mind that, given the phenotypic differences between RAR and nociceptive fibres, the mechanisms resulting in changes in RAR excitability will likely be different from those involved in excitability changes in airway nociceptors.

*Vanilloid receptor (TRPV1) mechanisms.* Vagal afferent nociceptors (C-fibres and Aδ-fibres) innervating the airways express the capsaicin receptor, a member of the transient receptor potential family, currently referred to as TRPV1 [13,14]. This receptor was previously termed vanilloid receptor 1 (VR1). TRPV1 is not expressed by RAR-type fibres in guinea-pig airways [24], and therefore the extent to which capsaicin can lead to RAR activation *in vivo* is likely through indirect means.

TRPV1 is an ionotropic receptor that upon activation serves as a non-selective cation channel resulting in membrane depolarization [25]. In addition to vanilloid compounds, TRPV1 is activated by endogenous lipid mediators including anandamide and arachidonic acid metabolites of various lipoxygenase enzymes [25,26]. Certain metabotrophic receptors may also activate TRPV1 through intracellular signal transduction mechanisms. For example, evidence from both somatosensory neurones and airway afferent C-fibres supports the hypothesis that bradykinin activates sensory nerves, at least in part, through production of lipoxygenase products of arachidonic acid and the subsequent activation of TRPV1 (see below) [26]. TRPV1 can be stimulated by heat, but the temperature required (>40°C) is unlikely to be relevant to cough physiology. More relevant to airways physiology is the fact that hydrogen ions can activate TRPV1 (pH ~ 6 at 37°C) [25].

A unique feature of TRPV1 is its ability to integrate disparate stimuli—i.e. action of one TRPV1 agonist potentiates the action of the other [25]. For example, hydrogen ions were found to potentiate TRPV1-mediated responses to vanilloids and heat. On the other hand, increases in temperature increase the TRPV1-mediated responses to vanilloids and lipid mediators. Integration is likely to be an important mechanism of increased sensitivity of nociceptive airway afferents involved in cough. Under various pathological conditions one or more TRPV1 agonists may accumulate in the airway wall. For example, airway inflammation in asthma could lead to TRPV1-mediated responses by increased concentration of hydrogen ions (i.e. decreasing the pH in the airway wall), bradykinin and certain lipid mediators.

Biophysical studies on sensory cell bodies show

that inflammatory mediators that stimulate classical G-protein-coupled receptors can increase conductance through TRPV1. Agonists of Gq-coupled receptors have been shown to increase TRPV1 conductance secondary to phospholipase C (PLC) activation and subsequent phosphorylation of TRPV1 by protein kinase C (PKC) [27]. In addition, activation of PLC has been shown to release TRPV1 from phosphatidylinositol [12,13] phosphate inhibition [28]. This mechanism appears to contribute to increases in TRPV1 activity secondary to nerve growth factor (NGF) stimulation of trk-A receptors and also bradykinin activation of $B_2$ receptors. One might speculate that bradykinin $B_2$-receptor activation (a classical Gq-coupled receptor) may both activate the nerve via lipoxygenase-dependent gating of TRPV1, and increase the excitability of the nociceptor via induction of prostaglandin production and PKC-dependent phosphorylation of TRPV1.

The amplitude of the TRPV1-mediated generator potential may also be increased by Gs-coupled receptors. Elevation in cAMP increases capsaicin-induced conductance in rat nociceptive neurones by a mechanism that can be inhibited by inhibitors of protein kinase A (PKA) [29]. This mechanism likely contributes to the observation that $PGE_2$ increases the capsaicin-induced action potential discharge in rat pulmonary nociceptors [21]. The generator potential evoked by TRPV1 agonists could in theory also be increased by changes in the number of TRPV1 receptors. Neurotrophins such as NGF have been found to increase the expression of TRPV1 in rat sensory neurones [30]. Although the relative expression of TRPV1 in nociceptors found in normal and diseased airways has not been studied, it is known that NGF can be elevated at sites of airway inflammation [31].

Inflammatory mediators may affect nociceptor excitability by mechanisms that do not involve TRPV1. Non-TRPV1 mechanisms likely contribute to excitability changes in RAR fibres as well as nociceptors. Various inflammatory mediators have been shown to decrease the threshold for mechanical stimulation of airway afferent nerves [21,23]. The mechanisms underlying this response are unknown but likely involve modulation of various ion channels.

*Potassium channels.* There are a large number of different types of potassium channels in sensory nerve fibres [32]. In general, inhibition of potassium channels

leads to an increase in excitability. Antigen challenge and mediators such as histamine have been found to inhibit resting potassium current in vagal sensory neurones [33]. Inhibiting potassium channels that are open under resting condition leads to an increase in membrane resistance and this could lead to an increase in the amplitude of the generator potential. Increased membrane resistance can also increase the efficacy of electrotonic conduction of the terminal membrane.

Other potassium channels play a key role in determining the refractory period of the nerve. One such channel is found in vagal sensory neurones and causes a slow hyperpolarization following the action potential, referred to as the 'slow afterspike hyperpolarization' (AHPslow) [34]. This channel is opened by calcium that enters the cell during the action potential through voltage-gated N-type calcium channels. Inhibiting these channels increases the peak frequency at which the sensory nerve can fire action potentials. In nodose ganglion neurones, antigen challenge, bradykinin, $PGD_2$ and $PGI_2$ effectively inhibit the AHPslow [34,35]. In addition, any process that leads to elevations in cAMP or inhibition of N-type calcium channels will inhibit the AHPslow current.

Potassium channels underlying the so-called maxi-K current may also affect the excitability of afferent nerves in the airways. Pharmacological opening of these channels with drugs such as NS1619 inhibits afferent nerve activity [36]. Similarly, there are various voltage-gated potassium channels in the airway afferent endings. Drugs that block some of these channels, such as 4-aminopyridine and certain dendrotoxins, can lead to increases in excitability of the nerve endings, or even to overt activation [37]. However, there is little information on how the process of airway inflammation affects these channels.

*Sodium channels.* The number and activity of voltage-gated sodium channels can affect the threshold for action potential generation, as well as peak frequency of action potential discharge. Indeed, long before veratrum alkaloids were known to act by increasing sodium channel activity (by inhibiting their inactivation), they were used to stimulate airway afferent nerves. There are a large number of different voltage-gated sodium channels expressed in mammalian nerves. Based on the sensitivity to tetrodotoxin (TTX), these channels have been pharmacologically divided into two families, the TTX-sensitive (potently blocked by TTX) and

TTX-resistant sodium channels. Sodium channels of each category are present in airway afferent nerves [32]. However, TTX-resistant channels may be particularly relevant to regulation of excitability because of their modulation by inflammatory mediators [38]. In addition, certain TTX-resistant sodium channels are preferentially localized to afferent nerves. These 'sensory nerve specific' (SNS) channels are found mainly in small-diameter (nociceptor-like) neurones. The nomenclature of SNS sodium channels is confusing, with SNS1 also referred to as PN3, while SNS2 is sometimes referred to as the NaN channel. Christian and Togo noted that the vast majority of neurones in guinea-pig jugular ganglia (source of nociceptive fibres innervating the airways), have sufficient TTX-resistant sodium channels to support action potential generation [39]. The sodium channels in airway afferent nerves have not been characterized in detail; however, preliminary data from our laboratory have shown that airway-specific jugular neurone cell bodies have sufficient TTX-resistant current to support action potential formation [32]. Current through the SNS TTX-resistant channels can be amplified by inflammatory mediators. For example, $PGE_2$, adenosine and 5-hydroxytryptamine (5-HT) are effective in enhancing TTX-resistant sodium current in somatosensory neurones [38]. The extent to which inflammatory mediators found in the airways modulate this current remains to be determined.

### Neurotransmitter plasticity

Sensory C-fibres innervating airways characteristically contain neuropeptides in their peripheral and central terminals. The most often studied sensory neuropeptides are substance P and related tachykinins, but other peptides are likely to be found in C-fibres including calcitonin gene-related peptide (CGRP), secretoneurin and various opioid peptides.

A hallmark of inflammatory disease is the up-regulation in production of various sensory neuropeptides. This has been seen both in animal models of inflammation and in numerous inflammatory diseases, including COPD [40]. This is often found to be secondary to increases in the expression of the preprotachykinin gene in the sensory neurones [41,42]. It remains unknown as to how inflammation within the airway wall sends signals to the distant cell body in the relevant sensory ganglia to induce the transcription of neuropeptide synthesizing enzymes. A likely mechanism, however, involves the action of various neurotrophins. Neurotrophins are known to interact with specific tyrosine kinase-linked receptors (trk receptors) to evoke signals in the cell body. The neurotrophin–trk receptor complex is thought to be transported from the nerve terminals to the cell body via axonal transport mechanisms, and therein to affect transcriptions of various genes including those involved in the synthesis of neuropeptides [43]. Adding to the evidence that neurotrophins may be involved in the up-regulation of neuropeptide synthesis in airway diseases are the observations that neurotrophins such as nerve growth factor (NGF) and brain-derived neurotrophin factor (BDNF) are found in the airways, and their production may be increased at sites of allergic inflammation [31].

Sensory neuropeptides are synthesized in the cell body and transported to both the peripheral and central terminals [1]. Neuropeptides can be released from the peripheral terminals of afferent nerves by a process referred to as the axon reflex. In addition, chemical mediators such as TRPV1 agonists and trypsin can cause neuropeptide release independent of action potential discharge and reflex activity. Neurokinins released in the airways can participate in the inflammatory reaction by causing vasodilatation, plasma extravasation and in some species bronchial smooth muscle contraction [44]. In the guinea-pig these processes may indirectly activate RAR nerves and thereby contribute to the tussigenic activity of these agents [44,45].

Neuropeptides are released from the central terminal in the brainstem as a result of action potential invasion of the central release sites [1]. It is the release of neurokinins from the central terminals that likely plays an important role in regulating cough reflex sensitivity. Neurokinins released in the synapse between primary and secondary vagal afferent neurones in the nucleus of the solitary tract can cause an increase in synaptic transmission. Typically neurokinins cause slow excitatory postsynaptic potentials and/or increases in input impedance [1]. These events can lead to changes in synaptic efficacy and neurotransmission in the NTS. There is evidence that, at least in some instances, central terminals of RAR fibres converge on the same secondary neurones as nociceptive C-fibres [46]. This fact, considered with the electrophysiological effects of neurokinins on postsynaptic membranes, provides the conceptual framework for the process referred to as 'central sensitization' [1]. This term is used to denote the process by which one type of nerve input (e.g. nociceptive C-fibre) enhances the synaptic transmission of another type of input (e.g. RAR fibres). This could lead to a substantive decrease in the amount of RAR input to the central nervous system (CNS) required to trigger cough. Moreover, such synergy provided by disparate converging inputs in the brainstem might explain, for example, how activation of nociceptive-type nerves in the oesophagus could affect the threshold for cough evoked by activation of airways-specific afferent nerves.

The increase in sensory neuropeptides associated with inflammation is thought to be secondary to induction of preprotachykinin genes in nociceptive neurones. However, recent studies in both the somatosensory and vagal sensory systems support the hypothesis that inflammation may also lead to phenotypic changes in the neuropeptidergic innervation [24,47,48]. Accordingly, exposure to respiratory allergen or virus infection increased the amount of sensory neurokinins in the airway afferent neurones in guinea-pigs [24,42,48]. Interestingly, however, the preprotachykinin gene expression and neurokinin production were found to be increased in neurones that project non-nociceptive fibres into the airway. The neurones induced by inflammation to produce neuropeptides were large-diameter neurones located in the nodose ganglia and had physiological characteristics consistent with the RAR phenotype. At sites of inflammation, therefore, neuropeptidergic innervation may consist of not only nociceptive C-fibres but also RAR fibres. In addition, histological evidence supports the hypothesis that the neuropeptides produced in response to airway inflammation are also transported to central terminals of the RAR neurones [24]. This raises the possibility that in allergic inflammation or respiratory virus infection, mechanical activation of the RAR fibres would lead to neurokinin release in the brainstem. Unlike nociceptors, many RAR fibres are activated during the breathing cycle. This could lead to central sensitization during breathing *independently of nociceptive stimulation*. In the somatosensory system an analogous phenotypic switch in neuropeptide innervation has been reported to play a role in painful sensation to non-painful stimuli termed allodynia [47]. It is tempting to speculate that this process in the airways could contribute to inappropriate or 'allotussive' cough sensations, i.e. the urge to cough in the absence of anything in the airway to productively cough up. The mechanism

underlying this inflammation-induced phenotypic switch in the neurochemistry of RAR has not been worked out; however, this effect of allergen challenge or virus exposure can be mimicked by local injection of NGF into the airway wall [49].

Changes in the neurotransmitter content in central terminals of primary afferents, combined with increases in afferent nerve excitability and activity, may lead to substantive changes in the synaptic input to secondary neurones (neurones receiving input from sensory afferents) in the central nervous system. This, in turn, can cause changes in the excitability of the secondary neurones. This is referred to as 'use-dependent' plasticity and has been extensively studied in the somatosensory system where activation of nociceptive afferent fibres results in increases in excitability of secondary neurones in the spinal cord, sensitizing them to noxious as well as innocuous stimuli [50]. The mechanisms of use-dependent excitability changes in secondary neurones are not clear, but several receptors and second messenger cascades may be involved [50]. With respect to cough-mediating pathways it is interesting to note that exposing the lungs of non-human primates repeatedly to allergen resulted in increases in excitability of secondary sensory neurones in the nucleus of the solitary tract [51]. These observations are consistent with the hypothesis that allergen inhalation-induced activation of primary airway afferent nerves can result in use-dependent changes in excitability of secondary neurones in the brainstem.

## Changes in nerve fibre density

The density of sensory innervation can change in response to its environment [52]. Tissue damage or release of various growth factors can lead to increased nerve fibre growth and fibre sprouting. The question as to whether increases in afferent nerve density may participate in increased cough sensitivity has not been extensively studied. To our knowledge only one study has addressed this issue as it relates to cough [53]. This elegant study was designed such that the nerve density was determined in biopsies taken from the carina of the right upper lobe and a subsegmental carina of the right lower lobe. The tissue was obtained from patients with persistent idiopathic cough who had increased cough sensitivity to capsaicin and from controls. There was no difference in the density of epithelial nerve fibres as quantified using the non-specific nerve marker PGP

CHAPTER 18

9.5, but patients with chronic cough had a higher density of CGRP-positive nerves compared with the control subjects. This supports the hypothesis of neurotransmitter plasticity contributing to cough sensitivity but does not favour a role for an increased nerve sprouting and density. Whether there is a higher nerve density in the submucosa plexus or near cough regions such as in the trachea or larynx was not investigated.

Extraneuronal effects

Most afferent nerves in the airways are mechanically sensitive, and the lungs are exposed to extensive mechanical forces during breathing [13,14]. Each breath causes discharge in various populations of afferent mechanosensors. As discussed above, the action potential discharge depends on the amplitude and duration of the generator potential. It is likely that the amplitude of the generator potential evoked by mechanical forces in the lungs will depend not only on the terminal membrane, but also on the viscoelastic properties of the lung tissue. In airway diseases such as COPD and asthma, airway tissue destruction and remodelling will likely affect the extent to which distension of the tissue in the microenvironment of the mechanosensors is transduced to a generator potential. Cough reflexes could be increased if changes in airway structure lead to increases in mechanotransduction of cough-inducing fibres (e.g. RAR-type fibres), or if they lead to decreases in activity in mechanosensors that are normally inhibitory to the cough reflex. The hypothesis that changes in airway structure that accompanies airway diseases alters the properties of airway mechanosensors has been studied as it pertains to COPD, but little information is available as regards cough [54].

## Conclusions

Excessive coughing accompanies many diseases including asthma, respiratory infections, lung cancer, bronchitis, COPD and gastro-oesophageal reflux disease. The increase in coughing in many cases is likely due to the production of tussigenic stimuli in the large airways. In addition, however, it is recognized that patients with chronic cough often present with an increase in the cough reflex sensitivity to tussigenic stimuli. Rational strategies for the treatment of chronic cough may

consider therefore both a reduction in the amount of tussigenic stimuli and a reduction in the heightened sensitivity of the cough reflex. Regrettably, short of nonspecific centrally acting drugs, there are no drugs that are aimed at decreasing the increased sensitivity of cough. This is likely because relatively little is known about the mechanisms underlying this process. The available data gathered from research on vagal sensory and somatosensory systems indicate that multiple mechanisms may lead to hypersensitivity of reflexes such as cough. These include increases in the excitability of the afferent terminals, changes in the neurotransmitter content and consequent changes in synaptic transmission in the brainstem, and extraneuronal changes that may lead to changes in the efficiency of mechanotransduction in afferent nerves. Adding to the complexity of this issue is the notion that at least two disparate types of afferent nerves may participate in cough reflexes (RARs and nociceptors). Inasmuch as these nerve subtypes are phenotypically distinct, it is likely that mechanisms resulting in increases in their activity will also be distinct. Finally, adding height to the hurdle in front of our understanding of this issue, is the difficulty in quantifying cough sensitivity in humans. At present most studies in this area have used classical nociceptive stimuli to study changes in cough sensitivity. This leaves open the question of the extent to which the sensitivity of RAR-driven cough is affected in various disease states. A combined effort from studies at the research bench and bedside will be required before some semblance of understanding of this complex area emerges.

## References

1 Woolf CJ, Salter MW. Neuronal plasticity: increasing the gain in pain. *Science* 2000; **288**: 1765–9.
2 Choudry NB, Fuller RW. Sensitivity of the cough reflex in patients with chronic cough. *Eur Respir J* 1992; **5** (3): 296–300.
3 Pounsford JC, Birch MJ, Saunders KB. Effect of bronchodilators on the cough response to inhaled citric acid in normal and asthmatic subjects. *Thorax* 1985; **40** (9): 662–7.
4 Chang AB, Phelan PD, Robertson CF. Cough receptor sensitivity in children with acute and non-acute asthma. *Thorax* 1997; **52** (9): 770–4.
5 Chang AB, Phelan PD, Sawyer SM, Del Brocco S, Robertson CF. Cough sensitivity in children with asthma,

recurrent cough, and cystic fibrosis. *Arch Dis Child* 1997; **77** (4): 331–4.

6 Doherty MJ, Mister R, Pearson MG, Calverley PM. Capsaicin responsiveness and cough in asthma and chronic obstructive pulmonary disease. *Thorax* 2000; **55** (8): 643–9.

7 Fujimura M, Sakamoto S, Kamio Y, Matsuda T. Cough receptor sensitivity and bronchial responsiveness in normal and asthmatic subjects. *Eur Respir J* 1992; **5** (3): 291–5.

8 Ferrari M, Olivieri M, Sembenini C, Benini L, Zuccali V, Bardelli E *et al*. Tussive effect of capsaicin in patients with gastroesophageal reflux without cough. *Am J Respir Crit Care Med* 1995; **151**: 557–61.

9 Wong CH, Morice AH. Cough threshold in patients with chronic obstructive pulmonary disease. *Thorax* 1999; **54** (1): 62–4.

10 O'Connell F, Thomas VE, Studham JM, Pride NB, Fuller RW. Capsaicin cough sensitivity increases during upper respiratory infection. *Respir Med* 1996; **90** (5): 279–86.

11 Empey DW, Laitinen LA, Jacobs L, Gold WM, Nadel JA. Mechanisms of bronchial hyperreactivity in normal subjects after upper respiratory tract infection. *Am Rev Respir Dis* 1976; **113** (2): 131–9.

12 Widdicombe JG. Receptors in the trachea and bronchi of the cat. *J Physiol Lond* 1954; **123**: 71–104.

13 Riccio MM, Kummer W, Biglari B, Myers AC, Undem BJ. Interganglionic segregation of distinct vagal afferent fibre phenotypes in guinea-pig airways. *J Physiol* 1996; **496** (2): 521–30.

14 Fox A. Airway nerves: in vitro electrophysiology. *Curr Opin Pharmacol* 2002; **2** (3): 278–9.

15 Hunter DD, Undem BJ. Identification and substance P content of vagal afferent neurons innervating the epithelium of the guinea pig trachea. *Am J Respir Crit Care Med* 1999; **159** (6): 1943–8.

16 Fontaine-Perus J, Chanconie M, Le Douarin NM. Embryonic origin of substance P containing neurons in cranial and spinal sensory ganglia of the avian embryo. *Dev Biol* 1985; **107** (1): 227–38.

17 Fain GL. *Molecular and Cellular Physiology of the Neurons*. Cambridge: Harvard University Press, 1999.

18 Choudry NB, Fuller RW, Pride NB. Sensitivity of the human cough reflex: effect of inflammatory mediators prostaglandin E2, bradykinin, and histamine. *Am Rev Respir Dis* 1989; **140** (1): 137–41.

19 Fox AJ, Lalloo UG, Belvisi MG, Bernareggi M, Chung KF, Barnes PJ. Bradykinin-evoked sensitization of airway sensory nerves: a mechanism for ACE-inhibitor cough. *Nat Med* 1996; **2** (7): 814–7.

20 Liu Q, Fujimura M, Tachibana H, Myou S, Kasahara K, Yasui M. Characterization of increased cough sensitivity after antigen challenge in guinea pigs. *Clin Exp Allergy* 2001; **31** (3): 474–84.

21 Ho CY, Gu Q, Hong JL, Lee LY. Prostaglandin E(2) enhances chemical and mechanical sensitivities of pulmonary C fibers in the rat. *Am J Respir Crit Care Med* 2000; **162**: 528–33.

22 Lee LY, Gu Q, Gleich GJ. Effects of human eosinophil granule-derived cationic proteins on C-fiber afferents in the rat lung. *J Appl Physiol* 2001; **91** (3): 1318–26.

23 Riccio MM, Myers AC, Undem BJ. Immunomodulation of afferent neurons in guinea-pig isolated airway. *J Physiol* 1996; **491** (2): 499–509.

24 Myers AC, Kajekar R, Undem BJ. Allergic inflammation-induced neuropeptide production in rapidly adapting afferent nerves in guinea pig airways. *Am J Physiol Lung Cell Mol Physiol* 2002; **282** (4): L775–81.

25 Caterina MJ, Julius D. The vanilloid receptor: a molecular gateway to the pain pathway. *Annu Rev Neurosci* 2001; **24**: 487–517.

26 Shin J, Cho H, Hwang SW, Jung J, Shin CY, Lee SY *et al*. Bradykinin-12-lipoxygenase-VR1 signaling pathway for inflammatory hyperalgesia. *Proc Natl Acad Sci USA* 2002; **99** (15): 10150–5.

27 Premkumar LS, Ahern GP. Induction of vanilloid receptor channel activity by protein kinase C. *Nature* 2000; **408**: 985–90.

28 Chuang HH, Prescott ED, Kong H, Shields S, Jordt SE, Basbaum AI *et al*. Bradykinin and nerve growth factor release the capsaicin receptor from PtdIns(4,5)P2-mediated inhibition. *Nature* 2001; **411**: 957–62.

29 Lopshire JC, Nicol GD. The cAMP transduction cascade mediates the prostaglandin E2 enhancement of the capsaicin-elicited current in rat sensory neurons: whole-cell and single-channel studies. *J Neurosci* 1998; **18** (16): 6081–92.

30 Michael GJ, Priestley JV. Differential expression of the mRNA for the vanilloid receptor subtype 1 in cells of the adult rat dorsal root and nodose ganglia and its downregulation by axotomy. *J Neurosci* 1999; **19** (5): 1844–54.

31 Virchow JC, Julius P, Lommatzsch M, Luttmann W, Renz H, Braun A. Neurotrophins are increased in bronchoalveolar lavage fluid after segmental allergen provocation. *Am J Respir Crit Care Med* 1998; **158** (6): 2002–5.

32 Carr MJ, Undem BJ. Ion channels in airway afferent neurons. *Respir Physiol* 2001; **125** (1–2): 83–97.

33 Undem BJ, Hubbard W, Weinreich D. Immunologically induced neuromodulation of guinea pig nodose ganglion neurons. *J Auton Nerv Syst* 1993; **44** (1): 35–44.

34 Cordoba-Rodriguez R, Moore KA, Kao JP, Weinreich D. Calcium regulation of a slow post-spike hyperpolarization in vagal afferent neurons. *Proc Natl Acad Sci USA* 1999; **96** (14): 7650–7.

35 Undem BJ, Weinreich D. Electrophysiological properties and chemosensitivity of guinea pig nodose ganglion neurons in vitro. *J Auton Nerv Syst* 1993; **44** (1): 17–33.

36 Fox AJ, Barnes PJ, Venkatesan P, Belvisi MG. Activation of large conductance potassium channels inhibits the afferent and efferent function of airway sensory nerves in the guinea pig. *J Clin Invest* 1997; **99** (3): 513–9.

37 McAlexander MA, Undem BJ. Potassium channel blockade induces action potential generation in guinea-pig airway vagal afferent neurones. *J Auton Nerv Syst* 2000; **78** (2–3): 158–64.

38 Gold MS, Reichling DB, Shuster MJ, Levine JD. Hyperalgesic agents increase a tetrodotoxin-resistant Na+ current in nociceptors. *Proc Natl Acad Sci USA* 1996; **93** (3): 1108–12.

39 Christian EP, Togo JA. Excitable properties and underlying Na+ and K+ currents in neurons from the guinea-pig jugular ganglion. *J Auton Nerv Syst* 1995; **56** (1–2): 75–86.

40 Tomaki M, Ichinose M, Miura M, Hirayama Y, Yamauchi H, Nakajima N *et al.* Elevated substance P content in induced sputum from patients with asthma and patients with chronic bronchitis. *Am J Respir Crit Care Med* 1995; **151**: 613–7.

41 Hunter DD, Castranova V, Stanley C, Dey RD. Effects of silica exposure on substance P immunoreactivity and preprotachykinin mRNA expression in trigeminal sensory neurons in Fischer 344 rats. *J Toxicol Environ Health A* 1998; **53** (8): 593–605.

42 Fischer A, McGregor GP, Saria A, Philippin B, Kummer W. Induction of tachykinin gene and peptide expression in guinea pig nodose primary afferent neurons by allergic airway inflammation. *J Clin Invest* 1996; **98** (10): 2284–91.

43 Klesse LJ, Parada LF. Trks: signal transduction and intracellular pathways. *Microsc Res Tech* 1999; **45** (4–5): 210–6 [p. ii].

44 Advenier C, Emonds-Alt X. Tachykinin receptor antagonists and cough. *Pulm Pharmacol* 1996; **9** (5–6): 329–33.

45 Joad JP, Kott KS, Bonham AC. Nitric oxide contributes to substance P-induced increases in lung rapidly adapting receptor activity in guinea-pigs. *J Physiol* 1997; **503** (3): 635–43.

46 Mazzone SB, Canning BJ. Synergistic interactions between airway afferent nerve subtypes mediating reflex bronchospasm in guinea pigs. *Am J Physiol Regul Integr Comp Physiol* 2002; **283** (1): R86–R98.

47 Neumann S, Doubell TP, Leslie T, Woolf CJ. Inflammatory pain hypersensitivity mediated by phenotypic switch in myelinated primary sensory neurons. *Nature* 1996; **384**: 360–4.

48 Carr MJ, Hunter DD, Jacoby DB, Undem BJ. Expression of tachykinins in non-nociceptive vagal afferent neurons during respiratory tract viral infection in guinea pigs. *Am J Respir Crit Care Med* 2002; **165**: 1071–5.

49 Hunter DD, Myers AC, Undem BJ. Nerve growth factor-induced phenotypic switch in guinea pig airway sensory neurons. *Am J Respir Crit Care Med* 2000; **161** (6): 1985–90.

50 Willis WD. Role of neurotransmitters in sensitization of pain responses. *Ann N Y Acad Sci* 2001; **933**: 142–56.

51 Chen CY, Bonham AC, Schelegle ES, Gershwin LJ, Plopper CG, Joad JP. Extended allergen exposure in asthmatic monkeys induces neuroplasticity in nucleus tractus solitarius. *J Allergy Clin Immunol* 2001; **108** (4): 557–62.

52 Stead RH. Nerve remodelling during intestinal inflammation. *Ann N Y Acad Sci* 1992; **664**: 443–55.

53 O'Connell F, Springall DR, Moradoghli-Haftvani A, Krausz T, Price D, Fuller RW *et al.* Abnormal intraepithelial airway nerves in persistent unexplained cough? *Am J Respir Crit Care Med* 1995; **152**: 2068–75.

54 Mansoor JK, Hyde DM, Schelegle ES. Contribution of vagal afferents to breathing pattern in rats with lung fibrosis. *Respir Physiol* 1997; **108** (1): 45–61.

# 19 Motor mechanisms and the mechanics of cough

*Giovanni A. Fontana*

'*Tussis est offendiculum spiritus in trachea arteria*' (Matteo Plateario, Scuola Medica Salernitana, 12th century)

## Introduction

Cough is a modified respiratory act that can be produced voluntarily but, in most instances, it represents a reflex action evoked by the activation of laryngeal and/or tracheobronchial receptors. Its main functions are protecting the lungs against aspiration and helping in the removal of excessive bronchial secretions. Coughing does not normally occur in healthy individuals, and persistent cough is one of the cardinal signs of respiratory disease. In health, mucociliary clearance and alveolar macrophages satisfactorily control minor insults from exogenous noxious agents. However, when these systems fail or become overloaded with foreign matter or excessive bronchial secretions, cough intervenes as a supplemental mechanism to the mucociliary escalator.

In his 1937 paper, Coryllos [1] provided a detailed description of the cough cycle, and noted that 'cough is not a simple expiratory act but is composed of three distinctive phases: inspiratory, compressive and expulsive'. He likened the phases of the cough cycle to the deflagration of a gun: the preparatory inspiration to the loading of the gun, the compressive phase to the blazing of the powder and production of gas under high pressure, and the expulsive phase to the ejection of the bullet from the barrel of the gun.

The purposes of this chapter are to describe the motor characteristics of cough and outline the princi-

pal aspects of respiratory mechanics that are relevant to the genesis of the high flow rates and gas velocities of cough. Some related topics will be mentioned, while others, which are presented elsewhere in this book, will be omitted.

## Description of cough

When cough is performed voluntarily or initiated by stimulation of tracheobronchial receptors, it usually begins with the inhalation of a variable volume of air. However, if coughing is triggered by stimulation of afferents from the vocal folds, the preparatory inspiration may be absent: this has also been considered a separate reflex, i.e. the so called 'expiration reflex' [2]. Next, the glottis is closed and the expiratory muscles contract intensely, leading to the build-up of high intrathoracic and abdominal pressures. The glottis is then actively reopened, and the inspired air volume forcefully expelled by the sustained contraction of the expiratory muscles. At the same time the central airways within the thorax are compressed and, for any given expiratory flow rate, the reduction in their cross-sectional area results in higher gas linear velocities than would have occurred had there been no bronchial narrowing. There may be a fourth phase mainly characterized by the cessation of expiratory muscle activity and the appearance of some antagonistic activity [3].

During spontaneous coughing, several expiratory thrusts may follow one another with replication of the above-mentioned events or with minor variations such as those characterized by the absence of glottis closure. The principal muscular and mechanical events that

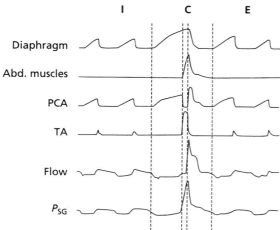

**Fig. 19.1** Diagrammatic representation of the motor pattern of a typical cough effort. The inspiratory (I), compressive (C) and expiratory (E) phases of cough are delimited by the dashed lines, and are preceded and followed by periods of normal breathing. PCA, posterior cricoarytenoid muscle (laryngeal abductor); TA, tyroarytenoid muscle (laryngeal adductor); $P_{SG}$, subglottic pressure. On some occasions (see [41]), diaphragmatic activity may extend into the early stages of the expiratory phase. Reprinted with permission from [17].

characterize a single cough effort are diagrammatically illustrated in Fig. 19.1.

## Inspiratory phase

As with most inspiratory acts, the first event of the inspiratory phase of cough is the contraction of the abductor muscles of the arytenoid cartilage leading to complete opening of the glottis and facilitating subsequent inhalation of a variable air volume [4]. The inspired air volume may range from a fraction of to several times the eupnoeic tidal volume.

Studies in which subjects were instructed to cough voluntarily suggest a high degree of volitional control over inspired volume, the latter being related to the anticipated forcefulness of the subsequent cough effort. In a group of normal subjects performing a series of 'single gentle coughs' [5], the mean duration of the inspiratory phase varied from 0.45 to 1.00 s, with an average value of 0.75 s. The corresponding inspiratory volume ranged from 0.09 to 0.53 L (mean 0.39 L), and was found to correlate with the duration of the preparatory inspiration [5]. In the study by Ross *et al.* [6], in which

subjects were instructed to perform maximum voluntary cough efforts, the mean duration of the inspiratory phase was 0.65 s, and resulted in a mean air intake of about 2.5 L.

Little is known regarding the regulation of inspiratory volume and flow during the inspiratory phase of reflex cough. It may be, however, that the magnitude of the inspired volume is related, at least in part, to the intensity of the stimulus causing cough (author's unpublished observations).

During mechanical stimulation of dog trachea, the typical sequence of cough's motor acts is often preceded by a sustained apnoeic period during which the diaphragm shows only minimal activation, and lung volume does not appreciably change [4].

Whatever the regulatory mechanism(s), the augmentation of the inspiratory volume may enhance the mechanical efficiency of the subsequent expiration by different means. At high lung volumes, the tension–length relationship of the expiratory muscles is optimized [7,8], thus allowing them to produce greater intrathoracic and abdominal pressures. Furthermore, activation of pulmonary stretch receptors by lung distension leads to central facilitation of cough [9].

## Compressive phase

Closure of the glottis by adduction of the ventricular folds and covering of the laryngeal inlet by the epiglottis marks the onset of the compressive phase of cough. Contraction of the expiratory muscles against a closed glottis leads to the development of high abdominal, pleural, alveolar and subglottic pressures. When pleural pressure increases, the alveolar gas is compressed and lung volume decreases. Glottis closure, rather than gas compression within the respiratory system, is regarded as the phenomenon that mostly differentiates coughing from a forced expiration. Indeed, marked increases in abdominal and intrathoracic pressures leading to compression of the alveolar gas are known to occur during expiratory thrusts with an open glottis due to the resistive properties of the tracheobronchial tree. Expiratory muscle contraction during the compressive phase is accompanied by the coactivation of the diaphragm [10] and other inspiratory muscles opposing further development of positive pleural and alveolar pressures [3].

Since the glottis remains closed for only 0.2 s, although with considerable variability, the rate of change in alveolar pressure over this brief interval is remarkably high. At the end of the compressive phase, alveolar pressure may exceed 20 kPa [11,12], i.e. values 50–100% higher than during other expulsive manoeuvres in which the glottis is open. Thus, the corresponding rate of change in alveolar pressure would approximate 100 kPa/s. Given the relationship between gas pressure and volume changes as dictated by Boyle's law, if one assumes a lung volume of 5 L at the end of the inspiratory phase, and an alveolar pressure of 20 kPa at the end of the compressive phase (i.e. ~ +20% of the atmospheric value), the corresponding reduction in lung volume will be ~ 1 L. The rate of change in lung volume during compression would then approximate to 5 L/s. The augmentation of pleural pressure during the compressive phase, as compared to other expiratory manoeuvres, may be related to a reflex increase in agonist and decreased antagonist muscle activity, presumably brought about by glottis closure [13], and/or optimization of the force–length–velocity relationships of the expiratory muscles [3].

As is the case for all other skeletal muscles, the force developed by the contracting expiratory muscles is proportional to their length and inversely related to their velocity of shortening [8]. Thus, there are mechanically advantageous conditions contributing to force development during the compressive phase of cough. In fact, glottis closure prevents significant decreases in lung volume, except for those produced by gas compression, thus allowing the expiratory muscles to express their maximal force during contraction at the length determined by the lung volume attained following the preceding inspiratory phase. In fact, due to the relatively small changes in lung volume during compression, the shortening velocity of the expiratory muscles is minimal, and muscle contraction nearly isometric.

Although glottic closure is generally considered a prerequisite for development of the high intrathoracic pressures of cough, some lines of evidence seem to deny this. For instance, the study of Gal [14] showed that, in subjects who performed maximum voluntary cough efforts prior to and following tracheal intubation, cough pressures were the same or even greater after intubation. Furthermore, neither glottic closure nor high pressures appear to be crucial to effective coughing: tracheostomized and intubated patients can still expectorate, and even normal subjects need not close the glottis for airway clearing [15].

## Expiratory phase

This is the phase of the cough cycle during which the airways are cleared of secretions, debris and foreign material. It is initiated by rapid (20–40 ms) abduction of the arytenoid cartilages, an active phenomenon involving muscle recruitment [4]. Opening of the glottis at the onset of expiration is associated with passive oscillations of gas and tissues causing the characteristic noise of cough and setting up pressure fluctuations that may play a role in shaking loose secretions. Pressure within central airways rapidly falls to nearly atmospheric values (Fig. 19.1), while pleural and alveolar pressures still continue to rise for about 0.5 s. The total duration of the expiratory phase is variable, but generally comprises between 0.5 and 1.0 s [5,16].

In normal subjects performing a maximum voluntary cough effort starting from near total lung capacity, expiratory flow sharply rises up to values of more than 10 L/s [17], and the central intrathoracic airways collapse. Airway compression causes rapid, transient displacement of the airway gas volume, and generates high supramaximal flow rates that superimpose on the airflow coming from the alveolar spaces. More detailed accounts of the mechanisms contributing to the generation of flow transients during maximum expiratory efforts will be given in a subsequent section. The time required to achieve these high flow transients (i.e. the time to peak flow) is approximately 30 ms [17]. After this short time interval, flow rate falls to much lower values, approximately 50% of the cough peak flow, which may be sustained for several milliseconds, up to half the total duration of the expiratory phase [5,16]. Lung volume and flow rate then decrease exponentially with time, with a time constant of ~ 0.5 s [3]. During the last stage of expiration, flow rapidly drops to zero and expulsion terminates.

The violent muscular activity associated with the expirations of cough may have noxious effects, including trauma of the larynx and airways, rib fractures and barotrauma. Indeed, costal fractures and abdominal muscle tears are well-known complications of intense cough, but have never been reported to occur with other expulsive efforts [3,18,19].

## Cessation

The cessation phase is associated with relaxation of expiratory muscle and perhaps onset of antagonistic muscle activity with a fall in pleural and abdominal pressures. In most instances, the glottis narrows and the laryngeal structures gradually return to their inspiratory position [5]. The compressed central airways re-expand.

## Mechanics of cough

The development of an effective cough as a clearing mechanism is thought to be critically dependent upon the linear velocity of the gas molecules travelling down the airway lumen [3,20]. It appears that the cough mechanism is designed to maximally increase the gas velocity by both generating high expiratory flow rates and dynamically compressing the airways to reduce their cross-sectional area. In this section, we will review the mechanisms implicated in the regulation of the rate and velocity of flow during the expulsive phase of cough. Excellent and more detailed descriptions of the mechanical events of cough, as well as of cough as a clearing mechanism, can be found in the literature [3,6,12,20,21].

### Regulation of expiratory flow

The high intrathoracic pressures that are generated during the nearly isometric expiratory muscle contraction of the cough compressive phase are suddenly released when the glottis opens at the onset of the expiratory phase. Pressure at the airway opening rapidly falls to atmospheric values, while alveolar and pleural pressures remain constant or may continue to rise for a short period [3,20]. Sustained expiratory muscle contraction and concomitant cessation of antagonist action of the inspiratory muscles allowing full transmission of expiratory muscle force to the pleural and alveolar spaces are the likely contributing mechanisms [3]. Due to the elastic recoil of the lungs, alveolar pressure is always greater than pleural pressure, while the pressure surrounding the outer wall of the airways, the peribronchial pressure, closely approximates that of the pleural space [22]. The pressure within the airways, the intrabronchial pressure, progressively diminishes as air travels down the airways from the alveolus to the airway opening. This pressure drop is the result of the energy expenditure that is required to accelerate flow as the total airway cross-sectional area decreases and airway resistance increases, as well as the result of laminar

and turbulent energy dissipation in the flow [23]. At some point along the tracheobronchial tree, at the *equal pressure point* (EPP), the decrease in intrabronchial pressure equals the elastic recoil of the lung (Fig. 19.2). Thus, the EPP divides the intrathoracic airways into two segments arranged in series, respectively, located upstream (i.e. toward the alveoli) and downstream of the EPP. In the upstream segment, the intrabronchial pressure is greater than peribronchial pressure, and the airways are distended. In the downstream segment, pressure within the airways becomes lower than the pressure surrounding them, and the airways tend to collapse. Once the maximum expiratory flow has been achieved, further expiratory efforts only cause more compression of the downstream segment, but do not affect flow through the upstream segment. In fact, since the pressure drop in the upstream segment equals the elastic recoil, the rate of flow in the upstream segment is dictated by the ratio between the elastic recoil of the lungs ($P_{EL}$) and the resistance ($R$) of the upstream (US) segment:

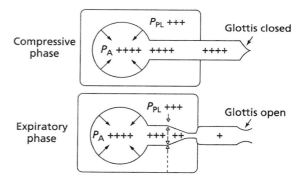

Fig. 19.2 Description of the principal mechanical events of cough by means of a model of the respiratory system. During the compressive phase, expiratory muscle activation increases pleural pressure ($P_{PL}$) that becomes markedly positive with respect to atmosphere. Alveolar pressure ($P_A$) is always greater than $P_{PL}$ due to the elastic recoil of the lung (arrows). Since the glottis is closed, intrabronchial pressure is similar to $P_A$ throughout the airways. When the glottis opens at the beginning of the expiratory phase, air starts to flow rapidly down the pressure gradient from the alveoli to the mouth. Thus, there must be a point along the airways at which the intrabronchial pressure and $P_{PL}$ pressures are equal: the equal pressure point (EPP). Downstream of the EPP, the airways are distended; upstream of the EPP the intrathoracic airways are compressed. Reprinted with permission from [17].

$$\dot{V} = P_{EL}/R_{US}.$$

This phenomenon, called *flow limitation* or *autoregulation of flow*, is the basic mechanism that sets up the upper limits to flow during both a forced expiration and the expiration of cough. It has been likened to the behaviour of a Starling resistor or a waterfall. The flow of water upstream of the waterfall depends on the slope of the terrain that delivers water to the waterfall, but is independent of the height of the waterfall or the conditions downstream to it. Thus, under conditions of flow limitation, changes in downstream pressure do not affect flow. When the intrathoracic pressures generated by the expiratory muscle contraction exceed the modest level necessary to attain maximal expiratory flow, the excess pressure markedly compresses the downstream segment of the intrathoracic airways, but does not affect flow. However, narrowing of the downstream airways augments flow velocity and kinetic energy, and this may increase the effectiveness of cough as a clearing mechanism.

An additional explanation for flow limitation is based on principles of the wave speed theory [24]. According to this theory, an elastic tube cannot carry a fluid at a mean velocity greater than the speed at which pressure waves will propagate along the tube, i.e. the tube wave speed. By analogy, this is the velocity at which pulse propagates in the arteries. At the site where the linear velocity of flow equals the velocity of propagation of pressure waves, a 'choke point' develops, and prevents further increases in flow rate. The tube wave speed depends on the gas density ($\rho$), the tube (i.e. airway) cross sectional area ($A$) and the specific elastance of the tube wall ($A\,\delta P/\delta A$). Then, maximum flow ($\dot{V}$) can be expressed as:

$$\dot{V} = A\,[\rho^{-0.5}\,(A\,\delta P/\delta A)]^{0.5}.$$

Actual $\dot{V}$, however, cannot be determined by using this equation, since values of $A$ and ($A\,\delta P/\delta A$) vary with choke point location, the latter depending on airway geometry and elasticity, and on lung volume. During an expiratory thrust performed at a large lung volume, the choke point resides in the central airways. As lung volume diminishes, the choke point moves in the upstream direction. In both humans and experimental animals, simultaneous measurements of pleural and intrabronchial pressures made it possible to estimate that, above functional residual capacity, the choke point is located at the level of lobar or segmental bronchi

[20,22]. At lung volumes near residual volume, the choke point moves down to the fifth- to sixth-generation branches [20,25]. Thus, when a series of coughs is initiated at a high lung volume, secretions are initially cleared from the larger airway; secretions are then moved from the small to the larger airway as lung volume progressively diminishes.

## Expiratory flow velocity

Given that in any condition flow is the same throughout the airway, flow velocity must be increased at the level of the compressed downstream segment. In fact, for any given flow, the velocity of flow is inversely related to the airway cross-sectional area:

Velocity = flow/cross-sectional area.

In theory, for a forced expiratory flow of 8 L/s through an uncompressed tracheal segment with a cross-sectional area of 2.0 cm, the linear velocity of gas would be approximately 2500 cm/s. Since dynamic airway compression may reduce the tracheal cross-sectional area by up to one-sixth of its normal value [6], the linear velocity would increase to over 14 000 cm/s. *In vivo* measurements of linear velocities in the human trachea [22] have demonstrated velocities close to 12 000 cm/s. The kinetic energy of a moving airstream increases as the square of the velocity. Thus, in the example shown, the force available to remove secretions from the compressed regions of the airways would be approximately 15 times greater than that available in uncompressed regions.

## Supramaximal flow

Dynamic airway compression not only plays a crucial role in limiting the expiratory flow, but is also implicated in the genesis of the flow transients that characterize the onset of both coughs and forced expirations (Fig. 19.3). The origin of such flow transients has been clearly understood since the work by Dayman in the early 1950s [26]. However, only the use of more advanced, fast response devices allowed quantitative analysis of the flow events generated by manoeuvres such as maximum voluntary cough, forced expirations and coughs triggered by the rapid release of a solenoid shutter valve placed at the mouth. Knudson *et al.* [17] were able to demonstrate that, during a series of maximum voluntary or triggered expiratory efforts performed from

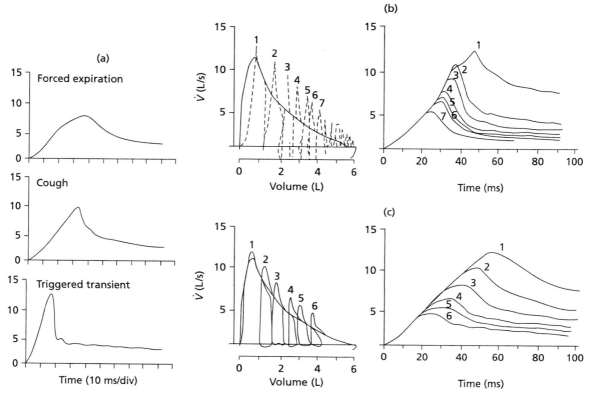

**Fig. 19.3** (a) Flow–time representations of forced expiration, cough and triggered transients performed at the same lung volume in a normal subject. (b) On the left is the flow–volume representation of a series of voluntary coughs beginning at total lung capacity and progressing sequentially down the vital capacity, superimposed on the subject's maximum expi-ratory flow–volume curve. On the right, the numbered coughs are represented as flow in time. (c) A series of brief, rapid expiratory efforts are depicted in the same manner as the coughs. Same subject provided all data shown. Reprinted with permission from [27].

near total lung capacity to near residual volume, two distinct components having different sites of origin, different time courses and mechanics contribute to the initial expiratory flow: the airway and the pulmonary components. The moment at which alveolar pressure exceeds mouth pressure, air begins to flow from the lung parenchyma, and this flow represents the pulmonary component. At the same time, since pleural pressure is greater than that within the central airways, these are subjected to dynamic compression and collapse abruptly. The flow produced by sudden displacement of the airway gas volume represents the airway component. This may be detected as a transient flow 'spike' at the beginning of the expiratory phase of each cough or forced expiration (Fig. 19.3), and is referred to as supramaximal expiratory flow, superimposed on more sustained flow from lung parenchyma. Transient peak flow rates, that are particularly evident at low lung volumes and in patients with airway obstruction [17], considerably exceed the limits imposed by the standard maximum expiratory flow–volume (MEFV) curve. If the expiratory effort is sustained, however, flow rapidly falls back to within the limits of the MEFV curve. Thus, with the exception of the initial supramaximal transients, the mechanisms limiting flow during forced expiration also operate to limit flow during cough.

The study by Arora and Gal [11] performed in normal curarized subjects demonstrated that expiratory muscle weakness markedly decreased inspiratory lung volume and the lung's ability to generate high pleural pressures during voluntary coughing. However, the decreased pleural pressure during cough following curarization had minimal effects on the pulmonary component of flow, whereas it markedly reduced airway compression as judged by the loss of flow transients in coughs initiated at the highest achievable lung volume [11].

The air volume displaced by dynamic compression is small, i.e. between 50 and 150 mL, also depending on the location of the EPP [17]. Volume acceleration (the ratio of peak flow to the time to peak) during cough and forced expiration may attain values as high as 300 L/s$^2$. Volume acceleration values of 1200 L/s$^2$ could be attained when coughing was triggered by a shutter at the mouth [17,27].

An additional phenomenon occurring during airway compression is that airway walls undergo substantial radial acceleration that may facilitate the interaction between flow and mucus (see below). As Leith *et al.* consider in their review on cough [3], during collapse the airways may behave in a manner similar to a rug being shaken in the wind. If the airways shake with full force, as in the case of intense cough or shutter-triggered coughs, more mucus can be shaken from the airways into the rapidly moving airstream of the cough, thus improving cough effectiveness. However, the possibility that supramaximal flow enhances cough clearance has recently been denied by Bennet and Zeman [27]. By using radiolabelled aerosols and gamma camera analysis, they compared the efficacy of voluntary coughs, forced expirations without glottis closure ('huffs') and shutter-triggered coughs for clearing mucus from the airways of patients with chronic airway obstruction. It was found that increasing supramaximal flow during coughing did not enhance mucus clearance, and that voluntary coughing was as effective as huffing in airway clearing [27]. Harris and Lowson [21] have evaluated the mechanical effectiveness of successive voluntary coughs in healthy young adults by simultaneously recording flow at the airway opening and changes in tracheal cross section by cine-radiography. They were able to show that peak flow occurred before maximum tracheal narrowing, so that maximum linear velocities were achieved during the period of more sustained but lower-rate flow which occurs after peak flow had subsided. They concluded that measurements of sustained flow rates during coughing might be of greater importance than measurements of peak flow for assessing the 'scrubbing action' of cough. In the light of these findings [21,27], it appears that both the time at which cough expiratory flow attains the highest velocity and the actual relevance of flow velocity to mucus removal need to be more clearly established.

### Flow–mucus interactions

In the airways flow can be either laminar (i.e. obeying Poiseuilles's law) or non-laminar (turbulent). Whether flow is laminar or turbulent can be predicted by the Reynolds number (*Re*), a dimensionless variable which depends upon $\dot{V}$, gas density ($\rho$) and viscosity ($\eta$), and the airway radius ($r$):

$$Re = 2\dot{V}\rho/\pi r\eta.$$

Turbulence is more likely to occur when *Re* is high, as is the case in the central airways, particularly the trachea. Conversely, laminar flow patterns occur only in the small peripheral airways. When an airway is lined with mucus, laminar flow exerts only a negligible shearing force on the lining. However, once flow becomes turbulent, it exercises a force on the lining layer, setting ripples and eventually shearing the mucus off the airway walls. In such conditions, where airflow exerts a mechanical influence on the mucus lining the airways, then it is said to be the *two-phase cocurrent flow* [3,25,28]. This refers to flow of gas and liquid (mucus) in the same direction within a conduit. For a gas density about that of air and a liquid viscosity similar to that of mucus, four main two-phase cocurrent flow regimes exist (Fig. 19.4). The bubble or aerated flow, in which the gas is dispersed as fine bubbles throughout the liquid, occurs for gas velocities below 60 cm/s. The piston or slug flow, in which the gas flows as large plugs, occurs for gas velocities from 60 to 1000 cm/s. The annular or film flow, in which the liquid is pumped up the airways as an annulus and the gas flows as a core, occurs for gas velocities over 1000 cm/s. Finally, for gas velocities over 2500 cm/s, the liquid is carried as fine drops in the gas phase: the mist flow, probably the most effective one [25]. Which types of mucus pumping occur in what parts of the airway depends on the linear velocity of gas which, as outlined above, is a function of flow rate and airway cross-sectional area. Air speeds sufficient to shear mucus from the airway wall typically occur in the collapsed airway segments downstream from the EPP. When the lungs are filled to vital capacity, the EPP is at

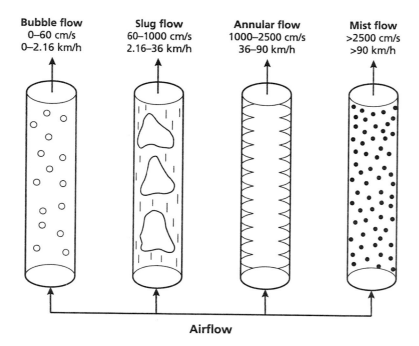

**Bubble flow**
0–60 cm/s
0–2.16 km/h

**Slug flow**
60–1000 cm/s
2.16–36 km/h

**Annular flow**
1000–2500 cm/s
36–90 km/h

**Mist flow**
>2500 cm/s
>90 km/h

**Airflow**

Fig. 19.4 The four basic regimens in two-phase cocurrent flow. The range of associated gas velocities is taken from engineering literature (see [32] for references) for large rigid conduits and Newtonian liquids. Reprinted with permission from [17].

the level of the trachea, and moves progressively upstream to segmental and smaller bronchi as the lungs empty. Since flow rate decreases at low lung volumes, it is doubtful whether the velocity of flow in the smaller bronchi is high enough to shift mucus, and theoretical analysis suggests that mist flow is unlikely to occur beyond the sixth-generation branches or for flow rates lower than 5 L/s [25].

## Cough motor mechanisms

The efferent outflows of cough are numerous, the most important ones being those to the airway smooth muscle, the upper airway and respiratory muscles, and the mucus-secreting apparatus. The mechanisms subserving mucus secretion during cough will be reviewed in Chapter 20 of this book.

### Airway smooth muscle

Cough and bronchoconstriction can be regarded as a defensive and protective reflex, respectively, for the respiratory tract [29]. Stimuli to the larynx and the tracheobronchial tree that cause coughing also cause reflex bronchoconstriction ([30] and references therein). Both these reflex responses appear to be mediated by the same type of receptor but their afferent neural pathways may be separate, since they can be induced individually and suppressed selectively by drugs [29]. In cats, mechanical stimulation of the larynx and tracheobronchial tree causes an increase in total lung resistance that closely corresponds with the inspiratory and expiratory motoneurone discharge [10]. A simultaneous recording of bronchoconstrictor fibre activity and of total lung resistance also reveals considerable correlation in time and magnitude [10].

The physiological meaning of cough-related bronchoconstriction is uncertain. It may, however, enhance both the sensory and the motor components of cough. Animal studies [31] have shown that airway rapidly adapting irritant receptors are stimulated or sensitized by smooth muscle contraction, and desensitized by muscle relaxants. Presumably, cough-related bronchoconstriction may also help to limit the progression of inhaled noxious substances into the lungs, or to stabilize the airway wall during the violent movements of coughing. In addition, constricted airways are more rigid than in the relaxed state, and this may prevent their total collapse when intrabronchial pressure falls below peribronchial pressure. This phenomenon might contribute to shifting the EPP upstream, and help to clear the smaller airways [32].

## Upper airway and respiratory muscles

The motor pattern of coughing involves the coordinated activation of several muscles, all having a prevailing respiratory function and exerting their mechanical action on the chest wall or upper airways. Simultaneous activation of muscles with an inspiratory or expiratory discharge pattern during normal breathing occurs during coughing [10]. For clarity, however, their functions will be analysed separately. Upper airway muscles do not contribute directly to airflow, but their activation needs to be synchronized with that of the respiratory muscles in the production of the normal pattern of breathing and the cough motor output. To ensure patency of the upper airways, muscles of the oral and nasal passageways are also recruited during coughing. They include the alae nasi muscles, muscles lowering the jaws to open the mouth, and soft palate muscles to close the nasopharynx. The genioglossus muscle may also be activated [33].

### Laryngeal muscles

The participation of individual laryngeal muscles in cough has been the object of several endoscopic analyses of the glottal chink [13]. In contrast, the analysis of laryngeal muscle activation has received considerably less attention. In humans, invasive electromyographic (EMG) recordings demonstrated intense activation of the adductor muscles occurring prior to the onset of the typical cough sounds, the magnitude of such activation being greater than that of both normal breathing and vocalization [34]. The abductor muscle contracted in reciprocal order to that of the adductors [34].

The study of the temporal relationships between the pattern of laryngeal muscle activation and the ongoing mechanical events during cough has recently been undertaken in anaesthetized dogs [4]. These authors recorded the EMG activity of the laryngeal abductor and adductor muscles, along with subglottic and intrathoracic pressure changes, during coughing elicited by mechanical stimulation of the tracheobronchial tree. The posterior cricoarytenoid (PCA) is the laryngeal abductor muscle, while the thyroarytenoid (TA) and arytenoid (AR) muscles are adductors. The role of the cricothyroid (CT) is still controversial, but its pattern of activation during cough closely resembles that of the abductor muscle [4]. During the inspiratory phase of cough, the PCA and the CT were activated, causing a reduction in upper airway resistance and promoting inspiratory flow. During glottal narrowing, the TA and AR were recruited, while both the PCA and CT displayed minimal activity. No consistent correlation was found between the magnitude of TA and RA EMG activity and intrathoracic and subglottic pressures, suggesting the intervention of additional mechanisms besides adductor muscle activation in the control of laryngeal resistance. Finally, during the expiratory phase, the PCA was recruited and the adductors were suppressed. These phenomena would open the glottis and, along with the activation of expiratory muscles, promote expulsion of air from the lung. Interestingly, this pattern of motor activation turned out to be unaffected by both isolating the larynx from the intrathoracic airways and sectioning of the internal branches of the superior laryngeal nerves. Therefore, the well-coordinated activation of laryngeal abductor and adductor muscles during tracheobronchial cough appears to be an entirely centrally preprogrammed event that is uninfluenced by the route of breathing and laryngeal sensory feedback [4].

### Diaphragm and other inspiratory muscles

Studies in cats have demonstrated that, compared with normal breathing, the EMG activity of the costal and crural diaphragm, along with that of the parasternal intercostals, is markedly increased during the inspiratory phase of coughing [35]. Large preparatory inspirations may optimize the precontractile lengths of the expiratory muscle, which is likely to be an advantageous situation for dynamic airway compression and high gas velocities during the subsequent expulsive phase of cough. The electrical activity of these inspiratory muscles also persists into the early expiratory portion of most mechanically induced cough efforts [10,34]. Tomori and Widdicombe [10] found that, at the beginning of the expiratory phase, the intensity of diaphragmatic activity exceeded that of the preceding inspiratory phase, lasted 0.1–0.2 s, and terminated prior to the attainment of peak positive intrapleural pressure. This pattern of diaphragmatic activation during cough may serve to counterbalance the simultaneous, intense activation of the expiratory musculature or delay the transmission of pressure from the abdomen to the thorax [10].

*Intercostal muscles*

The conventional view of intercostal muscle actions maintains that, because of muscle fibre orientation, the external intercostals (EIC) have an inspiratory action, whereas the internal intercostals (IIC) have an expiratory action ([34] and references therein). Indeed, recent human studies confirmed that the EIC in many areas of the rib cage shorten during passive inflation, whereas the IIC lengthen [36]. Thus, in agreement with Hamberger's theory ([36] and references therein), the EIC have an inspiratory advantage, while the IIC have an expiratory advantage. However, the magnitude of such mechanical advantages is such that the inspiratory advantage of the EIC is greatest at the rostral interspaces, and the expiratory advantage of the IEC is greatest at the ventral portion of the caudal interspaces [36]. The inspiratory effect of the EIC muscles is maximal at the level of the dorsal half of the second interspace, but decreases rapidly in the caudal direction and is reversed into an expiratory effect in the ventral half of the sixth and eighth interspaces. The IIC muscles in the ventral half of the sixth and eighth interspaces have large expiratory effects that decrease dorsally and cranially [36].

Previous EMG studies performed in experimental animals have demonstrated major differences in the control of intercostal muscles at different thoracic levels. In anaesthetized cats making respiratory efforts against an occluded airway, the EIC of the sixth costal interspace fired during inspiration and the IIC during expiration. However, both the EIC and the IIC of the third interspace discharged during inspiration, and those of the ninth space during expiration [37]. During coughing elicited by electrical stimulation of the superior laryngeal nerves in the decerebrate cat, midthoracic external and internal intercostal muscles discharged synchronously with the diaphragm and the abdominal muscles, respectively [38]. However, caudal external and internal intercostals discharged synchronously with the abdominal muscles [38].

*Abdominal and other expiratory muscles*

The principal expiratory muscles with significant respiratory function in humans lie in the ventrolateral aspect of the abdominal wall. The triangularis sternii also functions as an expiratory muscle. The abdominal muscles include the transversus abdominis muscle, the externus and internus obliquus muscles, and the rectus abdominis muscle [8].

The abdominal muscles have an important postural function as rotators and flexors of the trunk. As expiratory muscles, their contraction pulls the abdominal wall inward and increases abdominal pressure. As a result, the diaphragm is pushed cranially, lung volume decreases and pleural pressure increases. Due to their insertions on the rib cage, contraction of the abdominal muscles contributes to expiration by lowering the lower ribs. In humans breathing at rest, the abdominal muscles are silent in the supine position. In the standing posture, they often display a tonic activity unrelated to the phases of respiration [8]. Phasic expiratory contraction of these muscles occurs when ventilation reaches very high levels, or when the expiratory pressure is higher than 1 kPa [7].

In both humans and experimental animals, intense activation of the abdominal muscles is an essential component of cough. When triggered by appropriate afferent inputs, the respiratory network generating the cough motor pattern conveys an excitatory drive not only to the caudal expiratory neurones and, hence, to the major respiratory motoneurone pools, but also to the lower lumbar and sacral cord where pudendal motoneurones (nucleus of Onuf) innervating the external urethral and anal sphincters are located ([39] and references therein). Thus, an excitatory drive to caudal expiratory neurones may play a role also in preventing incontinence when abdominal pressure is raised by abdominal muscle activation during cough [39].

Tomori and Widdicombe [10] systematically investigated the motor pattern of a single abdominal muscle during coughing in cats, and showed that the rectus abdominis was strongly activated during this reflex and that such activation was associated with large intrathoracic pressures. Electromyographic recordings performed in humans during either voluntary or capsaicin-induced cough also documented strong activation of the rectus abdominis ([40] and references therein). The pattern of activation of the anterolateral abdominal muscles during coughing induced by mechanical stimulation of the tracheobronchial or laryngeal lumen has recently been studied in anaesthetized cats [40]. During cough, all four abdominal muscles proved to be simultaneously and vigorously activated and, unlike during expiratory threshold loading, the patterns of activation were very similar to one another [40]. In contrast, by means of surface EMG recordings performed in humans during voluntary coughing, Floyd and Silver [41] demonstrated substantial activation of both the internus and externus obliquus muscles that was associated with relative inactivity of the rectus abdominis muscle. Accordingly, a subsequent study by Strohl et al. [42] also showed greater activation of the upper and lower ventrolateral abdominal muscles compared with the rectus abdominis muscle during voluntary cough efforts in humans. Measurement of static expiratory airway pressure during spinal cord stimulation, performed before and after ablation of different expiratory muscle groups in the anaesthetized dog, confirmed that the oblique muscles make the largest mechanical contribution to pressure generation, and that the rectus abdominis muscle minimally contributes to pressure generation [43].

Non-invasive recordings of EMG activity of human abdominal muscle activity, particularly the obliquus externus muscle, have been used to assess the intensity of coughs elicited by inhalation of tussigenic agents [16,44,45]. Cox et al. [44] were the first to demonstrate that the sum of the electrical activity generated by each expiratory muscle contraction (i.e. the 'true' integrated EMG activity) correlated with the volume, flow and noise of coughs elicited by citric acid inhalation. More recently, the 'moving average' integrated EMG activity of the obliquus externus muscle has been used to evaluate the intensity of voluntary and reflex cough efforts [16,45]. These studies showed that the peak and rate of rise of the obliquus externus integrated EMG activity correlates with both the intensity of the cough stimulus [45] and the cough maximum expiratory flow [16,45].

In dogs, both the triangularis sternii and the transversus abdominis are active during normal breathing, and the peak activity of both these muscles increases approximately threefold during coughing [46]. De Troyer et al. [47] found that the triangularis sternii, an expiratory rib cage muscle, is active during the expiratory phase of coughing in humans. In tetraplegic subjects, contraction of the clavicular portion of the pectoralis major plays an important expiratory role during coughing [48].

## Cardiovascular implications of coughing

The intrathoracic pressure generated during both compression and the subsequent expiratory phase may be high enough to have important cardiovascular effects ([18] and references therein). If these high pressures are sustained, as may be the case in patients with bronchial obstruction, venous return, right and left cardiac filling and afterloads, systemic arterial flow distribution and vascular reflexes are markedly influenced. In consequence, cardiac output and systemic blood pressure are reduced, while systemic venous pressure rises. The reduction in blood pressure results in a decreased cerebral perfusion pressure that, along with the rise in cerebrospinal fluid pressure associated with the augmented thoracic and abdominal pressures, may eventually cause loss of consciousness [3,18]. The increase in venous pressure may result in rupture of subconjunctival, nasal and anal veins. Cough may also be accompanied by a reflex increase in vagal tone, also leading to bradycardia and heart blocks [18]. Cough has thus been used as a form of cardiopulmonary resuscitation to restore a more normal cardiac rhythm in patients with potentially lethal arrhythmia [18].

## References

1 Coryllos PN. Action of the diaphragm in cough. Experimental and clinical study on the human. *Am J Med Sci* 1937; **194**: 523–35.

2 Korpas J, Tomori Z. Cough and other respiratory reflexes. In: Herzog H, ed. *Progress in Respiratory Research*, Vol. 12. Basel: Karger, 1979: 94–105.

3 Leith DE, Butler JP, Sneddon SL, Brain JD. Cough. In: Fishman AP, Macklem PT, Mead J, Geiger SR, eds. *Handbook of Physiology. The Respiratory System. Mechanics of Breathing*, Sect. 3, Vol. III, Part 1. Bethesda, MD: American Physiological Society, 1979: 315–36.

4 Sant'Ambrogio G, Kuna ST, Vanoye CR, Sant'Ambrogio F. Activation of intrinsic laryngeal muscles during cough. *Am J Respir Crit Care Med* 1997; **155**: 637–41.

5 Yanagihara N, Von Leden H, Werner-Kukuk E. The physical parameter of cough: the larynx in a normal single cough. *Acta Otolaryngol* 1966; **61**: 495–510.

6 Ross BB, Graniak R, Rahn H. Physical dynamics of the cough mechanism. *J Appl Physiol* 1955; **8**: 264–8.

7 Agostoni E. Action of respiratory muscles. In: Fenn WO, Rahn H, eds. *Handbook of Physiology*, Vol. 1, Sect. 3, Chapter 12, *Respiration*. Washington, DC: American Physiological Society, 1964: 377–86.

8 De Troyer A, Loring SH. Action of respiratory muscles. In: Fishman AP, Macklem PT, Mead J, Geiger SR, eds. *Handbook of Physiology. The Respiratory System. Mechanics of Breathing*, Sect. 3, Vol. III. Bethesda, MD: American Physiological Society, 1986: 1–67.

9 Hanáček J, Davies A, Widdicombe JG. Influence of lung stretch receptors on the cough reflex in rabbits. *Respiration* 1984; **45**: 161–8.

10 Tomori Z, Widdicombe JG. Muscular, bronchomotor and cardiovascular reflexes elicited by mechanical stimulation of the respiratory tract. *J Physiol* 1969; **200**: 25–49.

11 Arora NS, Gal TJ. Cough dynamics during progressive expiratory muscle weakness in healthy curarized subjects. *J Appl Physiol* 1981; **51**: 494–8.

12 Lavietes MH, Smeltzer SC, Cook SD, Modak RM, Smaldone GC. Airway dynamics, oesophageal pressure and cough. *Eur Respir J* 1988; **11**: 156–61.

13 Von Leden H, Isshiki N. An analysis of cough at the level of the larynx. *Arch Otolaryngol* 1965; **81**: 616–25.

14 Gal TJ. Effects of endotracheal intubation on normal cough performance. *Anaesthesiology* 1980; **52**: 324–9.

15 Young S, Abdul-Settar N, Caric D. Glottic closure and high flows are not essential for productive cough. *Bull Eur Physiopathol Respir* 1987; **23** (Suppl. 10): 11s–17s.

16 Fontana GA, Pantaleo T, Lavorini F, Polli G, Pistolesi M. Coughing in laryngectomized patients. *Am J Respir Crit Care Med* 1999; **160**: 1578–84.

17 Knudson RJ, Mead J, Knudson DE. Contribution of airway collapse to supramaximal expiratory flow. *J Appl Physiol* 1974; **36**: 653–67.

18 Irwin RS, Boulet LP, Cloutier MM *et al.* Managing cough as a defence mechanism and as a symptom. A Consensus Panel Report of the American College of Chest Physicians. *Chest* 1998; **114**: 113s–81s.

19 Fontana GA, Lavorini F, Pantaleo T, Pistolesi M. Fisiologia della tosse. In: *La Tosse. Fisiopatologia e Clinica*. Pisa: Primula Multimedia, 2001: 14–43.

20 Macklem PT. Physiology of cough. *Ann Otol* 1974; **83**: 761–8.

21 Harris RS, Lawson TV. The relative mechanical effectiveness and efficiency of successive voluntary coughs in healthy young adults. *Clin Sci* 1968; **34**: 569–77.

22 Macklem PT, Wilson NJ. Measurement of intrabronchial pressure in man. *J Appl Physiol* 1965; **20**: 653–63.

23 Hyatt RE. Expiratory flow limitation. *J Appl Physiol* 1983; **55**: 1–8.

24 Dawson SV, Elliot EA. Wave-speed limitation on expiratory flow—a unifying concept. *J Appl Physiol* 1977; **43**: 498–515.

25 Leith DE. Cough. *J Am Phys Ther Assoc* 1968; **48**: 439–47.

26 Dayman H. Mechanics of airflow in health and emphysema. *J Clin Invest* 1951; **30**: 1175–90.

27 Bennet WD, Zeman KL. Effect of enhanced supramaximal flows on cough clearance. *J Appl Physiol* 1994; **77**: 1577–83.

28 Clarke SW, Jones JG, Oliver DR. Resistance to two-phase gas–liquid flow in airways. *J Appl Physiol* 1970; **29**: 464–71.

29 Karlsson J-A, Sant'Ambrogio G, Widdicombe JG. Afferent neural pathways in cough and reflex bronchoconstriction. *J Appl Physiol* 1988; **65**: 1007–23.

30 Widdicombe JG. Respiratory reflexes and defense. In: Brain JD, Procter DF, Reid LM, eds. *Respiratory Defense Mechanisms*, Part II. New York: Marcel Dekker, 1977: 593–630.

31 Mills JE, Sellick H, Widdicombe JG. Epithelial irritant receptors in the lungs. In: Porter R, ed. *Breathing, Hering-Breuer Centenary Symposium*. London: Churchill, 1970: 77–92.

32 Olsen CF, Stevens AE, Iroy MB. Rigidity of the trachea and bronchi during muscular contraction. *J Appl Physiol* 1967; **23**: 27–34.

33 Tatar M, Webber SE, Widdicombe J. Lung C-fibre receptor activation and defensive reflexes in dogs. *J Physiol* 1988; **402**: 411–20.

34 Faaborg-Andersen KL. Electromyographic investigation of intrinsic laryngeal muscles in humans: an investigation of subjects with normally movable cords and patients with vocal cord paresis. *Acta Physiol Scand* 1957; **41**: 1–148.

35 Van Lunteren E, Daniels R, Chandler Deal R, Haxhiou M. Role of costal and crural diaphragm and parasternal intercostals during coughing in cats. *J Appl Physiol* 1989; **66**: 135–41.

36 Wilson TA, Legarnd A, Gevenois P-A, De Troyer A. Respiratory effects of the external and internal intercostal muscles in humans. *J Physiol* 2001; **530.2**: 319–30.

37 Le Bars P, Duron B. Are the external and internal intercostal muscles synergist or antagonist in the cat? *Neurosci Lett* 1984; **51**: 383–6.

38 Iscoe S, Grelot L. Regional intercostal activity during coughing and vomiting in decerebrate cats. *Can J Physiol Pharmacol* 1992; **70**: 1195–9.

39 Bongianni F, Mutolo D, Fontana GA, Pantaleo T. Discharge patterns of Bötzinger complex neurons during cough in the cat. *Am J Physiol* 1988; **274**: R1015–R1024.

40 Bolser DC, Reier PJ, Davenport PW. Responses of the anterolateral abdominal muscles during cough and expiratory threshold loading in the cat. *J Appl Physiol* 2000; **88**: 1207–14.

41 Floyd WF, Silver PHS. Electromyographic study of patterns of activity of the anterior abdominal wall muscles in man. *J Anat* 1950; **84**: 132–45.

42 Strohl KP, Mead J, Banzett RB, Loring S, Kosch P. Regional differences in abdominal muscle activity during various maneuvres in humans. *J Appl Physiol* 1981; **51**: 1471–6.

43 Di Marco AF, Romaniuk JR, Kowalski KE, Supinski G. Mechanical contribution of expiratory muscles to pressure generation during spinal cord stimulation. *J Appl Physiol* 1999; **87**: 1433–9.

44  Cox ID, Wallis PJW, Apps MCP, Hughes DTD, Empey DW, Osman RCA, Burke CA. An electromyographic method of objectively assessing cough intensity and use of the method to assess effects of codeine on the dose–response curve to citric acid. *Br J Clin Pharmacol* 1984; **8**: 377–82.

45  Fontana GA, Pantaleo T, Lavorini F, Boddi F, Panuccio P. A non-invasive electromyographic study on threshold and intensity of cough in humans. *Eur Respir J* 1997; **10**: 983–9.

46  Van Lunteren E, Haxhiu MA, Cherniack NS, Arnold SJ. Role of triangularis sterni during coughing and sneezing in dogs. *J Appl Physiol* 1988; **65**: 2440–5.

47  De Troyer A, Ninane V, Gilmartin JJ, Lemerre C, Estenne M. Triangularis sterni muscle use in supine humans. *J Appl Physiol* 1987; **62**: 919–25.

48  Estenne M, De Troyer A. Cough in tetraplegic subjects: an active process. *Ann Intern Med* 1990; **112**: 22–8.

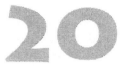

# 20 Mucus hypersecretion and mucus clearance in cough

*W. Michael Foster*

## Introduction

The tracheobronchial airways of the human lung are largely covered by a liquid lining of mucus. The mucus is a viscoelastic secretion that serves as a barrier for entrapment of microorganisms and xenobiotic material and protects the underlying mucosal tissues from dehydration. This fluid lining also acts as an extracellular surface for immunological and enzymatic action, and can absorb and neutralize toxic gases [1]. The airway lining fluid is hyperosmolar and relatively acidic, with high concentrations of calcium, sodium and potassium [2,3]. Current understanding is that the liquid lining is a two-phase model in which the superficial layer is a viscoelastic (mucins, tangled network of high molecular weight polymers) gel phase that overlays a periciliary sol phase (serous). The serous layer is approximately 2–4 μm in thickness and bathes the cilia that protrude from the epithelial surface, and thus the mucus layer with an estimated depth between 1 and 6 μm is thought to be propelled by ciliary beating and flows above the serous layer [1,4]. Recent *in vitro* studies suggest that perhaps the periciliary layer is not stationary but may move unidirectionally via ciliary activity [5]. The velocity of mucus layer transport can be fairly rapid in the tracheal airway, i.e. velocities observed in humans range between 4 and 21 mm/min [6], and appears related in part to the transfer rates of the mucus layer from the peripheral lung and dependent bronchi into the lower trachea [7]. Mucociliary transport and replacement of the mucus layer is influenced by several factors, e.g. secretion rate and viscoelasticity of the mucus, and synchrony and beat frequency of the cilia. Cough is a significant stimulus to mucus secretion in

health and a physical adjunct to mucociliary clearance in hypersecretory airway disease [8,9].

## Sources of airway mucus

In humans cellular sources of the mucin component of the airway liquid layer are the serous and mucous cells of the submucosal glands, the epithelial goblet cells and perhaps Clara cells. Submucosal glands are present throughout the lower respiratory tract in the airways containing cartilage; whereas goblet cells are located within all airways and extend to the level of the alveolar ducts, at which site Clara cells are found. Submucosal glands, due to their prominence in airway histological section, are considered to secrete the major contribution of mucus to airway surface liquid. Reid [10] had estimated that the volume of the glands in the airway mucosa was 40 times greater than the volume of goblet cells. This calculation was based on several assumptions and thus the current interpretation is that relative contributions of goblet cells and glands to the mucin component of airway mucus are uncertain and likely to vary with airway level and disease state. The normal daily output of tracheobronchial secretions does not exceed 0.5 mL/kg body weight under physiological conditions [11].

## Control of mucus secretion and transport

Due to the heterogeneity in the cell types that release secretory products onto the airway surface, control factors are not fully defined for the rate(s) of secretion or for the composition of products secreted by each cell type. Mechanisms that regulate the quality and volume of the respiratory secretions involve, for example, the transepithelial secretion of the chloride ion across the airway epithelium with passive diffusion of water, the stimulation of secretion by a number of mediators such as arachidonic acid metabolites, and the overall stability in the numbers of mucus-secreting epithelial cells present in the airways [12]. The final product, respiratory mucus, can be complex, with differing degrees of hydration and composition of ion and sugar content, as well as variation in amino acid, glycoprotein and lipid moities. Mucin proteins, the major constituents of airway mucus produced by goblet cells and submucosal glands, are a high molecular weight mixture of gene products. At least seven *MUC* genes are expressed in the human airways, but three predominate: *MUC5B*, *MUC1*, and *MUC5AC* [13]. Mucin glycoproteins are the major determinants for viscoelastic and adhesive properties of mucus [14]. Once synthesized, the mucin glycoproteins are stored within cytoplasmic membrane-bound granules; and upon appropriate stimulation, these granules are released via an exocytotic process in which the granules translocate to the cell periphery and fuse with the plasma membrane, followed by mucin release onto the epithelial surface. Intracellular protein kinases (protein kinase C and gCMP-dependent protein kinase) appear to be key determinants in the exocytotic release of mucin [15]. Three of the potential pathologies or airway lesions that lead to excess mucus are: (i) increased synthesis of mucus as a result of overexpression of mucin genes; and (ii) enhanced production of mucus secondary to hyperplasia, hypertrophy or even metaplasia of the secretory cells; or (iii) hypersecretion of stored mucin granules from surface goblet cells and submucosal glands.

A wide variety of agents and inflammatory/humoral mediators can provoke mucin secretion. In healthy subjects, the peripheral airways contain few goblet cells, but goblet cell metaplasia may occur in respiratory disorders. It is also recognized that surface goblet cells can quickly discharge vast quantities of mucus in response to an acute insult; although integral to defence, this outcome may also precipitate airway diseases associated with hypersecretion of mucus, including bronchitis [16]. Smokers with chronic bronchitis have been shown to have greater inflammation around gland ducts in bronchi larger than 4 mm in diameter. One hypothesis is that neutrophil infiltration of the airway epithelium may mediate hypersecretion by direct interaction with mucus-producing cells. This concept is supported by explants of human tracheal tissue in which integrin binding of neutrophils was required to induce degranulation of mucus cells [17]. A uniform airway response following exposure to respirable irritants, e.g. oxidants or acid aerosols, is a neural-mediated increase in the rate or volume of secretions from epithelial cells and/or submucosal glands [18]. In part this is a reflex defence mechanism to enhance the depth of the airway mucus layer and modify the sensitivity of airway irritant receptors and ameliorate bronchoconstrictive responses [18–20]. In addition to stimulation of neural reflexes, toxic agents can often interact with secretions directly. For example, an oxidant gas like ozone will react with the cross-linking bonds that hold glycoproteins together and lower viscosity [21]. Changes in the composition of secreted glycoproteins (either neutral or acid, depending upon specific sugars in their oligosaccharide side chains) may also alter the rheological properties of mucus; for example, an increase in the acidic glycoprotein content of mucins is associated with an increase in mucus viscosity.

## Control of mucociliary clearance

The mucociliary transport system is innervated predominantly by the parasympathetic nervous system; efferent postganglionic parasympathetic fibres have been identified in association with submucosal glands [22]. Airway surface epithelial cells and submucosal gland cells express muscarinic receptors [23–25]. There is also a high density of β-adrenergic receptors on surface epithelial cells and submucosal glands [26,27]. Submucosal glands also express α-adrenergic receptors which are localized mainly to serous cells [26]. Peptidergic receptors (for vasoactive intestinal peptide (VIP) and substance P) have also been identified on the airway epithelial cells [28,29]. Mucous glands preserved from bronchial surgical specimens of smokers with chronic bronchitis demonstrate a significant increase in the density of nerve fibres immunoreactive for VIP [30] and support the hypothesis for involvement of neuropeptides in hypersecretion of airway mucus [31]. Mucociliary transport does not appear to be under autonomic control; although it is known that atropine, a muscarinic antagonist that apparently does not change the rheological properties of mucus, can significantly reduce the rate of lung mucus transport in humans [32,33]. Both vagal and sympathetic nerve stimulation increase the rate of glandular secretion in several species; and direct stimulation of the airway surface by exogenous agonists, i.e. adrenergic and cholinergic, and mediators such as histamine, alter transepithelial secretory processes [1,16] and in humans increase airway mucociliary clearance [7,34,35].

Cough can be considered as a respiratory reflex with defensive capabilities and in general its presence is a sentinel of an abnormal condition or an irritant exposure. For example, an important role in epithelial membrane homeostasis and continuous effective clearance of the airway liquid layer is the interaction between mucus viscosity, periciliary fluid and the ciliary beating. Cough can signal dysfunction of these components, especially in chronic bronchitis, and may serve as a back-up and/or adjunct to the mucociliary clearance system. High intrathoracic pressures generated during cough serve to compress intrathoracic airways, thereby giving rise to high gas velocities within the airway. These high velocities of airflow supply the shearing forces necessary to dislodge material adherent to the airway epithelial surfaces. It appears likely that two-phase gas–liquid flow can occur in the human airway under certain conditions. During coughing and rapid breathing (such as with exercise) and maximal flow manoeuvres the Reynolds numbers in the large airways will be sufficiently high to result in gas–liquid interaction if the thickness of the mucus layer at the epithelial surface is in excess of approximately 300 μm [36]. These depths of mucus are believed to occur in hypersecretory airway disease [36] and, although the pathophysiology of persistent cough remains obscure, cough can be a manifestation of hypersecretory airway disease [37].

Cough is a rare occurrence in health (except for episodes of acute respiratory infection), and only a few investigations have evaluated the influence of cough on mucociliary clearance in subjects with normal pulmonary function. In fact, based upon mechanical principles, it has generally been presumed that voluntary cough manoeuvres are ineffective in the normal airway where moderate depths of the mucus layer (<20 μm) exist as compared to the excessive airway secretions and mucus layer thickness found in bronchitis (>200 μm) [8,38]. Camner et al. [38] observed no abrupt changes in airway clearance of a radiomarker during periods of short vigorous coughing (1–2 min). In similar fashion, Yeates and coworkers [39] demonstrated that voluntary coughing had no effect on tracheal velocities of mucus flow in healthy subjects. However, based upon a physical model with a turbulent stream of airflow through a straight tube and a non-Newtonian pseudoplastic fluid, Scherer and Burtz have proposed that cough-related ciliary mucus velocity can be enhanced down to about a 12th airway generation, even in a healthy individual [40]. In this connection, Bennett and colleagues have investigated the effects of cough on mucociliary clearance in healthy subjects during the performance of respiratory manoeuvres (cough-like expiratory, vs. rapid inspiratory, breathing) [8]. Their objective was to explore the influence of voluntary breathing manoeuvres on the clearance of airway secretions using respiratory efforts designed to generate directionally opposite, but instantaneous, airflow rates (peak mean airflow measured at the mouth of 7–10 L/s). The influence of these rapid breathing manoeuvres on lung mucociliary clearance is compared with respective control clearance curves in Fig. 20.1. Somewhat as expected, the cough-like expiratory manoeuvre significantly increased lung mucociliary clearance as compared with control clearance (Fig. 20.1a). However, surprisingly, the rapid inspiratory breathing pattern likewise had a stimulatory influence on transporting mucus out of the lung (Fig. 20.1b). Wolff et al. [41] have shown that both exercise and resting eucapnic hyperpnoea can enhance the rate of airway mucociliary clearance in normal subjects, though exercise provided for a more intense effect. However, the results with hyperpnoea are consistent with the results observed by Bennett and colleagues, i.e. independent of the direction of airflow, airway mucus clearance was stimulated by high velocity of airflow. Tracheobronchial neuronal reflexes may be responsible, whereby the velocity of airflow through large central airways could serve to be a stimulus via rapidly adapting receptors whose terminals lie within and under the epithelium of the larger bronchi and which respond to changes in lung volume (inflation and deflation). Following excitation of these receptors responses include cough or deep inspirations, bronchoconstriction, mucus secretion and airway vasodilatation [42]. Thus this integrated system is well suited as a neurophysiological line of defence that limits epithelial injury from respirable irritants. For example, following rapid lung inflation or deflation or exposure to a respirable irritant (dust, ozone, smoke, capsaicin) mucus release

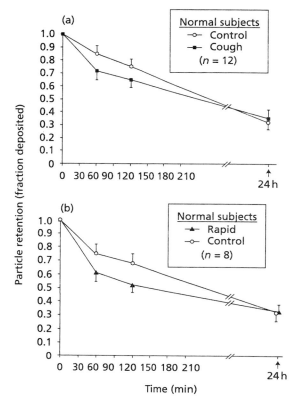

Fig. 20.1 Effect of voluntary respiratory manoeuvres on lung mucociliary clearance. (a) Comparison of high expiratory airflow (Cough) manoeuvre to relaxed breathing (Control); (b) Comparison of high inspiratory airflow (Rapid) manoeuvre to relaxed breathing (Control). Number of subjects studied as indicated and data represent mean and error bars as ±SEM. Assessment of mucociliary clearance on Control, Cough and Rapid study days; respiratory manoeuvres (high expiratory and inspiratory airflow rates, respectively) were performed voluntarily at 10-min intervals during the first hour of assessment of mucociliary clearance. Final measure of radiolabel retention assessed at 24 h post deposition of radiomarker.

from submucosal glands onto the epithelial surface would not only act to dilute the specific activity of a deposited irritant, but would serve to thicken the gel mucus layer and favour annular-type radial flow of the mucus layer during the expiratory phase through bronchoconstricted airways (undergoing increased airflow velocity, secondary to reduced airway diameter). Animal model studies support stimulation of tracheo-bronchial gland secretion in response to rapid deflation; an action that is abolished by vagal cooling, vagal section or anticholinergic treatment [43]. Thus during expiratory directed airflow (Fig. 20.1) the stimulatory action on mucociliary clearance may be reflex in nature and dependent upon cholinergic mechanisms. Support for this hypothesis arises from a study of stable, chronic airflow-obstructed patients who had demonstrable increases in mucociliary clearance during voluntary cough manoeuvres. However, pretreatment of these patients with a cholinergic antagonist that ablated vagal cholinergic efferent innervation of the airway and reflex responses prevented the cough-related augmentation of mucociliary clearance [44]. Thus during cough and near-maximal expiratory airflow mucociliary clearance becomes enhanced due to a combination of factors, i.e. neurally mediated mucus secretion coupled with radial transport of the gel–mucus layer out of the lung as a result of two-phase gas–liquid interaction [36,40].

## Control of mucociliary clearance in patients with chronic obstructive pulmonary disease

The significance of spontaneous cough or its frequency with regard to the kinetics of mucociliary clearance within tracheobronchial airways of patients with airflow obstruction is not completely understood [45]. Recently, in patients with chronic spontaneous cough exposure to isotonic alkaline salt solution that contained bicarbonate ions significantly enhanced airway mucociliary clearance as assessed with radiomarker technique [46]. It was hypothesized that replacement of $Cl^-$ by $HCO_3^-$ facilitated secretion of $Cl^-$ into the airway lumen and promoted hydration of the airway surface layer that favoured efficiency of cough clearance. Involuntary (spontaneous) cough is essential for clearance of secretions from the tracheobronchial airways in elderly (over 60 years) patients with obstructive lung disease [47]. For example, using airway clearance of an insoluble radiolabelled marker over a 4-h period as a gauge of lung mucus transport, mucociliary clearance in a small cohort of 16 patients (characterized by the half-time $T_{50}$, i.e. time to attain 50% clearance of the radiolabel) had a mean value of 145 min. Based upon the $T_{50}$ index and frequency of spontaneous cough during the 4-h measurement period the patients were divided into three groupings: (i) six patients had $T_{50} < 75$ min and over the 4 h averaged 23 coughs; (ii) three patients had $T_{50} > 75$ and $< 150$ min and averaged 13 coughs; and (iii) seven patients had $T_{50} > 150$ and $< 300$ min and averaged 4 coughs. There were no associations between indices of mechanical lung function of the patients, i.e. $FEV_1$ or FVC, and the $T_{50}$ index or the frequency of cough. These findings suggest that for elderly patients with obstructive airway disease the frequency of spontaneous cough is associated with effective clearance of airway mucus. Thus for patients with good preservation of their expiratory flow rates, spontaneous cough is an effective adjunct to mucociliary clearance of mucus from the lung. Submucosal inflammation, a common feature of obstructive airway disease, is a stimulus for cough [37,48]. Understanding the linkage in obstructive lung disease between inflammatory cells, mucosal injury, genesis of cough and efficient clearance of airway secretions will require further study [17,30,44].

Recent epidemiological studies have raised interest in risk assessment of patients with asthma, chronic obstructive pulmonary disease (COPD) and cystic fibrosis, and the presence of airway mucus hypersecretion is now considered to be a risk factor for increased morbidity. In general, hypersecretion of mucus within stem bronchi is usually related to cough and sputum; whereas inflammation and excess mucus discharge in the distal peripheral airway contribute to airflow obstruction and, as shown by morphological examination of airways (excised or postmortem), correlate with *in vivo* tests of small airways function [49,50]. Particularly for COPD patients, chronic hypersecretion of mucus is a major manifestation of their disease; however, its role in the development of chronic airflow obstruction is unclear. Peto and coauthors suggested that among males with similar initial airflow obstruction, age-specific COPD death rates were not significantly related to initial mucus hypersecretion, and supported the concept that airflow obstruction and mucus hypersecretion are largely independent disease processes [51]. However, recent support for a role of mucus hypersecretion in the development of chronic airflow limitation was documented by the Copenhagen City Heart Study [52], an 11-year follow-up study of over 12 000 men and women, that found chronic sputum production to be associated with both an excessive $FEV_1$ decline and an increased risk of hospitalization due to COPD.

Guided by clinical and therapeutic interests, mucociliary clearance has often been studied mechanistically in respiratory disease states (chronic bronchitis, COPD) to determine whether mucus hypersecretion is indeed correlated to indices of lung function, i.e. delays in clearance and thickening of the liquid lining layer contribute to airflow dysfunction. An examination of extremes (little or no functional impairment vs. severely obstructed) in these disease states provides insight for the hypothesis that hyperproduction of mucus is associated with airflow limitation. For example, asymptomatic bronchitis patients with short smoking histories and functional values in the predicted normal range for $FEV_1$ and peak expiratory flow have been shown to have normal values of mucus transport velocity within central airways (trachea and stem bronchi); and it was the peripheral bronchi that were first observed to exhibit delays and non-continuous clearance of airway mucus [53]. This peripheral abnormality in mucus transport was reversible with $\beta_2$-adrenergic therapy, but its presence is consistent with epithelial remodelling, changes in mucosal permeability and inflammatory cellular infiltrates, the triad of abnormal pathology commonly found in the lung periphery and respiratory bronchioles of young smokers [54]. By contrast, in patients with advanced airway obstruction, i.e. diagnosis of COPD, and severely reduced expiratory flow rates, delays in mucociliary clearance of airway secretions are predominantly found within airways of central lobar and stem bronchi. For example (Fig. 20.2), Smaldone and coauthors [55] using regional lung analysis techniques found that patients with chronic airflow obstruction and flow limitation, i.e. collapse of major bronchi during the expiratory phase of a tidal exhalation, exhibited significant slowing of mucus clearance within central airways. The patients were compared with normal subjects without airway obstruction and sufficient expiratory flow reserve, i.e. capable of increasing expiratory flow rates during tidal breathing. Mucociliary clearance was also significantly reduced in the peripheral airways of the patients (Fig. 20.2), although not so impaired as within the central airway. Although the flow-limited (expiratory) patients coughed at random during the clearance measures, due to their severe flow-limitation and low expiratory flow rates, cough likely would have been an ineffective adjunct to the mucociliary clearance process. Thus these patients exhibited a pattern of mucus stasis in the lung that was opposite to the normal situation: central air-

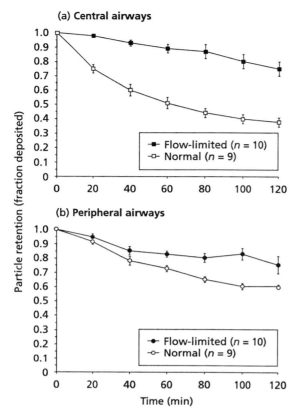

**(a) Central airways**

**(b) Peripheral airways**

Fig. 20.2 Regional mucociliary clearance in the lung. Average central (a) and peripheral (b) lung clearance of insoluble radiolabelled marker in healthy subjects and expiratory air-flow-limited COPD patients. Number of subjects studied as indicated and data represent mean and error bars as ±SEM. Lung regions located by radio-gas ventilation scan and divided into central (inner, 30% of total region and centred over large central airways) and peripheral (outer, remaining 70% of total region) airways. Time zero was at the time point immediately following inhalation and deposition of the radiomarker.

ways, that in the healthy airway clear most rapidly and are assisted by cough and two-phase gas–liquid transport, became rate-limiting. Previous investigations [56,57] have shown reduced whole-lung clearance in COPD; however, these studies did not try to assess whether clearance deficiencies were of a global or a regional nature. In COPD, which diffusely affects lung parenchyma and airways, there is no reason to suspect *a priori* that a rate-limiting clearance defect would be located in central bronchi. Thus the results of the

Smaldone report, disproportionate reduction of mucus clearance centrally in the lung, certainly support speculation that the prolonged retention and thickening of the mucus layer may reduce airway diameter and contribute to the mechanical effects causing airflow obstruction as suggested by the Copenhagen City Heart Study [52]. These findings do not imply that clearance abnormalities are confined to central airways in COPD, as significant evidence of peripheral impairment was also apparent (Fig. 20.2). However, the changes in the periphery were small as compared with the marked slowing found centrally where the effects of ineffective cough may be superimposed on a generalized increase in synthesis and release of mucin proteins onto the airway surface [17].

Therefore in the healthy airway, lung inflation/deflation reflexes, and perhaps shearing forces at the airway surface during airflow at high velocity, are significant stimuli for enhancing mucociliary clearance [8,42]. However, in the early stages of smoke-related airway pathology and mucus hypersecretion in which epithelial remodelling is extended over time, deficiencies in the mucociliary clearance system seem to predominate at least initially in the smaller peripheral airways [53]. If there is preservation of expiratory airflow rates then even with continued exposure to environmental irritants and cigarette smoke, mucociliary clearance remains effective when assisted by cough and two-phase, gas–liquid interactions [47,58]. However, for patients with advanced airway obstruction and incapable of generating forceful expiratory flows, i.e. expiratory flow limitation, cough is ineffective and mucociliary clearance is now disparate with markedly slowed mucus layer transport within central airways [55]. For irritant-induced mucus hypersecretion and the later stages of progressive airway obstruction, improving clearance of airway secretions may largely depend upon mucoactive and mucolytic therapies designed to limit viscous airway secretions, increase cough clearance, and improve ventilation [46,59,60].

## Control of mucociliary clearance in asthma

In bronchial asthma the mucous glands are distributed throughout the cartilaginous airways as they are in the normal lung, but also may extend into peripheral bronchioles where normally they are absent. Hypertrophy of the submucosal gland mass is thought to contribute to the presence of excessive mucus production found in fatal asthma. Frequently on pathological examination, there is dilatation of the secretory ducts leading from the submucosal glands into the bronchial airway lumen. An increase in the number of epithelial goblet cells also contributes to the excess of secretions within the airway in severe asthma [61] and the excessive secretions present in the larger bronchi may overwhelm the normal clearance mechanisms and undergo retrograde flow and/or aspiration into smaller airways. When mucus secretions are in excess, as in status asthmaticus, mucus plugs may extend from the larger second-generation bronchi into the smaller bronchioles [62].

Marked pathophysiological changes in mucociliary transport in bronchial asthma have been observed. Mucociliary transport has been found to be depressed in experimental as well as human asthma; during acute antigen challenge, a further reduction in mucociliary transport is observed. The abnormal mucociliary transport may contribute to physiological abnormalities in airways function. Cough and residual airways dysfunction found to be present in asthma patients in remission is partly related to the presence of excessive mucus in the peripheral airway. This is usually easily observed in scintigraphy studies of asthma patients by inhomogeneities of radioaerosol deposition in the larger bronchi and with poor penetration of micron-sized aerosol into the peripheral airway [63,64].

Fahy and coauthors [14] have recently addressed the question of whether excessive mucus is an important cause of morbidity in moderate and mild asthmatic subjects (severity characterized by $FEV_1$). Based upon airway epithelial biopsy of mainstem bronchi the epithelial mucin stores were increased in mild and moderate asthma and this increase was attributable to goblet cell hyperplasia (not hypertrophy). Induced sputum collected in the patients suggested that secreted mucin was increased only in the moderate asthmatics [65]. An interesting observation in the diathesis of asthma is the finding of a broad range of airway mucociliary clearance rates. Thus, for example, in severe asthma (mean $FEV_1 < 50\%$ of FVC) mucus clearance velocities in central airways are markedly reduced as compared to non-asthma subjects; and the patients (Fig. 20.3) in fact only exhibit measurable velocities of mucus transport within mainstem bronchi and tracheal airways when stimulated by a β-adrenergic agonist [66]. A corresponding increase in whole-lung clearance was also observed in the patients following β-adrenergic aerosol treatment, e.g. on average 53% of the mucus marker was removed with treatment as compared with 22% on a control day without treatment. This represented a 1.5-fold increase in lung mucus clearance and transport of the airway mucus layer was now comparable with lung clearance observed in unstimulated healthy subjects [53,66]. However, rapid rates of lung mucociliary clearance have been observed in stable asthma patients with mild to moderate airflow obstruction (mean $FEV_1$ of 66% FVC) in which over 40% of the airway mucus marker was cleared within the initial 30 min of assessment and on average 60% cleared after a 1-h time period [67]. These supranormal rates of airway mucus clearance in mild to moderate asthmatics are consistent with observations by other laboratories for

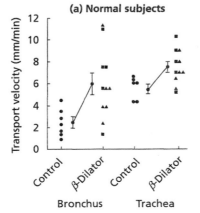 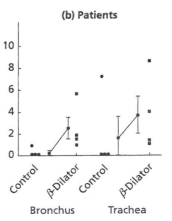

Fig. 20.3 Bronchial and tracheal mucus transport velocity. (a) Healthy subjects; (b) asthma patients. Individual values and means ± SEM of these values are shown for control (●) velocities and after β-adrenergic aerosol stimulation: isoproterenol (■), or isoetharine (▲). Increases in velocity were significant compared with control tracheal and bronchial mucus velocities; $P < 0.01$.

non-symptomatic patients at the time of their mucus clearance evaluation [68,69]. Although in mild asthma lung mucus clearance can become impaired and be severely compromised during a period of acute exacerbation that requires hospitalization, after recovery and hospital discharge, a repeat evaluation of lung mucociliary clearance demonstrated remarkable improvement [70] although at recovery it is difficult to separate out influences of rescue medications and therapeutic (β-adrenergics, theophylline, corticosteroids) intervention on mucus clearance. The patients voluntarily resisted coughing during the assessment periods, so clearly physical adjuncts to therapy were not responsible for the return of normal clearance at recovery. Therapeutic approaches [71] to prevent exacerbation in bronchial asthma are based on long-term control medications and include corticosteroids, sodium cromoglycate and nedocromil sodium, long-acting $\beta_2$ adrenoceptor agonists and methylxanthines, all of which enhance the efficiency of mucociliary function [72]. As new information becomes available on mechanisms of goblet cell synthesis and release of mucin granules [15] novel strategies are expected to evolve to limit factors related to secretion, i.e. inflammatory cells such as neutrophils [17], or inhibit growth receptors [73] located on epithelial cells and that are key to secretory cell metaplasia and secretagogue activity.

## Conclusions

1 The airway surface of the lower respiratory tract is largely protected by a liquid lining layer composed of a periciliary phase, adjacent to the luminal surface of the epithelial lining cells, and a gel phase superimposed on top. The thickness of this layer depends on transepithelial secretion of $Cl^-$ across the epithelial lining cells with passive diffusion of water, steady-state and stimulated mucin secretion, and overall stability in the numbers of mucus-secreting epithelial cells.

2 Effective transport of the gel phase to the larynx limits residence time, and removes secretions and xenobiotic materials from the epithelial surface. Transport results from coordinated ciliary activity of the epithelial lining cells. Lung inflation/deflation reflexes and shearing forces at the airway surface during high-velocity airflow, i.e. cough, are stimulatory factors for increasing mucociliary clearance. Thus in health and airway disease, spontaneous and/or voluntary cough is a powerful adjunct to mucociliary activity for clearance of airway secretions.

3 In hypersecretory airway disease like bronchitis, tracheal mucus velocities are normal but mucus layer transport is deficient within the peripheral airways. In severe stages of COPD, mucus clearance is preferentially impaired within central dependent bronchi. Cough is an effective adjunct for clearance of secretions when high velocities of expiratory airflow are preserved and gas flow and airway liquid interaction favours cough clearance of secretions.

4 In bronchial asthma, severity of disease in large measure determines whether airway clearance of secretions is: (i) supranormal; (ii) capable of therapeutic up-regulation; or (iii) ineffective during states of exacerbation and hypersecretion of mucus.

5 As new information develops on control mechanisms for mucin synthesis and mucin granule release, therapeutic measures likewise are expected to evolve to fortify mucociliary clearance and ameliorate mucus hypersecretion.

*Acknowledgements*

Preparation of this chapter was supported in part by awards from National Heart Lung and Blood Institute: HL-62641 and HL-68072 (Washington, DC, USA).

## References

1 Kaliner M, Shelhamer JH, Borson B *et al.* Human respiratory mucus. *Am Rev Respir Dis* 1986; **134**: 612–21.

2 Robinson NP, Kyle H, Webber SE *et al.* Electrolyte and other chemical concentrations in tracheal airway surface liquid and mucus. *J Appl Physiol* 1989; **66**: 2129–35.

3 Knowles M, Gatzy J, Boucher R. Ion composition of airway surface liquid of patients with cystic fibrosis as compared to normal and disease-control subjects. *J Clin Invest* 1997; **100**: 2588–95.

4 Widdicombe J. Airway and alveolar permeability and surface liquid thickness: theory. *J Appl Physiol* 1997; **82**: 3–12.

5 Matsui H, Randell SH, Peretti SW *et al.* Coordinated clearance of periciliary liquid and mucus from airway surface. *J Clin Invest* 1998; **102**: 1125–31.

6 Wolff RK. Mucociliary clearance. In: Parent RA, ed. *Comparative Biology of the Normal Lung*. Boca Raton, FL: CRC Press, 1992: 659–80.

7 Foster WM, Langenback EG, Bergofsky EH. Measurement of tracheal and bronchial mucus velocities in man:

relation to lung clearance. *J Appl Physiol* 1980; **48**: 965–71.

8  Bennett WD, Foster WM, Chapman WF. Cough-enhanced mucus clearance in the normal lung. *J Appl Physiol* 1990; **69**: 1670–5.

9  Groth ML, Macri K, Foster WM. Cough and mucociliary transport of airway particulate in chronic obstructive lung disease. *Ann Occup Hyg* 1997: **41** (S): 515–21.

10  Reid L. Measurement of the bronchial mucous gland layer a diagnostic yardstick in chronic bronchitis. *Thorax* 1960; **15**: 132–41.

11  Toremalm NG. The daily amount of tracheo-bronchial secretions in man. *Acta Otolaryngol* 1960: **158** (S):43–53.

12  Jacquot J, Hayem A, Galabert C. Functions of proteins and lipids in airway secretions. *Eur Respir J* 1992; **5**: 343–58.

13  Rose MC, Gendler SJ. Airway mucin genes and gene products. In: Rogers DF, Lethem DI, eds. *Airway Mucus: Basic Mechanisms and Clinical Perspectives*. Boston: Birkhauser-Verlag, 1997: 41–66.

14  Fahy JV. Airway mucus and mucociliary system. In: Middleton E, Reed CE, Busse WW, eds. *Allergy Principles and Practice*. St Louis, MO: CV Mosby, 1998: 520–31.

15  Li Y, Martin LD, Spizz G *et al*. MARCKS protein is a key molecule regulating mucin secretion in human airway epithelial cells *in vitro*. *J Biol Chem* 2001; **276**: 40982–90.

16  Rogers DF. Airway goblet cell: responsive and adaptable front-line defenders. *Eur Respir J* 1994; **7**: 1690–706.

17  Nadel JA. Role of neutrophil elastase in hypersecretion during COPD exacerbations, and proposed therapies. *Chest* 2000; **117**: 386S–89S.

18  Costa DL, Schelegle ES. Inhaled air pollutants. In: Swift DH, Foster WM, eds. *Air Pollutants and the Respiratory Tract*. New York: Marcel Dekker, 1999: 119–45.

19  King M, Kelly S, Cosio M. Alteration of airway reactivity by mucus. *Respir Physiol* 1985; **62**: 47–59.

20  Kim CS, Eldridge MA, Wanner A. Airway responsiveness to inhaled and intravenous carbachol in sheep: effect of airway mucus. *J Appl Physiol* 1988; **65**: 2744–51.

21  Last JA. Mucus production and the ciliary escalator. In: Witschi H, Nettersheim P, eds. *Mechanisms in Respiratory Toxicology*, Vol. 1. Boca Raton, FL: CRC Press, 1982: 247–60.

22  Laitinen A. Ultrastructural organization of intraepithelial nerves in human airway tract. *Thorax* 1985; **40**: 488–92.

23  Barnes PJ, Nadel JA, Roberts JM, Basbaum CB. Muscarinic receptors in lung and trachea: autoradiographic localization using quinuclidinyl benzilate. *Eur J Pharmacol* 1983; **86**: 103–6.

24  Basbaum CB, Barnes PJ, Grillo M *et al*. Adrenergic and cholinergic receptors in submucosal glands in ferret trachea: autoradiographic localization. *Eur J Respir Dis* 1983; **64**: 433–5.

25  Basbaum CB, Grillo M, Widdicombe JH. Muscarinic receptors: evidence for a non-uniform distribution in tracheal smooth muscle and exocrine glands. *J Neurol Sci* 1984; **4**: 508–20.

26  Barnes PJ, Basbaum CB. Mapping of adrenergic receptors in mammalian trachea using an autoradiographic method. *Exp Lung Res* 1983; **5**: 183–92.

27  Kelsen SG, Mardini IA, Zhou S *et al*. A technique to harvest viable tracheo-bronchial epithelial cells from living human donors. *Am J Respir Cell Mol Biol* 1992; **67**: 66–72.

28  Carstairs JR, Barnes PJ. Visualization of vasoactive intestinal peptide receptors in human and guinea-pig lung. *J Pharmacol Exp Ther* 1986; **239**: 240–55.

29  Basbaum C. Innervation of the airway mucosa and submucosa. *Semin Respir Med* 1995; **308**: 313.

30  Lucchini RE, Facchini F, Turato G *et al*. Increased VIP-positive nerve fibers in the mucous glands of subjects with chronic bronchitis. *Am J Respir Crit Care Med* 1997; **156**: 1963–8.

31  Barnes PJ, Barianuk JN, Belvisi MG. Neuropeptides in the respiratory tract. I. State of art. *Am Rev Respir Dis* 1991; **144**: 1187–98.

32  Groth ML, Langenback EG, Foster WM. Influence of inhaled atropine on lung mucociliary function in humans. *Am Rev Respir Dis* 1992; **145**: 215–9.

33  Foster WM, Bergofsky EH, Bohning D *et al*. Effect of adrenergic agents and their mode of action on mucociliary clearance. *J Appl Physiol* 1876; **41**: 146–52.

34  Camner P, Strandberg K, Philipson K. Increased mucociliary transport by cholinergic stimulation. *Arch Environ Health* 1974; **29**: 220–4.

35  Mussato DJ, Garrard CS, Lourenco RV. The effect of inhaled histamine on human tracheal mucus velocity and bronchial mucociliary clearance. *Am Rev Respir Dis* 1988; **138**: 775–9.

36  Clarke SW, Jones JG, Oliver DR. Resistance to two-phase gas-liquid flow in airways. *J Appl Physiol* 1970; **29**: 464–71.

37  Banner AS. Cough: physiology, evaluation, and treatment. *Lung* 1986; **164**: 79–92.

38  Camner P, Mossberg M, Philipson K *et al*. Elimination of test particles from the human tracheobronchial tract by voluntary coughing. *Scand J Respir Dis* 1979; **60**: 56–62.

39  Yeates D, Aspin N, Levinson H *et al*. Mucociliary tracheal transport rates in man. *J Appl Physiol* 1975; **39**: 47–95.

40  Scherer P, Burtz L. Fluid mechanical experiments relevant to coughing. *J Biomech* 1978; **11**: 183–7.

41  Wolff RK, Dolovich MB, Obminski G, Newhouse MT. Effects of exercise and eucapnic hyperventilation on bronchial clearance in man. *J Appl Physiol* 1977; **43**: 46–50.

**215**

42 Widdicombe JG. Neurophysiology of the cough reflex. *Eur Respir J* 1995; **8**: 1193–202.

43 Yu J, Schultz HD, Goodman JC, Coleridge JCG, Coleridge HM, Davis B. Pulmonary rapidly adapting receptors reflexly increase airway secretion in dogs. *J Appl Physiol* 1989; **67**: 682–7.

44 Bennett WD, Chapman WF, Mascarella JM. The acute effect of ipratropium bromide bronchodilator therapy on cough clearance in COPD. *Chest* 1993; **103**: 488–95.

45 Irwin RS, Curley FJ, French CL. Chronic cough: spectrum and frequency of causes, key components of the diagnostic evaluation, and outcome of specific therapy. *Am Rev Respir Dis* 1990; **141**: 640–7.

46 Haidl P, Schonhofer B, Kohler D. Inhaled isotonic alkaline versus saline solution and radioaerosol clearance in chronic cough. *Eur Respir J* 2000; **16**: 1102–8.

47 Groth ML, Macri K, Foster WM. Cough and mucociliary transport of airway particulate in chronic obstructive lung disease. *Ann Occup Hyg* 1997; **41**(S1): 515–21.

48 Linden M, Ramussen JB, Piitulainen E *et al.* Airway inflammation in smokers with nonobstructive and obstructive chronic bronchitis. *Am Rev Resp Dis* 1993; **148**: 1226–32.

49 Wright JL, Lawson LM, Pare PD *et al.* The detection of small airways disease. *Am Rev Respir Dis* 1984; **129**: 989–94.

50 Peto R, Speizer FE, Cochrane AL *et al.* The relevance in adults of air-flow obstruction, but not of mucus hypersecretion, to mortality from chronic lung disease. *Am Rev Respir Dis* 1983; **128**: 491–500.

51 Cosio M, Ghezo H, Hogg JC *et al.* The relationship between structural changes in small airways and pulmonary function tests. *N Engl J Med* 1978; **298**: 1277–81.

52 Vestbo J, Prescott E, Lange P. Copenhagen City Heart Study Group. Association of chronic mucus hypersecretion with $FEV_1$ decline and chronic obstructive disease mortality. *Am J Respir Crit Care Med* 1996; **153**: 1530–5.

53 Foster WM, Langenback EG, Bergofsky EH. Disassociation of mucociliary function in central and peripheral airways of asymptomatic smokers. *Am Rev Respir Dis* 1985; **132**: 633–9.

54 Niewoehner DE, Kleinerman J, Rice DB. Pathologic changes in the peripheral airways of young cigarette smokers. *N Engl J Med* 1974; **153**: 629–32.

55 Smaldone GC, Foster WM, O'Riordan TG *et al.* Regional impairment of mucociliary clearance in chronic obstructive pulmonary disease. *Chest* 1993; **103**: 1390–6.

56 Camner P, Mossberg B, Philipson K. Tracheobronchial clearance and chronic obstructive lung disease. *Scand J Respir Dis* 1978; **54**: 272–81.

57 Mossberg B, Strandberg K, Philipson K *et al.* Tracheobronchial clearance and beta agonist stimulation in patients with chronic bronchitis. *Scand J Respir Dis* 1976; **57**: 281–9.

58 Puchele E, Zahm JM, Girard F *et al.* Mucociliary transport *in vivo* and *in vitro*: relations to sputum properties in chronic bronchitis. *Eur J Respir Dis* 1980; **61**: 254–64.

59 Ziment I. Help for an overtaxed mucociliary system: managing abnormal mucus. *J Respir Dis* 1991; **12**: 21–33.

60 Poole PJ, Black PN. Oral mucolytic drugs for exacerbations of chronic obstructive pulmonary disease: systematic review. *Br Med J* 2001; **322**: 1271–83.

61 Shimure S, Andoh Y, Haraguchi M *et al.* Continuity of airway goblet cells and intraluminal mucus in the airways of patients with bronchial asthma. *Eur Respir J* 1996; **9**: 1395–401.

62 Sheehan JK, Richardson PS, Fung DC *et al.* Analysis of respiratory mucus glycoproteins in asthma: a detailed study from a patient who died in status asthmaticus. *Am J Respir Cell Mol Biol* 1995; **13**: 748–56.

63 Chopra SK, Taplin GV, Tashkin DP *et al.* Imaging sites of airway obstruction and measuring functional responses to bronchodilator treatment in asthma. *Thorax* 1979; **34**: 493–500.

64 Agnew JE, Bateman JRM, Pavia D *et al.* Radionuclide demonstration of ventilatory abnormalities in mild asthma. *Clin Sci* 1984; **66**: 525–31.

65 Ordonez CL, Khashayar R, Wong HH *et al.* Mild and moderate asthma is associated with airway goblet cell hyperplasia and abnormalities in mucin gene expression. *Am J Respir Crit Care Med* 2001; **163**: 517–23.

66 Foster WM, Bergofsky EH. Airway mucus membrane: effects of beta-adrenergic and anticholinergic stimulations. *Am J Med* 1986; **81** (S5A): 28–35.

67 Groth ML, Ackner V, Foster WM. Targeting of therapeutic aerosols in asthma: is poor penetration of aerosols associated with mucociliary dysfunction in central airways? *Am Rev Respir Dis* 1991; **143**: A634.

68 Mussato DJ, Chakravarthy VS, Masssey VJ *et al.* Computer generated scintigraphy and mucociliary clearance in healthy and asthmatic patients. *Am Rev Respir Dis* 1989; **139**: A142.

69 O'Riordan TG, Zwang J, Smaldone GC. Mucociliary clearance in adult asthma. *Am Rev Respir Dis* 1992; **146**: 598–603.

70 Messina MS, O'Riordan TG, Smaldone GC. Changes in mucociliary clearance during acute exacerbations of asthma. *Am Rev Respir Dis* 1991; **143**: 993–7.

71 Bousquet J, Jeffery PK, Busse WW *et al.* State of the art: asthma from bronchoconstriction to airways inflammation and remodeling. *Am J Respir Crit Care Med* 2000; **161**: 1720–45.

72 Wanner A, Salathe M, O'Riordan TG. State of the art: mucociliary clearance in the airways. *Am J Respir Crit Care Med* 1996; **154**: 1868–902.

73 Takeyama K, Fahy JV, Nadel JA. Relationship of epidermal growth factor receptors to goblet cell production in human bronchi. *Am J Respir Crit Care Med* 2001; **163**: 511–6.

# 21 Animal models of cough

*Maria G. Belvisi & David J. Hele*

## Introduction

The ultimate goal of an animal model is to provide a system to elucidate mechanisms and test putative drug candidates. The model needs to accurately reflect the disease in humans as closely as is possible. If treatments are available for the disease in humans then demonstrable activity of these treatments in the animal model of choice greatly enhances the credibility of that model.

Cough, a reflex defence mechanism, is an extremely common symptom of many inflammatory diseases of the airways such as asthma and chronic obstructive pulmonary disease [1]. At present there are no satisfactory treatments for acute cough as was outlined in a recent review [2] where over-the-counter (OTC) cough medicines were assessed. It was concluded that the currently available medicines could not be recommended, as there was no good evidence for their effectiveness.

It is therefore essential to develop animal models of cough, models that reflect the disease in humans. A reliable, robust and reproducible model of cough is essential to profile, and establish the efficacy of, novel antitussive therapies under development prior to testing in humans. The chosen model should also allow the study of the physiology of cough and the mechanisms and mediators that lead to cough or the exacerbation of cough.

Therefore a requirement of the animal of choice for the model is that the physiology should resemble as closely as possible that of humans, which in models used to study the cough reflex means not only the structure of the lungs but also the innervation of the trachea, bronchi and intrapulmonary airways.

## Physiology

The cough reflex can be evoked by mechanical or chemical stimuli or by changes in ion concentration or osmolarity in the local mucosal surface. The reflex composes three parts, the afferent system, which senses the cough-inducing stimulus, the central nervous system (CNS), which in turn stimulates the efferent system that produces the cough [3]. Interference with the afferent signal is thought to provide the best opportunity for pharmacological intervention as the cough centre in the brain has not yet been clearly identified and may be diffuse. Interference with the efferent signal may affect many other processes, i.e. the gut and cardiovascular system. The afferent nerves that are thought to play an important role in the cough reflex are the myelinated Aδ-fibres (also known as rapidly adapting stretch receptors, RARs) and the non-myelinated C-fibres.

## Model development

### Species

In an attempt to accurately reflect the disease in humans several different species have been used to provide a variety of models of cough. Most preclinical studies of neural pathways involved in the cough reflex and the pharmacological regulation of those pathways have been conducted in mice, rats, guinea-pigs, rabbits, cats and dogs [4], and more recently in conscious pigs [5].

In rodents the cough reflex is difficult to study in

anaesthetized animals as anaesthesia suppresses neuronal conduction and activity in the CNS. However, several investigators have used a conscious rat model of cough to study the effect of potential antitussive therapies. Although many studies have been performed in conscious rats, and cough sounds recorded [6], there is much scepticism regarding the ability of these animals to produce a cough that resembles the reflex seen in humans. In fact, it is thought that if cough can be elicited in rats it would appear that the main reflexogenic origin of the cough is the larynx rather than the tracheobronchial tree. Indeed, expulsive events originating from the larynx can include expiration reflexes, which are difficult to differentiate from cough. Furthermore, the two reflexes are regulated differently [7]. Other studies have described a murine model of cough [8] but again there are certain reservations regarding the use of this model given that mice do not have RARs (rapidly adapting receptors conducting in the Aδ range, the nerves traditionally believed, along with C-fibre afferents, to play an important role in the cough reflex) and have been found to be lacking in intraepithelial nerve endings and thus are thought to be without a cough reflex [8]. It has also been shown that mice cannot cough, as they cannot generate the energy needed to cough. It is therefore probable that investigators using the model are measuring an expiration reflex rather than a true cough.

The use of large animals such as cats, dogs and pigs involves a cost element, not only in their purchase price but also in the cost of feeding and housing and in the cost of producing large quantities of drug substance for screening purposes. Although the use of these animals is thus precluded for routine screening they may be of value for tertiary screening of a compound selected for development, and the cat, for example, has played a useful role in determining the physiology and mechanisms involved in the cough response.

The most useful and commonly used model for cough studies in recent years has been the conscious guinea-pig [9,10]. Much information has now been gathered in this model regarding the pharmacological modulation of the cough reflex. Various tussive stimuli have been examined, with the most commonly used being inhaled citric acid or capsaicin. In these experiments cough can be detected by putting the guinea-pig in a transparent perspex chamber, exposing it to aerosols of tussive stimuli and measuring changes in airflow, observing the characteristic posture of an

animal about to cough and recording the cough sound [11–14]. This method is described in detail below.

## Conscious vs. anaesthetized animals

As mentioned earlier, in rodents the cough reflex is difficult to study in anaesthetized animals as anaesthesia suppresses neuronal conduction and activity in the CNS. In some species (non-rodent), a suitable depth of anaesthesia, with respiratory reflexes being essentially intact, can be obtained and a tussive response easily measured [4]. An example of this is the anaesthetized cat, which has been utilized to analyse both the central effects of antitussives administered intracerebroventricularly [15] and the peripheral effects of compounds administered intravenously [16]. In these experiments cough in response to mechanical and chemical stimuli is characterized by a deep inspiration followed by an active expiratory effort. In other experiments cough has been defined in anaesthetized animals as a large burst of electromyogram activity in the diaphragm immediately followed by a burst of activity in the rectus abdominis muscle [17]. Interestingly, data recently presented by Canning et al. (unpublished) demonstrated that capsaicin and bradykinin (C-fibre stimulants) are totally ineffective at initiating and may actually inhibit the cough reflex in anaesthetized guinea-pigs even though the cough reflex initiated by mechanical stimuli (largely RAR selective) is entirely preserved in the anaesthetized state. However, these chemical agents do elicit a cough reflex in conscious guinea-pigs. These data illustrate the importance of accumulating evidence from different experimental settings before making firm conclusions with regard to the influence of certain fibre types and their role in respiratory reflexes. Furthermore, even if cough can be readily elicited in a given preparation, the work by Canning et al. supports the concept that the physiological state of the animal (i.e. anaesthetized or awake) may alter how this defensive reflex is regulated. This further suggests that perhaps anaesthesia is best avoided when studying the cough reflex in animal models.

## Tussive stimuli

The cough reflex can be elicited by electrical, mechanical (in anaesthetized animals) or chemical stimulation, as well as by changes in ion concentration or osmolarity in the mucosal surface fluid, or of sensory afferents (in the larynx, trachea or bronchial mucosa), or by stimulation of the CNS. More recent studies have utilized the irritant capsaicin and low pH solutions (e.g. citric acid) to study the cough response. Citric acid confers the advantage of allowing repeated cough measurements without the occurrence of tachyphylaxis whereas repeated exposure to capsaicin is known to result in tachyphylaxis thus preventing the production of a reproducible cough response in the same animal [18]. Different methods of stimulation may involve different populations of sensory afferent and there has been much discussion in the literature regarding the selectivity of agents for different fibre types, e.g. the use of capsaicin as a selective C-fibre stimulant [12,19].

## Different airway levels and the sensitivity of the cough reflex

The density and type of sensory nerves present at each airway level determines the sensitivity to tussive stimuli. The larynx of most species including cat, dog, guinea-pig and humans is particularly sensitive to mechanical stimulation and even the most gentle pressure in this region leads to strong expiratory efforts. In the dog both chemical and mechanical irritation are more potent tussive stimuli in the tracheobronchial tree than in the larynx, and C-fibre stimulants such as bradykinin and capsaicin have little effect when applied to the larynx which would be consistent with the sparse C-fibre innervation to the canine larynx. Furthermore, the cat intrapulmonary bronchi are much more sensitive to chemical irritation and less sensitive to mechanical stimulation than the larynx or trachea. Interestingly, studies have been performed in human subjects, which are in agreement with the studies performed in animal models in that the tracheobronchial tree is more sensitive to chemical stimuli than the laryngeal region [20].

# The guinea-pig model of cough

## Similarity to the human cough reflex

As stated above, many different species have been used to study the cough reflex, in both the anaesthetized and the conscious state. The electrophysiological and mechanical characteristics of the cough reflex appear to be conserved across species. The current animal of choice for studying pharmacological intervention in the cough

reflex is the guinea-pig. This animal has been utilized extensively, with cough being induced in conscious animals by inhalation of aerosols of either capsaicin or low pH solutions such as citric acid [11,14,21–23]. One caveat to the use of guinea-pigs is that they need to be pretreated with a β-adrenoceptor agonist to suppress bronchoconstriction to ensure that only the cough reflex is being studied. With this exception the guinea-pig provides a good model of the human cough reflex and this has been confirmed by a study showing the similarity in response to both citric acid and capsaicin in humans and guinea-pig [21]. Furthermore, recent *in vitro* data suggest that the isolated guinea-pig vagus nerve depolarizes in response to tussive stimuli in a similar manner to the human isolated vagus [24], again providing evidence in favour of using the guinea-pig cough model.

## Experimental design

Male or female guinea-pigs have been used. Animals should be housed under controlled conditions with frequent changes of bedding as the build-up of ammonia in cages has been shown to influence the cough response to citric acid [25]. Belvisi *et al.* (unpublished data) have shown that the cough response to a given stimuli varies greatly from guinea-pig to guinea-pig but that repeated assessments within the same animal are fairly reproducible. Therefore animals should be prescreened to assess their level of response to the stimuli of choice before being treated with test or standard compound. The same authors have not found it necessary to precondition guinea-pigs to accept aerosol exposure in the challenging box.

The assessment should take the form of a prescreening exercise, i.e. exposure to cough stimulus for 10 min, to establish the basal cough rate (expressed as number of coughs/min) for each individual animal to be used in a study. The entire group of animals should then be ranked by cough response and the non-responders excluded. The remaining animals should be blocked into high, medium and low responders and randomly assigned to groups from each block to ensure a spread of high, medium and low responders across the treatment groups. This process allows each animal to be compared with its own control (prescreening) level by paired analysis as well as allowing meaningful comparisons between treated groups at the post-treatment cough screening stage.

Once the prescreening is complete, animals should be 'rested' for at least 72 h before being re-exposed to the cough stimulant. Prior to the second exposure, treatment with test compound or compounds can be performed at a time and by a route determined by the pharmacokinetic profile (if available) of the compound or compounds under scrutiny. The most commonly used routes of administration in this model are oral, aerosol inhalation, intraperitoneal or subcutaneous. The intravenous route may be employed via the marginal ear vein but this route is not without difficulty. The aim should be to give test substances by a route that causes the least stress to the animal as any undue stress may affect the response to the cough stimuli.

## Methodology

The procedure for measuring cough in conscious guinea-pigs has been described and modified by several authors [9,12–14,21].

The protocol currently in common use involves pre-dosing the guinea-pig with terbutaline (0.05 mg/kg i.p.)

3 min prior to exposure to cough stimuli to inhibit bronchoconstriction and facilitate cough detection [14]. The guinea-pig is then placed in a small perspex box (approximately 1 L in volume) that allows free movement during exposure to aerosols. Airflow through the box is provided by compressed medical air via a flow regulator at 600 mL/min with changes in airflow induced by respiration and coughing detected by a pneumotachograph, amplified via a pressure transducer and recorded on a chart recorder (see Fig. 21.1). Cough sounds are amplified and recorded via a microphone sited in the cough chamber and recorded concurrently on the chart recorder (see Fig. 21.2). Tussive agents (capsaicin, citric acid, etc.) are delivered by aerosol using an ultrasonic nebulizer with an output of 0.4 mL/min and delivering a median particle diameter of 0.9 μm connected to the airflow port. The animal is exposed for a defined period, usually 10 min. A dose–response curve to the chosen stimuli should be constructed and a submaximal dose chosen for further studies.

Coughs are assessed and counted by a trained ob-

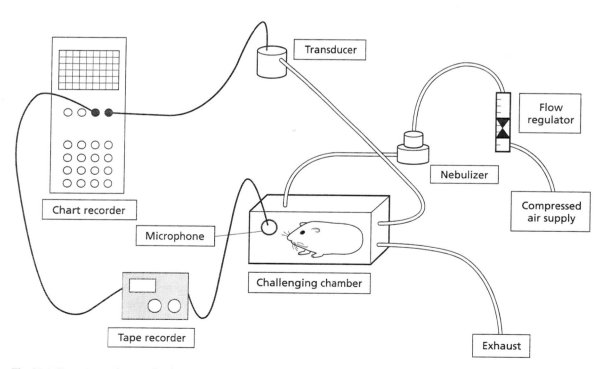

**Fig. 21.1** Experimental set-up for the evaluation of the cough response to aerosolized tussive stimuli in the conscious unrestrained guinea-pig.

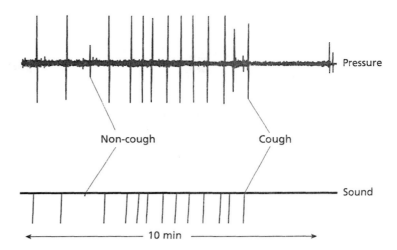

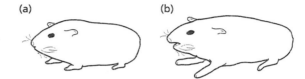

Fig. 21.2 A representative trace showing both airflow and sound recordings of the guinea-pig cough response over a 10-min period.

server using three different methods to ensure that only coughs are counted and that sneezes and augmented breaths are excluded. The three methods are as follows:
1 by observation, by an observer trained to differentiate between coughs and sneezes and to recognize the changes in posture (splaying of the front feet and forward stretching of the neck) and the characteristic opening of the mouth associated with cough (see Fig. 21.3);
2 by pressure changes, showing as full- or near full-scale deflections in both directions on the chart recorder (see Fig. 21.2), reflecting the deep inspiration and explosive expiration occurring during cough;
3 by sound, the characteristic sound of a guinea-pig cough.

Results can be expressed as coughs/10 min or as coughs/min and comparisons made with prescreening cough rate or with postscreening vehicle control treated animals.

## Conclusion

Cough, irrespective of which airways disease it is associated with, represents an unmet clinical need. There are no efficacious treatments available for cough and those that are available have been shown to be ineffective [2]. It is therefore essential to identify and develop new treatments for cough. To achieve this end it is necessary to develop and utilize an animal model of cough that accurately reflects the condition in humans.

The development of an animal model always re-

Fig. 21.3 The classic change in posture seen when a guinea-pig coughs in response to tussive stimuli. (a) Normal posture at rest; (b) cough posture with front feet splayed, body extended and mouth open.

quires the answering of key questions and cough is no exception. The key questions for a cough model are:
• The choice of species.
• The choice of tussive stimuli to elicit a functional response.
• Should the model employ conscious or anaesthetized animals?
• What should the end-point measurement be?
• Is the model reliable and reproducible?
• Does the model represent cough in humans?

It would appear that the 'citric acid-induced cough in guinea-pig' model answers most if not all of these questions. The guinea-pig shows distinct advantages over other small rodents in that it does cough to given stimuli in the conscious state and that the physiology of the cough response reflects that in humans. The tussive stimulus, citric acid, used to elicit cough in this model also causes cough in humans and acts on C-fibres and possibly RARs which are thought to be involved in the cough response pathway in humans. Citric acid also

**221**

has the advantage of producing reproducible cough responses in the same animal within a short period of time and unlike repeated administration of capsaicin does not result in tachyphilaxis. The end-point measurement in this model is cough and as this can be assessed in three different ways, by observed posture change, by pressure change and by sound, this adds to the reproducibility and reliability of the model.

In conclusion, citric acid-induced cough in the conscious guinea-pig provides a robust model in which to test and develop much needed putative treatments for cough in humans.

# References

1 Choudry NB, Fuller RW. Sensitivity of the cough reflex in patients with chronic cough. *Eur Respir J* 1992; **5**: 296–300.

2 Shroeder K, Fahey T. Systematic review of randomised controlled trials of over the counter cough medicines for acute cough in adults. *Br Med J* 2002; **324**: 1–6.

3 Widdicombe JG. Advances in understanding and treatment of cough. *Monaldi Arch Chest Dis* 1999; **54**: 275–9.

4 Karlsson J-A, Fuller RW. Pharmacological regulation of the cough reflex—from experimental models to antitussive effects in man. *Pulm Pharmacol Ther* 1999; **12**: 215–28.

5 Moreaux B, Beerens D, Gustin P. Development of a cough induction test in pigs: effects of SR 48968 and enalapril. *J Vet Pharmacol Ther* 1999; **22**: 387–9.

6 Kamei J, Hukuhara T, Kauya Y. Dopaminergic control of the cough reflex as demonstrated by the effects of apomorphine. *Eur J Pharmacol* 1987; **141**: 511–3.

7 Korpas J. Differentiation of the expiration and the cough reflex. *Physiol Bohemoslov* 1972; **21**: 677–80.

8 Karlsson J-A, Sant'Ambrogio G, Widdicombe J. Afferent neural pathways in cough and reflex bronchoconstriction. *J Appl Physiol* 1988; **65**: 1007–23.

9 Forsberg K, Karlsson J-A, Theodorsen E, Lundberg JM, Persson CGA. Cough and bronchoconstriction mediated by capsaicin-sensitive sensory neurons in guinea pigs. *Pulm Pharmacol* 1988; **1**: 33–9.

10 Fox AJ, Barnes PJ, Urban L, Dray A. An *in vivo* study of the properties of single vagal afferents innervating guinea pig airways. *J Physiol* 1993; **469**: 21–35.

11 Fox AJ. Modulation of cough and airway sensory fibres. *Pulm Pharmacol* 1996; **9**: 335–42.

12 Fox AJ, Lalloo UG, Belvisi MG, Bernareggi M, Chung KF, Barnes PJ. Bradykinin-evoked sensitization of airway sensory nerves: a mechanism for ACE-inhibitor cough. *Nature Med* 1996; **2**: 814–7.

13 Fox AJ, Barnes PJ, Venkatesan P, Belvisi MG. Activation of large conductance potassium channels inhibits the afferent and efferent function of airway sensory nerves in the guinea pig. *J Clin Invest* 1997; **99/3**: 513–9.

14 Lalloo UG, Fox AJ, Belvisi M, Chung KF, Barnes PJ. Capsazepine inhibits cough induced by capsaicin and citric acid but not by hypertonic saline in guinea pigs. *J Appl Physiol* 1995; **79**: 1082–7.

15 Bolser DC, Hey JA, Chapman RW. Influence of central antitussive drugs on the cough motor pattern. *J Appl Physiol* 1999; **86**: 1017–24.

16 Bolser DC, McLeod RL, Tulshian DB, Hey JA. Antitussive action of nociceptin in the cat. *Eur J Pharmacol* 2001; **430**: 107–11.

17 Bolser DC, Aziz SM, DeGennaro FC, Kreutner W, Egan RW, Siegel MI, Chapman RW. Antitussive effects of $GABA_B$ agonists in the cat and guinea pig. *Br J Pharmacol* 1993; **110**: 491–5.

18 Morice AH, Kastelik JA, Thompson R. Cough challenge in the assessment of cough reflex. *Br J Clin Pharmacol* 2001; **52**: 365–75.

19 Widdicombe JG. Sensory mechanisms. *Pulm Pharmacol* 1996; **9** (5–6): 383–7.

20 Karlsson J-A. The role of capsaicin-sensitive C-fibre afferent nerves in the cough reflex. *Pulm Pharmacol* 1996; **9**: 315–21.

21 Laude EA, Higgins KS, Morice AH. A comparative study of the effects of citric acid, capsaicin and resiniferatoxin on the cough challenge in guinea pig and man. *Pulm Pharmacol* 1993; **6**: 171–5.

22 Hay DWP, Giardina GAM, Griswold DE, Underwood DC, Kotzer CJ, Bush B, Potts W, Sandhu P, Lundberg D, Foley JJ, Luttmann MA, Grugni M, Raveglia LF, Sarau HM. Nonpeptide tachykinin receptor antagonists. III. SB 235375, a low central nervous system-penetrant, potent and selective neurokinin 3 receptor antagonist, inhibits citric acid-induced cough and airways hyper-reactivity in guinea pigs. *J Pharmacol Exp Ther* 2002; **300**: 314–23.

23 Emonds-Alt X, Advenier C, Cognon C, Croci T, Daoui S, Ducoux JP, Landi M, Naline E, Neliat G, Poncelet M, Proietto V, Van Broeck D, Vilain P, Soubrie P, Le Fur G, Maffrand JP, Breliere JC. Biochemical and pharmacological activities of SR 144190, a new potent non-peptide tachykinin NK2 receptor antagonist. *Neuropeptides* 1997; **5**: 449–58.

24 Belvisi MG, Venkatesan P, Barnes PJ, Fox AJ. A comparison of the chemosensitivity of the isolated guinea pig and human vagus nerves. *Am J Respir Crit Care Med* 1998; **157**: A487.

25 Moreaux B, Nemmar A, Beerens D, Gustin P. Inhibiting effect of ammonia on citric acid-induced cough in pigs: a possible involvement of substance P. *Pharmacol Toxicol* 2000; **87/6**: 279–85.

# Therapy

and cessation of spontaneous firing, This effect is caused by the activation of the G-protein-coupled inwardly rectifying $K^+$ (GIRK) channels. It has been shown that intracellular perfusion with guanosine 5'-o-(3-thiotriphosphate) (GTPγS) causes irreversible 5-$HT_{1A}$ receptor-mediated activation of the GIRK channels, in the conventional whole-cell recording mode. The irreversible activation of $K^+$ current by intracellular perfusion with GTPγS reminded us of the direct activation of $K^+$ channels by G-protein, and enabled us to determine whether GIRK channels could be blocked by Dex even in the absence of the agonist. As shown in Fig. 22.2(c), when we used a recording electrode filled with pipette solution containing GTPγS, brief application of 5-HT induced a continuous and almost irreversible inward $K^+$ current. Dex markedly inhibited the current activated by intracellular GTPγS in the absence of 5-HT [16], whereas spiperone, a 5-$HT_{1A}$ receptor antagonist, had no effect on this current. There appeared to be two possible explanations for the inhibition of the GTPγS-activated currents by Dex, because it has been reported that the activation of GIRK channels is mediated by the G-protein βγ subunit. One possible mechanism is blocking of the GIRK channel itself. The other mechanism is blocking the G-protein-mediated activation of the channel by inhibiting the action of the G-protein βγ subunits. Although the site of action of Dex is not clearly indicated by the available evidence, the fact that onset and termination of the Dex response were relatively rapid suggests that Dex may act at the level of the GIRK channel [16].

We felt it could be instructive to determine whether Dex also inhibits currents caused by activation of other neurotransmitter receptors coupled to G protein, because GIRK channels are coupled to other receptors, including adrenergic $α_2$-receptors and $GABA_B$ receptors. Therefore, we examined the effect of Dex on norepinephrine (NE)-induced current, which is mediated by $α_2$-adrenoceptors [17], in the locus coeruleus neurones. We found that Dex reversibly inhibits the NE-induced current, with rapid onset and termination. Although it is known that GIRK channels are heterotetrameric channels with two or more subunit isoforms, little is known about the isoforms of GIRK channels that are coupled with 5-$HT_{1A}$ receptors and $α_2$-adrenoceptors. The above results indicate that Dex has no specific effect on GIRK channels coupled to 5-$HT_{1A}$ receptors in DR neurones.

An important question is whether blocking of GIRK

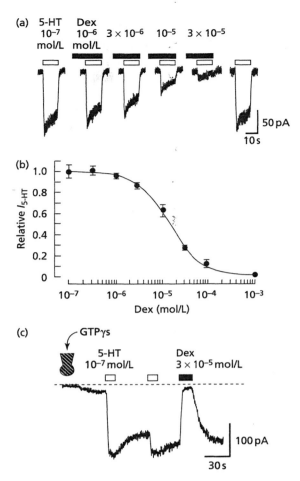

Fig. 22.2 Concentration-dependent suppression of $I_{5-HT}$ by dextromethorphan (Dex). (a) Representative current traces illustrating the effect of Dex on $I_{5-HT}$. All recordings were performed in external solution containing 20 mmol/L $K^+$ at a $V_H$ of −80 mV. (b) Concentration–inhibition relationship for the inhibitory effect of Dex on $I_{5-HT}$. Each point represents mean from five to seven neurones; vertical bars show SE mean. The continuous line was drawn according to the following equation: $I = 1 - C^n/(C^n + IC^n_{50})$ where $I$ is the maximalized current amplitude, $n$ is the Hill coefficient and $C$ is the concentration of Dex. (c) Effect of Dex on the $I_{5-HT}$ irreversibly activated by intracellular GTPγS. The neurones were intracellularly perfused with an internal solution containing 0.1 mmol/L GTPγS by using the conventional whole-cell patch recording mode. Current recording was performed in external solution containing 20 mmol/L $K^+$ at a $V_H$ of −80 mV.

**229**

channels by antitussives causes inhibition of coughing. Interestingly, all centrally acting antitussives that we studied inhibited $I_{5-HT}$ caused by 5-$HT_{1A}$ receptor activation. $IC_{50}$ values of various antitussives for the current caused by 0.1 µmol/L 5-HT ranged from 1 µmol/L to 10 µmol/L. Also, currents irreversibly activated by intracellular perfusion with GTPγS were also inhibited, suggesting inhibition of GIRK channels by these antitussives, which included narcotic antitussives. It may be significant that Dex inhibited GIRK channels, because only a few GIRK channel blockers are currently available.

Many antitussives have respiratory depressant action in experimental animals. Furthermore, it is well known that activation of serotonergic neurones in the brain depresses respiration. Unlike antitussives, pentobarbital-Na, which has potent respiratory depressant action, had little effect on 5-HT-induced current, suggesting that it had little effect on the GIRK channels. Thus, it is likely that inhibition of GIRK channels by antitussive drugs contributes to antitussive action, although the mechanism by which inhibition of GIRK channels affects coughing is not known.

As described above, the results obtained from pharmacological studies using 5-$HT_{1A}$ receptor agonists and antagonists suggest that direct activation of the 5-$HT_{1A}$ receptor may lead to inhibition of cough. However, a patch-clamp study using acutely dissociated single neurones revealed that Dex did not act directly on the 5-$HT_{1A}$ receptor but rather blocked GIRK channels coupled to 5-$HT_{1A}$ receptor and $\alpha_2$-adrenoceptor via G protein. Although these findings appear contradictory, the following discussion and findings may resolve this dilemma.

## Significance of inhibitory action on GIRK channels

Results of a competitive binding assay indicated that Dex had no effect on 5-$HT_{1A}$ receptors [18]. It is well known that serotonergic neurones often have autoreceptors that may have an inhibitory influence on the neurones. It has been reported that a subtype of autoreceptors in serotonergic neurones are 5-$HT_{1A}$ receptors. Furthermore, activation of 5-$HT_{1A}$ receptors is known to cause hyperpolarization in these neurones. Therefore, a reasonable working hypothesis is that the effect of Dex on GIRK channels coupled to 5-$HT_{1A}$ autoreceptors blocks feedback inhibition in serotonergic neurones, in turn augmenting release of 5-HT. In fact, it has

been reported that Dex and dihydrocodeine increase the release of 5-HT from slices prepared from the NTS, an important relay centre in the modulation of cough [19]. The agonist sensitivity of autoreceptors is also known to be rather higher than that of postsynaptic receptors.

It has also been reported that $GABA_B$ receptor agonists such as baclofen and 3-aminopropylphosphinic acid (3-APPi) have antitussive activity in cats and guinea-pigs. Based on their study of $GABA_B$ receptor antagonists and comparison of equieffective doses administered via veins and arteries, Bolser *et al.* concluded that baclofen inhibits cough by activating CNS $GABA_B$ receptors, whereas 3-APPi inhibits cough by acting at peripheral sites [7]. $GABA_B$ agonists that act on presynaptic receptors are known to inhibit glutamate exocytosis from synaptosomes, primary neuronal cultures and brain slices [20]. Here it is important to remember that N-methyl-D-aspartate (NMDA) receptor antagonists have antitussive action in experimental animals [21], although not all centrally acting antitussives block NMDA receptors. On the other hand, $GABA_B$ receptors are known to be coupled to GIRK channels. If antitussives inhibit GIRK channels coupled to $GABA_B$ receptors, they should affect the level of GABA in the brain, because $GABA_B$ receptors are also presynaptic autoreceptors. In turn, cough responses may be modulated via changes in GABA levels in the brain.

Recently, it has been reported that a δ-opioid receptor antagonist exerts antitussive action via a CNS mechanism [3]. However, Kotzer *et al.* have recently reported that the selective δ-opioid receptor agonist SB 227122 has an antitussive effect in guinea-pigs [22]. They have also reported that the selective δ-opioid receptor antagonist SB 244525 has little antitussive effect in guinea-pigs when administered alone. It has also been reported that the $\delta_1$-opioid receptor agonist DPDPE has little effect on experimentally induced cough in animals, but inhibited the antitussive effect of the µ-opioid receptor agonist DAMGO [23]. In contrast, the $\delta_2$-opioid receptor agonist [D-Ala$^2$] deltorphin II (DELT-II) potentiated the antitussive effect of DAMGO [23]. Studies of involvement of δ-opioid receptors in antitussive activity have produced some conflicting results. Surprisingly, in our preliminary study, the δ-opioid receptor antagonists naltrindole and naltriben, known to have antitussive action, both inhibited GIRK channels in single brain neurones.

There have been several reports suggesting involvement of σ-receptors in mechanisms of action of antitussive drugs [24]. It has also been reported that there is a high-affinity binding site for Dex on σ-receptors [25]. Other studies suggest that σ-receptors are associated with $K^+$ channels, because some σ-ligands modify $K^+$ conductances in some tissues. It has been reported that σ-ligands inhibit ligand-induced hyperpolarization mediated by $\alpha_2$-adrenoceptors and μ-opioid receptors in locus coeruleus (LC) neurones [26]. As described above, Dex inhibits not only $I_{5\text{-HT}}$ in DR neurones but also norepinephrine-induced currents in LC neurones. Furthermore, $\alpha_2$-adrenoceptors in LC neurones are known to be coupled to GIRK channels [17]. Therefore, it is possible that σ-ligands exert antitussive action at least partly through inhibition of GIRK channels. A patch-clamp study by Nguyen et al. revealed no correlation between binding affinities of antitussives at $\sigma_1$- or $\sigma_2$-binding sites and potency of inhibition of $K^+$ currents [27].

Coughing is regulated by higher brain areas, and is under voluntary control to some extent. It may be reasonable to speculate that action of antitussive drugs is facilitated, at least in part, by a placebo effect [28], since low doses of some antitussives suppress cough with a potency little greater than that of a placebo.

Recently, it has been reported that antitussive drugs may act, at least in part, at a cortical level. Our study also showed that microelectrophoretically applied antitussives inhibited spontaneous unit activities recorded from the pyramidal layer of the cerebral cortex of guinea-pigs in vivo (Fig. 22.3). To our knowledge, the mechanism of inhibition of unit activities in the cerebral cortex has not been studied. However, it is possible that inhibition of unit activities is the result of in-hibition of GIRK channels, because GIRK channels are found in various regions of the brain, including the cerebral cortex [29].

## NMDA and neurokinin 1 (NK$_1$) receptors

### NMDA receptor

Glutamate is often an excitatory neurotransmitter in primary afferent neurones. Netzer et al. were the first to report that Dex inhibited NMDA-induced currents in brain neurones [6]. We confirmed this, and demonstrated that Dex had no effect on kainate-induced current in single brain neurones. Interestingly, codeine and the non-narcotic antitussive eprazinone did not have an effect on this current, although Dex and codeine both have a morphinan structure. These findings indicate that blocking of NMDA receptors is not essential for antitussive effects.

### Substance P and its receptor

There is a high density of substance P (SP)-containing nerve terminals in the NTS [30], and there is a parallel distribution of SP receptors in the postsynaptic neurones of these nerve terminals in the NTS. Also, recent pharmacological and physiological studies using guinea-pigs have revealed that SP in the NTS augments bronchopulmonary C-fibre reflex output, causing bronchoconstriction and changes in respiration including coughing [31]. Although it is unknown whether clinically available centrally acting antitussives act on NK$_1$ receptors in the NTS, it seems likely that drugs

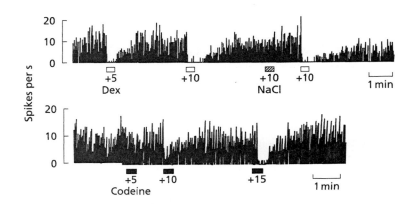

Fig. 22.3 Inhibitory effect of micro-electrophoretically applied antitussives on single neurone activities in the cerebral cortex of guinea-pigs. Dextromethorphan (Dex) and codeine inhibited single neurone activities in a concentration-dependent manner. Na$^+$ was applied to confirm that the inhibitory effect of antitussives was not due to the current applied. Numerals under each record represent the current intensity in nA.

**231**

which block $NK_1$ receptors in the NTS have antitussive action.

Sasaki *et al.* [32] reported that an increase in the level of SP significantly lowered the risk of pneumonia due to aspiration of oropharyngeal bacterial pathogens among older adults, apparently via recovery (or strengthening) of cough and swallowing reflexes. They also suggested that treatment with dopamine analogues or potentiating drugs such as amantadine may affect the incidence of pneumonia, because production of SP is regulated by dopaminergic neurones in the cerebral basal ganglia. SP is synthesized in the nodose and jugular ganglia, and has been shown to be transported peripherally and released in the airway. Increased release of SP is involved in cough and neurogenic inflammation in the airway. However, there is considerable morphological and physiological evidence that SP is also released at central synapses in the NTS [31]. This suggests that $NK_1$ receptors in the NTS could serve as target receptors for new antitussive drugs. Finally, studies of the $NK_1$ receptor and glycine receptor may provide useful data for development of a 'cough recovery' (or 'strengthening') drug for older adults with decreased cough and swallowing reflexes, which increase susceptibility to aspiration pneumonia.

## Opioid receptors and narcotic antitussives

It is clear that antitussive drugs derived from opium alkaloids act via opioid receptors, because (i) antitussive action of these drugs is effectively abolished by opioid receptor antagonists such as levallorphan and naloxone and (ii) the blocking action of opioid receptor antagonists occurs with a very short latency. Opioid receptors are classified into three receptor types: $\mu$, $\delta$ and $\kappa$, and $\mu$- and $\delta$-receptors are in turn divided pharmacologically into subtypes. Kamei *et al.* have reported a series of pharmacological findings on involvement of opioid receptor groups and subgroups in antitussive activities of opioid drugs. These findings can be summarized as follows: (i) selective agonists for $\mu$- and $\kappa$-receptors have significant antitussive action, but $\delta$-receptor agonists have little antitussive action [33,34]; (ii) antitussive action of $\mu$-agonists occurs via $\mu_2$- but not $\mu_1$-receptors [35,36]; (iii) antitussive action via $\mu_2$-receptors is depressed via $\mu_1$-receptors [37]; (iv) DPDPE, a $\delta_1$-receptor agonist, depresses the antitussive action of $\mu$- and $\kappa$-receptor agonists [34,38]; and (v) DELT-II, a $\delta_2$-receptor agonist, inhibits antitussive action that occurs via $\mu_2$-receptors, suggesting that the relationship between $\mu$- and $\delta$-receptors in antitussive action may be different from their relationship in analgesic action [23]. Although these findings are suggestive, some are controversial; for example, Kotzer *et al.* have recently reported that the selective $\delta$-receptor agonist SB 227122 has an antitussive effect in guinea-pigs [22].

As discussed above, action of narcotic antitussives such as codeine is thought to occur via opioid receptors. However, nothing is known about effects of these antitussives on opioid receptor-mediated responses in single neurones. Findings of several studies indicate that activation of opioid receptors inhibits excitability of neurones in various regions of the brain and spinal cord, while increasing excitability in a few neurones. In addition, there have been several findings regarding mechanisms of opioid receptor-mediated inhibition of excitability of single neurones. For example, it has been reported that a $\mu$-receptor agonist inhibits $Ca^{2+}$ currents in dorsal root ganglion (DRG) neurones [39]. This inhibition occurred via activation of a Gi- or G(o)-type G protein, but was independent of changes in adenylate cyclase activity [39]. On the other hand, a study using DRG neurones in organotypic cultures revealed that most $\mu$-, $\delta$- and $\kappa$-opioid agonists elicit dimodal excitatory as well as inhibitory modulation of the action potential duration (APD) of these neurones [40]. Excitatory opioid effects have been shown to be mediated by opioid receptors that are coupled via Gs to cyclic AMP-dependent ionic conductances that prolong APD, whereas inhibitory opioid effects are mediated by opioid receptors coupled via Gi/Go to ionic conductances that shorten APD [40]. A relatively recent study of dissociated neurones of the periaqueductal grey of rats has found that a $\mu$-opioid receptor agonist, DAMGO, inhibits high-voltage-activated (HVA) $Ca^{2+}$ current [41]. It has been confirmed that this effect is due to inhibition of N-type HVA $Ca^{2+}$ channels via pertussis toxin (PTX)-sensitive G proteins [13]. It has also been reported that $\mu$-opioid receptor stimulation causes activation of inward rectifying $K^+$ conductance in various brain regions [42]. Thus, signal transduction across cellular membranes by opioid receptors is mediated by coupling to G proteins. However, the actions and mechanisms of opioids in individual brain neurones appear to vary among different types of neurones. Also, recent evidence indicates that a single receptor type can interact with several G proteins [43], which in turn can couple to more than one effector [44]. In addition, studies of the $\alpha_2$-adrenergic receptor indicate that receptor/G-protein interactions are affected by receptor density [45]. Thus, actions of opioids in single neurones might be greatly influenced by the region of the brain that the neurones are from and the type of G protein involved in the signal transduction mechanism. This also seems to be the case for κ- and δ-opioid receptors. Therefore, when studying the actions of narcotic antitussives at the neurone level, it is important to use neurones that are involved in the cough reflex. Rhim *et al.* [46] found that, in neurones of the NTS, an important relay centre in the modulation of cough, activation of μ-opioid receptors inhibited both N- and P/Q-type $Ca^{2+}$ channels. Because they found that inhibition of $Ca^{2+}$ currents by DAMGO, a μ-receptor agonist, was reduced by treatment with PTX and by a conditioning prepulse to +80 mV, they suggested that a PTX-sensitive G protein was involved in inhibition of $Ca^{2+}$ currents by DAMGO. Also, they found that DAMGO-induced inhibition of $Ca^{2+}$ currents, unlike somatostatin-induced inhibition of $Ca^{2+}$ currents, was not attenuated by intracellular loading with an antiserum raised against the amino terminus of the α subunits of Go (Goα), suggesting that at least two different PTX-sensitive G-protein-mediated pathways are involved in receptor-mediated inhibition of $Ca^{2+}$ currents in NTS neurones.

As discussed above, narcotic antitussives such as codeine inhibit GIRK channel currents in brain neurones at relatively high concentrations. Accordingly, we have conducted a preliminary study of the actions of codeine on HVA $Ca^{2+}$ currents and delayed rectifier $K^+$ currents in acutely dissociated NTS neurones. A high concentration of 1 mmol/L was needed to inhibit both currents. In this context, it seems likely that the primary site of action of clinically available narcotic antitussives is in opioid receptors such as μ-opioid receptors, but not ionic channels such as HVA $Ca^{2+}$ and delayed rectifying $K^+$ channels. However, further study is needed to determine whether opioid receptor-mediated actions of narcotic antitussives inhibit cough directly or via changes in levels of other neurotransmitters. Several studies have found that μ-opioid receptors decrease GABA release presynaptically in the brain [47].

A recent study using expression of the Fos-like immunoreactivity (FLI) has revealed that many regions of the brain are involved in laryngeal-induced fictive cough in cats [48], including the interstitial and ventrolateral subdivisions of the nucleus of the tractus solitarius, the medial part of the lateral tegmental field, the internal division of the lateral reticular nucleus, the nucleus retroambiguus, the para-ambigual region, the retrofacial nucleus and the medial parabrachial nucleus. Furthermore, FLI in these regions was found to be significantly reduced by treatment with codeine [48]. Also, μ- and κ-opioid receptors are densely localized in the NTS and parabrachial nucleus [49]. However, δ-receptors do not distribute to those regions in which FLI increases after cough stimulation, although a very low density of δ-receptors was found in the NTS [49]. These findings seem to be consistent with findings that μ- and κ-agonists, but not δ-agonists, have antitussive actions in experimental animals. However, further studies are needed to clarify the neuronal mechanisms of the action of narcotic antitussives, because (i) μ-, δ- and κ-opioid receptors are widely distributed in the brain, including the cerebral cortex [49] and (ii) coughing is under the control of both lower and higher brain regions [1].

## Conclusions

The centrally acting antitussives currently available have been derived from various compounds that have different pharmacological actions, such as analgesic, anticholinergic and antihistaminergic actions. Because of this, antitussive drugs are diverse in chemical structure. For some time, researchers studying cough and antitussives have wondered whether centrally acting antitussives have a common mechanism or site of action in the brain, despite known differences between receptors for narcotic and non-narcotic antitussives. Our recent studies have shown that centrally acting antitussives have inhibitory actions on the strychnine-sensitive glycine receptor–ionophore complex and GIRK channels (Table 22.1). Inhibitory action on the glycine receptor does not appear to be important for the action of antitussives other than Dex, because relatively high concentrations are needed to inhibit glycine-induced current. However, blocking of GIRK channels appears to contribute at least partly to the action of centrally acting antitussives. As described above, GIRK channels are coupled to various receptors. A recent study has revealed that GIRK channels are also coupled to

**Table 22.1** Effects of antitussive drugs on receptor-mediated or ion channel-activated currents in single brain neurones.

| | Narcotic (codeine) | Non-narcotic | | |
|---|---|---|---|---|
| | | Dextromethorphan | Others* | δ-Antagonist or σ-agonist |
| $I_{gly}$ | ↓↓ | ↓↓↓ | ↓ | n.d. |
| $I_{GABA}$ | → | → | → | n.d. |
| $I_{NMDA}$ | → | ↓↓↓ | → | n.d. |
| $I_K$ | n.d. | → | n.d. | n.d. |
| $I_{5\text{-HT}}$ | ↓ | ↓↓↓ | ↓↓↓ | ↓↓ |
| $I_{NE}$ | n.d. | ↓↓↓ | n.d. | ↓↓ |
| GIRK channel | ↓ | ↓↓↓ | ↓↓↓ | ↓↓ |

A downward arrow indicates the magnitude of the inhibitory effect: the greater the number of arrows, the greater is the inhibitory action on the currents. $I_{Gly}$, $I_{GABA}$, $I_{NMDA}$, $I_K$, $I_{5\text{-HT}}$ and $I_{NE}$ are the currents induced by glycine, GABA, NMDA, kainate, 5-HT and norepinephrine, respectively.

n.d., not determined.

* For example, eprazinone.

μ-receptors in the cerebral cortex [29]. GIRK channels are tetramers, and exist as homo- and heteromeric complexes of the following four subunits: GIRK1, GIRK2, GIRK3 and GIRK4. However, it is not known whether GIRK channels coupled to different receptors each have a unique GIRK subunit composition. Detailed studies on the effects of antitussives on the GIRK channels coupled to various receptors may help clarify neuronal mechanisms of centrally acting antitussives, in particular, non-narcotic antitussives, because GIRK channels are coupled to receptors for many different transmitters, including acetylcholine, dopamine, 5-HT, GABA, somatostatin, norepinephrine, ATP and opioids, and because results of an FLI expression study suggest that multiple sites (even in the brainstem) are involved in the cough reflex and may be involved in antitussive action [48].

Narcotic antitussives inhibit various channels, including GIRK channels. However, their primary site of action appears to be opioid receptors such as μ- and κ-receptors, because high concentrations are needed to inhibit μ- and κ-receptor-mediated channels. It is likely that further understanding of central mechanisms of narcotic antitussives can be achieved by conducting studies using neurones that are primarily or secondarily involved in cough responses, and by using preparations such as cough response-related single neurones with synaptic buttons or brain slices containing neuronal circuits related to cough responses. The use of such methods may also help elucidate the mechanisms of action of non-narcotic antitussives.

*Acknowledgements*

The author thanks Professor T. Miyata and Drs H. Kai, Y. Isohama, H. Ishibashi and T. Shirasaki, Faculty of Pharmaceutical Sciences, Kumamoto University, for their collaboration. The author thanks the following graduate students for their assistance: H. Honda, H. Fukushima, M. Otsuka, S. Nagayama, Y. Terasako and F. Soeda, Department of Pharmacology, and K. Kuwano and K. Abe, Department of Hygienic Chemistry, Faculty of Pharmaceutical Sciences, Kumamoto University. The author sincerely thanks Emeritus Professor Y. Kase for his continuous encouragement.

## References

1 Kase Y, Kito G, Takahama K, Miyata T. Influence of cerebral cortex stimulation upon cough-like spasmodic expiratory response (SER) and cough in the cat. *Brain Res* 1984; **306**: 293–8.

2 Kase Y. Antitussive agents and their sites of action. *Trends Pharmacol Sci* 1980; **1**: 237–9.

3 Widdicombe J. Neuroregulation of cough: implications for drug therapy. *Curr Opin Pharmacol* 2002; **2**: 256–63.

4 Baekey DM, Morris K, Gestreau C, Li Z, Lindsey B, Shannon R. Medullary respiratory neurones and control

of laryngeal motoneurones during fictive eupnoea and cough in the cat. *J Physiol* 2001; **534**: 565–81.

5 Takahama K, Fukushima H, Isohama Y, Kai H, Miyata T. Inhibition of glycine currents by dextromethorphan in neurones dissociated from the guinea-pig nucleus tractus solitarii. *Br J Pharmacol* 1997; **120**: 690–4.

6 Netzer R, Pflimlin P, Trube G. Dextromethorphan blocks N-methyl D-aspartate-induced currents and voltage-operated inward currents in cultured cortical neurons. *Eur J Pharmacol* 1993; **238**: 209–16.

7 Bolser DC, DeGennaro FC, O'Reilly S, Chapman RW, Kreutner W, Egan RW, Hey JA. Peripheral and central sites of action of GABA-B agonists to inhibit the cough reflex in the cat and guinea pig. *Br J Pharmacol* 1994; **113**: 1344–8.

8 Fukushima K, Nagayama S, Otsuka M, Takahama K, Isohama Y, Kai H, Miyata T. Inhibition of glycine-induced current by morphine in nucleus tractus solitarii neurones of guinea pigs. *Methods Find Exp Clin Pharmacol* 1998; **20**: 125–32.

9 Honda H, Takahama K, Kawaguchi T, Fuchikami J, Kai H, Miyata T. Involvement of N-methyl-D-aspartic acid (NMDA) receptor in the central mechanism of cough reflex. *Jpn J Pharmacol* 1990; **52** (Suppl. I): 308P.

10 Kubo T, Kihara M. Evidence for the presence of GABAergic and glycine-like systems responsible for cardiovascular control in the nucleus tractus solitarii of the rat. *Neurosci Lett* 1987; **74**: 331–6.

11 Takahama K, Soeda F, Usui S, Isohama Y, Kai H, Miyata T. Is glycinergic transmission in the nucleus tractus solitarii (NTS) involved in cough reflex. *Naunyn-Schmiedeberg's Arch Pharmacol* 1998; **358** (Suppl. 1): R64.

12 Kamei J, Ogawa M, Kasuya Y. Monoamine and the mechanisms of action of antitussive drugs in rats. *Arch Int Pharmacodyn* 1987; **290**: 117–27.

13 Stone RA, Barnes PJ, Chung KF. Effect of 5-HT$_{1A}$ receptor agonist, 8-OH-DPAT, on cough responses in the conscious guinea pig. *Eur J Pharmacol* 1997; **332**: 201–7.

14 Kamei J, Mori T, Igarashi H, Kasuya Y. Effects of 8-hydroxy-2-(di-n-propylamino) tetralin, a selective agonist of 5-HT$_{1A}$ receptors, on the cough reflex in rats. *Eur J Pharmacol* 1991; **203**: 253–8.

15 Kamei J, Hosokawa T, Yanaura S, Hukuhara T. Effects of methysergide on the cough reflex. *Jpn J Pharmacol* 1986; **42**: 450–2.

16 Ishibashi H, Kuwano K, Takahama K. Inhibition of the 5-HT$_{1A}$ receptor-mediated inwardly rectifying K$^+$ current by dextromethorphan in rat dorsal raphe neurones. *Neuropharmacology* 2000; **39**: 2302–8.

17 Arima J, Kubo C, Ishibashi H, Akaike N. $\alpha_2$-Adrenoceptor-mediated potassium currents in acutely dissociated rat locus coeruleus neurones. *J Physiol (Lond)* 1998; **508**: 57–66.

18 Craviso GL, Musacchio JM. High affinity dextromethorphan binding sites in guinea pig brain, competition experiments. *Mol Pharmacol* 1983; **23**: 629–40.

19 Kamei J, Mori T, Igarashi H, Kasuya Y. Serotonin release in the nucleus of the solitary tract and its modulation by antitussive drugs. *Res Comm Chem Pathol Pharmacol* 1992; **76**: 371–4.

20 Nicholls DG, Sanchez-Prieto J. Neurotransmitter release mechanism. In: Stephenson FA, Turner AJ, eds. *Frontiers in Neurobiology 3, Amino Acid Neurotransmission*. London: Portland Press, 1998: 1–24.

21 Kamei J, Tanihara H, Igarashi H, Kasuya Y. Effects of N-methyl-D-aspartate antagonists on the cough reflex. *Eur J Pharmacol* 1989; **168**: 153–8.

22 Kotzer CJ, Hay DWP, Dondio G, Giardina G, Petrillo P, Underwood DC. The antitussive activity of δ-opioid receptor stimulation in guinea pigs. *J Pharmacol Exp Ther* 2000; **292**: 803–9.

23 Kamei J, Iwamoto Y, Suzuki T, Nagase H, Misawa M, Kasuya Y. Differential modulation of μ-opioid receptor-mediated antitussive activity by δ-opioid receptor agonists in mice. *Eur J Pharmacol* 1993; **234**: 117–20.

24 Kamei J, Iwamoto Y, Misawa M, Kasuya Y. Involvement of haloperidol-sensitive σ-sites in antitussive effects. *Eur J Pharmacol* 1992; **224**: 39–43.

25 Klein M, Paturzo JJ, Musacchio JM. The effects of prototypic σ-ligands on the binding of [$^3$H]dextromethorphan to guinea pig brain. *Neurosci Lett* 1989; **97**: 175–80.

26 Bobker DH, Shen K-Z, Surprenant A, William JT. DTG and (+)-3PPP inhibit a ligand-activated hyperpolarization in mammalian neurons. *J Pharmacol Exp Ther* 1989; **251**: 840–5.

27 Neuyen VH, Ingram SL, Kassiou M, Christie MJ. σ-Binding site ligands inhibit K$^+$ currents in rat locus coeruleus neurons in vitro. *Eur J Pharmacol* 1998; **361**: 157–63.

28 Eccles R. The powerful placebo in cough studies? *Pulm Pharmacol Ther* 2002; **15**: 303–8.

29 Ponce A, Bueno E, Kentros C, Vega-Saenz de Miera E, Chow A, Hillman D, Chen S, Zhu L, Wu MB, Wu X, Rudy B, Thornhill WB. G-protein-gated inward rectifier K$^+$ channel proteins (GIRK1) are present in the soma and dendrites as well as in nerve terminals of specific neurons in the brain. *J Neurosci* 1996; **16**: 1990–2001.

30 Kawai Y, Mori S, Takagi H. Vagal afferents interact with substance P–immunoreactive structures in the nucleus of the tractus solitarius: immunoelectron microscopy combined with an anterograde degeneration study. *Neurosci Lett* 1989; **101**: 6–10.

31 Mutoh T, Bonham AC, Joad JP. Substance P in the nucleus of the solitary tract augments bronchopulmonary C fiber reflex output. *Am J Physiol Regul Integr Comp Physiol* 2000; **279**: R1215–23.

32  Yamaya M, Yanai M, Ohrui T, Arai H, Sasaki H. Interventions to prevent pneumonia among older adults. *J Am Geriatr Soc* 2001; 49: 85–90.

33  Kamei J, Tanihara H, Kasuya Y. Antitussive effect of two specific κ-opioid agonists, U-50,488H and U-62,066E, in rats. *Eur J Pharmacol* 1990; 187: 281–6.

34  Kamei J, Tanihahara H, Kasuya Y. Modulation of μ-mediated antitussive activity in rats by a δ agonist. *Eur J Pharmacol* 1991; 203: 153–6.

35  Kamei J, Iwamoto Y, Kawashima N, Suzuki T, Nagase H, Misawa M, Kasuya Y. Possible involvement of $\mu_2$-mediated mechanisms in μ-mediated antitussive activity in the mouse. *Neurosci Lett* 1993; 149: 169–72.

36  Kamei J, Iwamoto Y, Suzuki T, Misawa M, Nagase H, Kasuya Y. The role of the $\mu_2$-opioid receptor in the antitussive effect of morphine in $\mu_1$-opioid receptor-deficient CXBK mice. *Eur J Pharmacol* 1993; 240: 99–101.

37  Kamei J, Saitoh A, Morita K, Nagase H. Antagonistic effect of buprenorphine on the antitussive effect of morphine is mediated via the activation of $\mu_1$-opioid receptors. *Life Sci* 1995; 57: 231–5.

38  Kamei J, Tanihahara H, Kasuya Y. Modulation of κ-mediated antitussive activity in rats by a δ agonist. *Res Comm Chem Pathol Pharmacol* 1992; 76: 375–8.

39  Moises HC, Rusin KI, Macdonald RL. μ-Opioid receptor-mediated reduction of neuronal calcium current occurs via a G(o)-type GTP-binding protein. *J Neurosci* 1994; 14: 3842–51.

40  Crain SM, Shen KF. Modulatory effects of Gs-coupled excitatory opioid receptor functions on opioid analgesia, tolerance, and dependence. *Neurochem Res* 1996; 21: 1347–51.

41  Kim CJ, Rhee JS, Akaike N. Modulation of high-voltage activated $Ca^{2+}$ channels in the rat periaqueductal gray neurons by μ-type opioid agonist. *J Neurophysiol* 1997; 77: 1418–24.

42  Loose MD, Kelly MJ. Opioids act at μ-receptors to hyperpolarize arcuate neurons via an inwardly rectifying potassium conductance. *Brain Res* 1990; 513: 15–23.

43  Laugwitz K, Offermanns S, Spincher K, Schultz G. μ and δ opioid receptors differentially couple to G protein subtypes in membranes of human neuroblastoma SH-SY-5Y cell. *Neuron* 1993; 10: 233–42.

44  Hescheler J, Rosenthal W, Trautwein W, Schutz G. The GTP-binding protein, Go, regulates neuronal calcium channels. *Nature* 1987; 325: 445–7.

45  Eason MG, Kurose H, Holt BD, Raymond JR, Liggett SB. Simultaneous coupling of $\alpha_2$-adrenergic receptors to two G proteins with opposing effects. *J Biol Chem* 1992; 267: 15795–801.

46  Rhim H, Toth PT, Miller RJ. Mechanism of inhibition of calcium channels in rat nucleus tractus solitarius by neurotransmitters. *Br J Pharmacol* 1996; 118: 1341–50.

47  Alreja M, Shanabrough M, Liu W, Leranth C. Opioids suppress IPSCs in neurons of the rat medial septum/diagonal band of Broca: involvement of μ-opioid receptors and septohippocampal GABAergic neurons. *J Neurosci* 2000; 20: 1179–89.

48  Gestreau C, Bianchi AL, Grelot L. Differential brainstem fos-like immunoreactivity after laryngeal induced coughing and its reduction by codeine. *J Neurosci* 1997; 17: 9340–52.

49  Mansour A, Khachaurian H, Lewis ME, Akil H, Watson SJ. Anatomy of CNS opioid receptors. *Trends Neurosci* 1988; 11: 308–14.

# 23 Pharmacology of peripherally acting antitussives

*Sandra M. Reynolds, Domenico Spina & Clive P. Page*

## Introduction

Cough is a common symptom of a variety of airway diseases, from upper respiratory tract infections to chronic illnesses such as asthma, chronic obstructive pulmonary disease (COPD) and bronchial carcinoma. Cough is also a protective reflex, which prevents entry of foreign bodies into the respiratory tract and also aids the expulsion of mucus. Chronic persistent non-productive cough that lasts for longer than a month, where no specific cause can be found, occurs in about 30–40% of patients [1], resulting in significant morbidity in terms of quality of life. Drugs currently used to treat cough are among the most widely used over-the-counter drugs in the world, despite a recent analysis suggesting that there is little evidence to suggest that such drugs produce any meaningful efficacy [2]. In 1999 alone $750 million was spent on antitussive medications in the US, Canada and Europe [2]. There is a current unmet need for the development of safe, effective antitussive therapeutic options in the treatment of persistent cough as alternatives to existing medications.

Antitussive drugs are broadly divided into two groups based on their site of action. Peripherally acting drugs act outside the central nervous system (CNS) to inhibit cough by suppressing the responsiveness of one or more types of sensory nerves that produce cough [3]. Central antitussive drugs act inside the central nervous system to suppress the responsiveness to one or more components of the central reflex pathway of cough [4]. This chapter will discuss existing knowledge of the peripherally acting antitussive medications that are currently used in the clinic and the development of novel antitussives in this area (Fig. 23.1).

## 'Sensory' regulation of the cough reflex

The cough reflex can be evoked by mechanical and/or chemical stimuli in the airways. There are four main groups of airway receptors which may initiate the cough reflex: the rapidly adapting stretch receptors (RARs), nociceptive Aδ-fibres, the pulmonary and bronchial C-fibre receptors, and the slowly adapting stretch receptors (SARs). All of these groups are located within the epithelial layer of the trachea and lower airways [5,6]. RARs and C-fibres have also been located in the larynx [7], and pulmonary C-fibres are located in the alveolar wall (Fig. 23.1).

It is well documented that RARs can cause cough as they are activated by the same stimuli that initiate coughing. Studies in experimental animals have demonstrated that impulse conduction in these nerves is activated by mechanical, chemical and osmotic stimuli that are all capable of inducing cough in humans [8–10]. SARs facilitate the cough reflex by activating RARs as shown in cats and rabbits via interneurones called 'pump cells', which are believed to open gates that either permit or augment the cough reflex due to RAR activity in the larynx and trachea [11]. They are not believed to be directly involved as their activity is not altered by stimuli evoking cough. The C-fibres (pulmonary or bronchial, depending on their location along the airways) are also activated by the same stimuli, but C-fibres are less sensitive to mechanical stimuli than are RARs. Non-myelinated C-fibre afferents contain neuropeptides such as substance P (SP), neurokinin A (NKA) and calcitonin gene-related peptide (CGRP) and may be indirectly involved in the cough reflex, by the release of these neuropeptides from peripheral

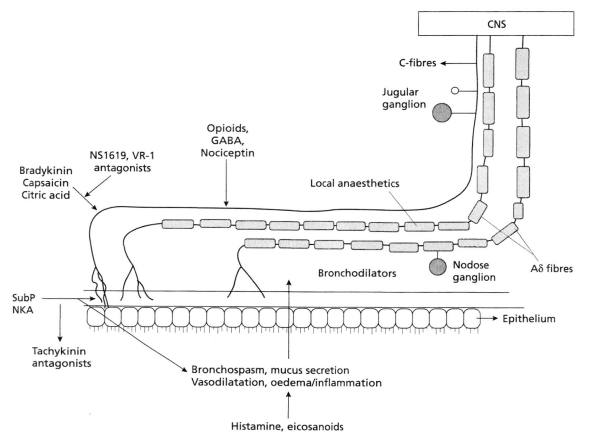

**Fig. 23.1** Representation of neuronal innervation of the airways and the potential drug targets in the treatment of cough. Modified from [6].

nerve terminals. The release of endogenous neuropeptides may also induce bronchospasm and oedema which indirectly stimulate RARs [4]. Most of the evidence for the direct involvement of C-fibres in cough has come from the fact that capsaicin, which was thought to be a selective stimulant of C-fibres, can evoke coughing in animals and humans [12,13] although there are also suggestions that stimulation of C-fibre receptors with capsaicin may actually inhibit cough [14]. However, it is now regarded that capsaicin is not selective for C-fibres as it has been reported to activate Aδ-fibres also [15]. In addition, recent work has shown that the vanilloid (VR1) receptor, which is activated by capsaicin, is also found in airway nerves not containing sensory neuropeptides [16–18]. The implication of these findings is that capsaicin can no longer

be considered selective for C-fibre afferents and that C-fibre involvement in the cough response is more complex than previously recognized.

## Opioids and opioid-like drugs

Opioids, especially morphine and codeine, have been shown to suppress cough in a number of animal models [19,20] and in humans [21,22] to a range of different stimuli including capsaicin and citric acid. Of the five receptor subtypes known, it is thought that the antitussive actions of these drugs is via stimulation of μ-opioid receptors. μ-Opioid receptors are found within the cough centres of the brain and traditionally it is believed that opioids exert their antitussive effects via a central action [21,23]. However, the possibility that opioids suppress cough also by a peripheral mechanism of action led to the development of BW443C, a novel peripherally acting μ-opioid receptor agonist for the treatment of cough.

In the guinea-pig BW443C (H–Tyr–D-Arg–Gly–Phe (4-NH4)) was shown to inhibit cough by a peripheral site of action as there appears to be little or no penetration of this drug into the CNS sufficient to cause respiratory depression, in comparison with codeine and morphine. Furthermore, the antitussive actions of BW443C were significantly reduced by N-methylnalorphine, a salt of nalorphine, and therefore designed not to penetrate the blood–brain barrier [20]. Follenfant *et al.* also showed that BW443C was unable to cross the blood–brain barrier in chemically induced writing models [24]. BW443C inhibits activity in airway sensory neurones originating from RARs and C-fibre receptors [3,4]. BW443C has not been tested as an antitussive in humans but it failed to significantly alter hyperresponsiveness in asthmatic subjects, although the possibility of enzymatic destruction following deposition on the epithelial surface may account for this result [25].

Nociceptin/orphanin FQ (N/OFQ), is an opioid-like peptide and is the endogenous ligand for the recently discovered ORL1 receptor now known as NOP1 [26]. Nociceptin also has low affinity for opioid receptors but it is not recognized as a member of the opioid group due to the fact that nociceptin does not have high binding affinity for opioid receptors and opioid antagonists such as naltrexone are unable to block the activity of nociceptin. Nociceptin has been located in the lung and has been found to inhibit the release of sensory neuropeptides following depolarization of C-fibres [27] and to inhibit bronchospasm in the guinea-pig. This latter effect could be due to the inhibition of the release of sensory neuropeptides from C-fibres [28]. More recently it has been shown that N/OFQ inhibited cough induced by mechanical and capsaicin stimuli in guinea-pigs and cats [29]. This suggests that NOP1 receptors are involved in the modulation of the cough reflex. N/OFQ is a peptide and probably does not cross the blood–brain barrier when administered by the intravenous route; it also has similar efficacy when delivered by the intracerebroventricular (i.c.v.) route [26,30]. N/OFQ-selective agonists that activate NOP1 show promise as potentially novel peripherally acting antitussives, that would be without the side-effects associated with classical opioid antitussives.

## Local anaesthetics

Local anaesthetics like lidocaine, benzonatate, bupivacaine and mexiletine have been used experimentally to block cough, and local anaesthetics are the most consistently effective antitussive medications but their use is controversial and they are often used as the drugs of last resort in patients with irritable cough. If local anaesthetics are applied locally they can reversibly inhibit pulmonary vagal afferent discharge [31]. The inhibition of action potential generation and transmission in afferent nerves is thought to be a result of a use-dependent inhibition of voltage-gated sodium channels.

Lidocaine given systemically is very effective at inhibiting cough in animal models and in humans, although it is subject to tachyphylaxis. However, high plasma concentrations are necessary for effective cough suppression in humans [32]. Lidocaine also has a quite rapid equilibration through the blood–brain barrier and therefore an inhibition of neural activity in the CNS may contribute to these antitussive effects when the drug is administered systemically [33,34]. Penetration within the CNS may be reduced by direct application to the lung. Thus, inhaled and topically administered lidocaine inhibited cough in humans presumably by an action on afferent nerves in the lung, but it also has a short duration of action. The duration of action may be improved following oral administration.

RSD 931 (carcainium chloride), a quaternary ammonium molecule, has been shown to inhibit citric acid and aerosolized capsaicin-induced cough in the guinea-pig, an effect not thought to be due to local anaesthetic activity [35]. RSD 931 almost completely inhibited citric acid-induced cough at the highest dose used. In rabbits that were pretreated with ozone in order to increase cough sensitivity to citric acid, this cough response was distinctly inhibited by RSD 931, an effect equivalent to intravenous codeine in rabbits. RSD 931 also inhibited histamine-evoked discharge in Aδ-fibres originating from RARs in the tracheobronchial tree of rabbits in a similar way to lidocaine, which suggests a peripheral site of action for this compound [35]. However, RSD 931 differs from lidocaine in that it does not inhibit the spontaneous and capsaicin-evoked discharges in pulmonary and bronchial C-fibres, which suggests a novel mechanism of action.

Mexiletine is an orally active local anaesthetic and a single oral dose reduced histamine-induced reflex bronchoconstriction to the same degree as intravenous lidocaine in subjects with mild asthma [36]. Furthermore, it has been shown that oral administration of mexiletine suppressed cough in humans induced by tartaric acid but not by capsaicin [37]. The implications of these findings are that these stimuli induce cough by different pathways which are differentially regulated by blockade of sodium channels. Interestingly it has been reported that carcainium chloride, which is structurally related to lidocaine and mexiletine but which lacks significant local anaesthetic effects, has a selective effect on RAR nerves in the rabbit and is considerably more effective than lidocaine as an antitussive drug [35]. Mexiletine could prove a more long-lasting antitussive as it has a longer equilibration period.

Bupivacaine administered by the inhaled route reduced cough that was generated by inhalation of citric acid in humans, an effect that was not observed following intravenous administration. This seems to suggest a local site of action for this drug [38]. Dyclonine failed to reduce the cough response to inhaled capsaicin at doses that did not cause bronchoconstriction in humans, despite adequately causing oral anaesthesia. This suggests that the inhibition caused by lidocaine may be due to the difference in rate of penetration of the two different anaesthetics through the airway mucosa [34].

## Tachykinin antagonists

Tachykinins are a group of small peptides, including SP, NKA and neurokinin B (NKB), found in the peripheral endings of capsaicin-sensitive primary afferent neurones (C-fibres) which innervate the lung. The local release of tachykinins following activation of C-fibres may stimulate RARs to enhance the cough reflex [39]. It has also been shown that substance P released from C-fibre afferents augments the stimulatory effect of mild pulmonary congestion on RAR activity, by enhancing hydraulically induced microvascular leak [40]. The actions of the tachykinins are mediated through $NK_1$, $NK_2$ and $NK_3$ receptors, which are located in both the central and peripheral nervous system. The predominant sites containing tachykinin peptides are

capsaicin-sensitive primary afferents that are found in various locations including the lung, skin and gastrointestinal tract [41,42]. There are now several potent tachykinin antagonists available which have proved effective against cough in a number of experimental conditions [43,44]. Substance P given at high concentrations does not evoke cough in guinea-pigs, pigs, healthy humans and asthmatics [45,46]. This may not be surprising since substance P is rapidly metabolized by neutral endopeptidase present in airway epithelium. However, substance P release seems to play a sensitizing role on the cough reflex in guinea-pigs through the stimulation of tachykinin $NK_1$, $NK_2$ and $NK_3$ receptors [46].

The antitussive effect of $NK_2$ antagonists has been observed in many studies. An $NK_2$ receptor antagonist (SR 48968) suppressed the cough reflex in a dose-dependent manner and was found to be more potent than codeine in the guinea-pig [47]. The actions of SR 48968 were not reversed by naloxone implying a lack of involvement of opioid receptors in the suppression of cough. Interestingly, both SR 48968 and codeine only partially inhibited the cough reflex when administered by the inhaled route [44,48]. Although there are conflicting views on the site of action of tachykinin receptor antagonists, a direct action on NK receptors on RARs would indirectly suppress the cough reflex, mediated following activation by NK receptors by endogenous tachykinins from stimulated C-fibres [39,48,49].

The antitussive effect of $NK_1$ antagonists is not clear. FK 888 and CP-99994 ($NK_1$ antagonists) have been shown to inhibit cough induced by tobacco smoke and citric acid in guinea-pigs and mechanical stimulation of the trachea in anaesthetized cats [48,49]. Another $NK_1$ antagonist SR 140333 was reported to have no inhibitory effect on cough, but when it was combined with SR 48968 it was noted that there was an inhibitory effect more marked than with SR 48968 alone [47]. The different effectiveness by these $NK_1$ antagonists may be reconciled with the findings that unlike CP-99994, SR 140333 does not penetrate the blood–brain barrier [50].

The role of $NK_3$ receptors in the cough reflex has received scant attention. The most widely studied $NK_3$ receptor antagonist SR 142801 has high affinity, and is a selective, reversible and competitive antagonist for the $NK_3$ receptor [51]. SR 142801 has also been shown to have an inhibitory effect on citric acid-induced cough in guinea-pigs and pigs although the possibility

68 Chapman RW, Hey JA, Rizzo CA *et al*. GABAB receptors in the lung. *Trends Pharmacol Sci* 1993; **14**: 26–9.

69 Dicpinigaitis PV, Dobkin JB. Antitussive effect of the GABA-agonist baclofen. *Chest* 1997; **111**: 996–9.

70 Bolser DC, Aziz SM, DeGennaro FC *et al*. Antitussive effects of GABAB agonists in the cat and guinea-pig. *Br J Pharmacol* 1993; **110**: 491–5.

71 Bolser DC, DeGennaro FC, O'Reilly S *et al*. Peripheral and central sites of action of GABA-B agonists to inhibit the cough reflex in the cat and guinea pig. *Br J Pharmacol* 1994; **113**: 1344–8.

72 Fox AJ, Barnes PJ, Venkatesan P *et al*. Activation of large conductance potassium channels inhibits the afferent and efferent function of airway sensory nerves in the guinea pig. *J Clin Invest* 1997; **99**: 513–9.

73 Poggioli R, Benelli A, Arletti R *et al*. Antitussive effect of K+ channel openers. *Eur J Pharmacol* 1999; **371**: 39–42.

74 Morita K, Kamei J. Involvement of ATP-sensitive K(+) channels in the anti-tussive effect of moguisteine. *Eur J Pharmacol* 2000; **395**: 161–4.

75 Ventresca PG, Nichol GM, Barnes PJ *et al*. Inhaled furosemide inhibits cough induced by low chloride content solutions but not by capsaicin. *Am Rev Respir Dis* 1990; **142**: 143–6.

76 Sant'Ambrogio FB, Sant'Ambrogio G, Anderson JW. Effect of furosemide on the response of laryngeal receptors to low-chloride solutions. *Eur Respir J* 1993; **6**: 1151–5.

77 Stone RA, Barnes PJ, Chung KF. Effect of frusemide on cough responses to chloride-deficient solution in normal and mild asthmatic subjects. *Eur Respir J* 1993; **6**: 862–7.

78 Morikawa T, Gallico L, Widdicombe J. Actions of mogu-isteine on cough and pulmonary rapidly adapting receptor activity in the guinea pig. *Pharmacol Res* 1997; **35**: 113–18.

79 Sant'Ambrogio G, Sant'Ambrogio FB. Action of moguis-teine on the activity of tracheobronchial rapidly adapting receptors in the dog. *Eur Respir J* 1998; **11**: 339–44.

80 Gallico L, Borghi A, Dalla RC *et al*. Moguisteine: a novel peripheral non-narcotic antitussive drug. *Br J Pharmacol* 1994; **112**: 795–800.

81 Barnabe R, Berni F, Clini V *et al*. The efficacy and safety of moguisteine in comparison with codeine phosphate in patients with chronic cough. *Monaldi Arch Chest Dis* 1995; **50**: 93–7.

82 Schwartz JC, Diaz J, Bordet R *et al*. Functional implications of multiple dopamine receptor subtypes: the D1/D3 receptor coexistence. *Brain Res Rev* 1998; **26**: 236–42.

83 Newbold P, Jackson DM, Young A *et al*. Dual $D_2$ receptor and β-adrenoceptor agonists for the modulation of sensory nerves. In: Hansel TT, Barnes PJ, eds. *New Drugs for Asthma, Allergy and COPD*. Basel: Karger, 2001: 68–71.

84 Trevisani M, Tognetto M, Amadesi S *et al*. $D_2$ dopamine receptor agonists inhibit neuropeptide release from human airway sensory nerves. *Am J Respir Crit Care Med* 2001; **163**: A905.

85 Jackson DM, Simpson WT. The effect of dopamine on the rapidly adapting receptors in the dog lung. *Pulm Pharmacol Ther* 2000; **13**: 39–42.

86 Birrell MA, Crispino N, Hele DJ *et al*. Effect of dopamine receptor agonists on sensory nerve activity: possible therapeutic targets for the treatment of asthma and COPD. *Br J Pharmacol* 2002; **136**: 620–8.

# 24 Current and potential future antitussive therapies

*Peter V. Dicpinigaitis*

## Introduction

Cough is usually distinguished in the medical literature as acute or chronic, the latter often being arbitrarily defined as cough of greater than 3 weeks' duration. Antitussive therapy is appropriately classified as specific therapy, which is aimed at an established or presumed specific aetiology of cough, and non-specific therapy, whose goal is to suppress the cough reflex.

The successful treatment of chronic cough is inextricably linked to the establishment of its aetiology. Multiple prospective studies have demonstrated that the use of a systematic diagnostic protocol will provide a diagnosis in the vast majority of patients [1–3]. A definite diagnosis will allow the initiation of specific antitussive therapy, which is highly effective [1–3]. Non-specific therapy, which does not address the underlying mechanism of a patient's cough, is often ineffective.

Acute cough, most commonly associated with an upper respiratory tract infection (URTI), is usually transient and self-limited. For patients seeking relief from bothersome acute cough, currently available options are less than satisfactory. Contributing to this therapeutic void are a dearth of adequately performed trials of non-prescription cough preparations [4], as well as a lack of consensus among clinicians regarding logical and appropriate treatment strategies for dealing with acute cough [5].

## Chronic cough

### Specific antitussive therapy (Table 24.1)

Prospective studies have shown that, in the vast majority of patients (> 80%) who are non-smokers, are not receiving angiotensin-converting enzyme (ACE) inhibitors, and who do not demonstrate acute pathology on chest radiograph, chronic cough is explained by one or more of three aetiologies: postnasal drip syndrome (PNDS), asthma and gastro-oesophageal reflux disease (GORD) [1–3,6]. Multiple causes of chronic cough are present simultaneously in approximately 25% of patients [1–3,6]. Therefore, the clinician must bear in mind that a partial response to specific antitussive therapy may indicate that only one of multiple aetiologies of cough has been eliminated.

### Postnasal drip syndrome

Multiple studies have demonstrated PNDS to be the most common cause of chronic cough in adults [1–3,6,7]. PNDS may be the result of various processes, including seasonal and perennial allergic rhinitis, perennial non-allergic rhinitis, vasomotor rhinitis, postinfectious (postviral) rhinitis and chronic bacterial sinusitis. Bacterial sinusitis distinguishes itself from the other causes of PNDS since it requires aggressive antibiotic therapy.

The combination of a first-generation antihistamine and decongestant is regarded as the most consistently effective sole form of therapy for PNDS-induced cough not due to sinusitis [8]. These older, potentially sedating antihistamine/decongestant preparations have been shown in prospective trials to be effective in treating chronic cough due to PNDS [1,2,9]. The newer, relatively non-sedating antihistamines, alone or in combination with a decongestant, have been shown to be ineffective antitussives in controlled trials evaluating cough due to the common cold [10–12]. The superior-

**Table 24.1** Specific antitussive therapy.*

*Postnasal drip syndrome*
Antihistamine/decongestant†
Nasal corticosteroids
Nasal cromolyn
Nasal ipratropium bromide

*Asthma-associated cough*
Inhaled bronchodilators ($\beta_2$-agonists)
Inhaled corticosteroids
Leukotriene receptor antagonists
Systemic (oral) corticosteroids

*Gastro-oesophageal reflux disease*
Proton pump inhibitors
$H_2$-receptor antagonists
Metaclopramide
Conservative (non-pharmacological) measures‡
Surgery (Nissen fundoplication)§

*Postinfectious cough*
Oral corticosteroids
Inhaled corticosteroids¶
Inhaled ipratropium bromide**

*Cough due to angiotensin-converting enzyme (ACE) inhibitors*
Cessation of ACE inhibitor††

* See text for discussion of supporting evidence.
† First-generation antihistamine/decongestant combination (see text).
‡ Including high-protein, low-fat diet; avoidance of coffee and tobacco; elevation of head of bed.
§ When aggressive medical antireflux therapy eliminates acid reflux, but cough persists; laparoscopic procedure preferred; surgery not uniformly effective (see text).
¶ Efficacy not demonstrated in adequately performed clinical trials.
** Efficacy demonstrated in one small randomized placebo-controlled trial (see text).
†† Numerous agents shown partially effective (see text).

ity of the first-generation antihistamines is presumably due to their greater anticholinergic potency and penetration into the central nervous system.

Because PNDS has been shown to be the most common cause of chronic cough [1–3,6,7], and, since cough may be the sole presenting symptom of PNDS [2], one therapeutic strategy shown to be successful is to empirically treat patients with a first-generation antihista-

mine/decongestant combination when they present with a chronic cough whose aetiology is not evident from initial history and physical examination [2]. In a prospective study employing this strategy, 36% of 45 patients achieved complete resolution, and 87% reported an improvement in cough [2]. Patients unresponsive or only partially responsive to initial, empirical PNDS therapy were further managed according to a stepwise diagnostic algorithm [2].

Other effective treatments for rhinitis include nasally administered corticosteroids, cromolyn, ipratropium bromide and decongestants, but studies evaluating the effect of these agents specifically on PNDS-induced cough are lacking.

*Cough associated with asthma*
In most asthmatics, cough is associated with other typical features of the disease, including dyspnoea and wheezing. In a subgroup of patients, however, cough is the predominant or sole symptom [13]. This condition has been termed cough-variant asthma (CVA).

In general, the therapeutic approach to CVA is similar to that of typical asthma. An initial, albeit partial, response is often seen after 1 week of therapy with an inhaled $\beta_2$-agonist [14]. Prospective studies have demonstrated inhaled corticosteroids to be efficacious in CVA, although up to 8 weeks of therapy may be necessary to achieve full resolution of cough [14,15]. Inhaled steroids are also effective in the treatment of eosinophilic bronchitis, a condition that causes chronic cough in association with sputum eosinophilia, but in the absence of bronchial hyperresponsiveness characteristic of asthma [16].

An important potential pitfall of inhaled steroid therapy is the possibility that the medication itself may induce or exacerbate cough, likely due to a constituent of the aerosol. For example, the more common occurrence of cough after inhalation of beclometasone dipropionate compared to triamcinolone acetonide is thought to be caused by a component of the dispersant in the former [17].

As with other conditions, there appears to exist a subgroup of CVA patients whose symptoms are particularly severe. Such patients, whose cough is refractory to inhaled steroids, have been described as having 'malignant cough-equivalent asthma' [18]. When cough is severe, or when inhaled steroid-induced cough is suspected, oral corticosteroid therapy (i.e. prednisone 40 mg or equivalent daily for 7–14 days), alone or followed by inhaled therapy [19], is appropriate.

The leukotriene receptor antagonists (LTRAs) represent the newest drug class available for the treatment of asthma. Initial anecdotal reports suggested that LTRAs appeared to be quite effective in asthma-associated cough [20,21]. Subsequently, a randomized double-blind placebo-controlled crossover study demonstrated that a 14-day course of oral zafirlukast, 20 mg twice daily, significantly improved subjective cough scores and diminished capsaicin-induced cough in a group of eight patients with CVA whose cough had been refractory to inhaled bronchodilators and, in five of eight patients, was refractory to inhaled steroids [22]. The ability of zafirlukast to suppress cough that had been refractory to inhaled bronchodilators and inhaled steroids suggests that, in subjects with CVA, the LTRAs more effectively modulate the inflammatory milieu of the afferent cough receptors within the airway epithelium. The mechanism by which this occurs remains to be elucidated.

Given these recent data, LTRAs appear to be an appropriate choice for asthmatic cough refractory to inhaled bronchodilators and steroids, before escalation of therapy to systemic steroids. Whether LTRAs should be used before inhaled steroids in CVA remains unclear. Subepithelial layer thickening, a pathological feature of airway remodelling, is present in CVA, although to a lesser extent than in typical asthma [23]. Therefore, chronic anti-inflammatory therapy may be beneficial in CVA as in typical asthma. Long-term comparisons of inhaled steroids and LTRAs in this setting are required.

Other agents shown in prospective trials to be effective in CVA include inhaled nedocromil sodium [24] (double-blind placebo-controlled study) and azelastine hydrochloride [25], a second-generation $H_1$-receptor antagonist (unblinded, uncontrolled study). The mechanism by which azelastine inhibits cough remains unclear. An antihistaminic effect is supported by the drug's ability to inhibit allergen-induced histamine release in nasal lavage fluid [26]. Furthermore, studies in guinea-pigs suggest that the antitussive effect of azelastine may be due to inhibition of substance P release from sensory nerves [27].

### Gastro-oesophageal reflux disease

The successful treatment of chronic cough due to GORD presents a challenge to the clinician since, in up to 75% of cases, no associated symptoms suggestive of

GORD are present [28]. Further complicating diagnosis and therapy of this condition is the prolonged interval that may be required in some patients before cough improvement and resolution occur.

Initial studies evaluating the treatment of GORD-induced cough employed conservative measures such as high-protein, low-fat diet, avoidance of coffee and tobacco, and elevation of the head while sleeping, in combination with pharmacological therapy consisting of histamine $H_2$-receptor antagonists and/or metaclopramide. This strategy led to resolution of cough in 70–100% of patients. In some cases, however, initial improvement did not occur for 2–3 months, and full resolution of cough required up to 6 months of therapy [8].

The subsequent appearance of more potent acid-suppressing medications in the form of proton pump inhibitors appears to have aided the clinician performing a diagnostic therapeutic trial of antireflux therapy for presumed GORD-induced chronic cough by more promptly and effectively achieving initial improvement and resolution of cough. For example, a regimen of omeprazole, 40 mg twice daily, has been shown, in a randomized double-blind placebo-controlled study, to achieve significant improvement in cough within 2 weeks [29]. In another placebo-controlled study, which employed a crossover design, therapy with a once-daily 40 mg dose of omeprazole led to significant improvement within 8 weeks [30].

In a subgroup of patients cough will persist despite documentation of total or near-total elimination of oesophageal acid with intensive medical therapy [31]. Since such refractory cough often improves after antireflux surgery (Nissen fundoplication), it appears likely that, at least in some patients, reflux-induced cough is due to non-acid mediators [31]. Surgical intervention is not uniformly effective, however. One study prospectively evaluating the results of antireflux surgery in 21 patients with reflux-induced cough refractory to intensive pharmacological therapy demonstrated postoperative improvement in 86%, and complete resolution of cough in 62%, with symptomatic improvement persisting after 1 year [32].

### Postinfectious cough

Although cough associated with an acute URTI is usually transient, in a subgroup of patients a dry cough may persist for weeks to months after resolution of other symptoms. Viral infections likely cause most cases of postinfectious cough; in adults, *Chlamydia pneumoniae*, strain TWAR, *Mycoplasma pneumoniae* and *Bordetella pertussis* have also been implicated [8].

The harsh, persistent, dry cough that may follow an acute URTI is a common stimulus for medical attention and eventual referral to a pulmonary specialist. Postinfectious cough can be particularly difficult to treat. Even codeine, which has been demonstrated to have antitussive activity in chronic and induced cough, was shown to be ineffective in the acute phase of URTI [33].

Since infection-induced, persistent airway inflammation is the likely cause of enhanced cough sensitivity during URTI [34], anti-inflammatory therapy with steroids for severe, debilitating cough seems logical. Although oral steroids have been shown to be effective in this setting [35], inhaled steroids, which are commonly prescribed for postinfectious cough, have not been properly evaluated in clinical trials. One study of non-asthmatic idiopathic chronic cough, though not specifically postinfectious cough, demonstrated a 2–4-week course of budesonide to be ineffective [36].

Inhaled ipratropium bromide has been shown in one small, randomized, placebo-controlled study to be effective in chronic postinfectious cough [37]. The combination of an oral $H_1$-antagonist, oxatomide, and dextromethorphan demonstrated antitussive activity in a small open-label study [38].

### Cough due to ACE inhibitors

The mechanism of ACE inhibitor-induced cough remains unclear. Possible mediators include bradykinin and substance P, which are degraded by ACE and therefore accumulate in lung tissue when the enzyme is inhibited. Prostaglandins, whose production may be enhanced by bradykinin, have also been implicated [39].

The only uniformly effective intervention for ACE inhibitor-induced cough is cessation of the offending agent. Numerous small studies evaluating various drugs have been performed. Agents demonstrating the ability to attenuate ACE inhibitor-induced cough in randomized double-blind placebo-controlled trials include sodium cromoglycate [40], theophylline [41], indometacin [42], the calcium channel antagonists amlodipine and nifedipine [42], the thromboxane receptor antagonist picotamide [43], and ferrous sulphate [44]. In open-label uncontrolled studies, drugs shown to suppress ACE inhibitor-induced cough include the GABA agonist baclofen [45], the thrombox-

ane synthetase inhibitor ozagrel [46], and aspirin (500 mg daily) [47].

The recently introduced drug class, the angiotensin II receptor antagonists, theoretically should not induce cough, since their mechanism of action does not involve inhibition of ACE with resultant elevation of tissue levels of bradykinin and substance P. Indeed, losartan, the first angiotensin II receptor antagonist approved for clinical use, has been associated with a low incidence of cough, similar to that of the diuretic hydrochlorothiazide [48]. Interestingly, multiple cases of angioedema associated with the use of angiotensin II receptor antagonists have been reported [49].

### Non-specific antitussive therapy

Because specific antitussive therapy is highly effective [1–3], an aggressive diagnostic evaluation aimed at determining the specific aetiology of a patient's chronic cough is always indicated. Non-specific antitussive therapy, whose goal is to suppress bothersome cough by inhibiting the cough reflex regardless of the cause of cough, is appropriate only under particular circumstances: (i) when the specific aetiology of cough cannot be established (idiopathic); (ii) when severe cough needs to be suppressed while awaiting the effect of specific antitussive therapy or the resolution of postinfectious cough; and (iii) when the aetiology of cough is known but the cause is irreversible, such as inoperable lung cancer or pulmonary fibrosis.

Non-specific antitussive agents are broadly classified as central or peripheral, based on their site of action (Table 24.2). The pharmacology of these agents is discussed in detail elsewhere in this text.

### Centrally acting agents

*Opioids.* Three narcotic opioids, codeine, hydrocodone and hydromorphone, are approved for use as antitussives. Codeine is the preferred narcotic antitussive because of its lower potential for abuse and more favourable side-effect profile. Nevertheless, codeine in antitussive doses can cause sedation, nausea, vomiting and constipation.

Codeine has been shown in randomized double-blind placebo-controlled studies to have antitussive activity against pathological cough [50,51] as well as induced cough in healthy volunteers [52,53]. However, as mentioned above, codeine has been demonstrated to

**Table 24.2** Non-specific antitussive therapy.*

*Centrally acting agents*
Opioids
  Codeine
  Dextromethorphan
Diphenhydramine

*Peripherally acting agents*
Benzonatate
Levodropropizine
Moguisteine

* Only agents demonstrated in controlled clinical trials to have antitussive activity against pathological cough are listed; see text for discussion of other agents.

be ineffective against cough associated with acute respiratory tract infections [33]. The minimal effective dose of codeine appears to be 20–30 mg.

Dextromethorphan is a non-narcotic opioid that lacks the sedative, analgesic and respiratory depressant effects of codeine, although it can cause confusion and irritability at antitussive doses. It is one of the most widely used antitussive agents worldwide, either alone or as a component of numerous non-prescription cough and cold preparations. The drug most commonly appears in a 20–30 mg dose.

Dextromethorphan has been shown, in randomized double-blind placebo-controlled studies, to be effective against pathological cough [50,51]. In a recent meta-analysis of six blinded placebo-controlled studies containing 710 subjects, a single 30 mg dose of dextromethorphan demonstrated antitussive efficacy against cough associated with URTI [54].

*Diphenhydramine.* Diphenhydramine, a first-generation histamine $H_1$-receptor antagonist, is believed to have central antitussive activity [55]. Placebo-controlled crossover studies have demonstrated the ability of diphenhydramine to suppress induced cough in healthy volunteers [56] as well as chronic pathological cough due to bronchitis [57]. A dose of 25 mg achieved an antitussive effect in both studies.

*Baclofen.* Baclofen is an agonist of γ-aminobutyric acid (GABA), a central inhibitory neurotransmitter. Animal studies initially demonstrated the drug's central antitussive mechanism [58]. Subsequently, baclofen

was shown, in randomized double-blind placebo-controlled studies, to inhibit capsaicin-induced cough in healthy human volunteers at doses as low as 20 mg daily [59,60]. Baclofen demonstrated antitussive activity when evaluated in a double-blind placebo-controlled manner in two patients with chronic idiopathic cough [61]. In an open-label study, baclofen effectively suppressed ACE inhibitor-induced cough [45]. Adequate clinical trials in patients with pathological cough are required to assess the potential therapeutic role of baclofen or other GABA agonists.

*Peripherally acting agents*

*Benzonatate.* Benzonatate (Tessalon™ perles), a long-chain polyglycol derivative chemically related to procaine, is an orally administered agent that may act through inhibition of stretch receptors [62]. Studies performed soon after the drug's release in the 1950s demonstrated its ability to inhibit induced cough as well as to attenuate subjectively measured pathological cough [55]. The benzonatate perle must be swallowed whole to prevent oral anaesthetic effects. Although more contemporary controlled trials are lacking, benzonatate was recently reported to suppress refractory opioid-resistant cough in three patients with advanced cancer [63].

*Levodropropizine.* Levodropropizine is a non-opioid agent whose peripheral antitussive action may be due to its modulation of sensory neuropeptides within the respiratory tract [64]. It has been shown to inhibit experimentally induced cough in healthy volunteers [65] and in subjects with obstructive lung disease [66]. In patients with pathological cough, levodropropizine has been shown to be superior to placebo [67], and comparable in antitussive activity to dextromethorphan [68] and dihydrocodeine [69] in randomized double-blind clinical trials.

*Moguisteine.* Moguisteine is a novel, non-opioid compound whose peripheral site of action [70], which may involve ATP-sensitive potassium channels [71], has been established in animal studies. In human trials involving patients with chronic cough, moguisteine was found to be superior to placebo in a randomized double-blind study [72], and demonstrated antitussive activity similar to that of codeine in a double-blind parallel-group comparison trial [73].

*Inhaled anaesthetics.* Nebulized lidocaine has been shown to inhibit experimentally induced cough in volunteers [74] and, in multiple case reports and small studies, to suppress chronic refractory cough [75–77], alone or in combination with nebulized bupivacaine [77]. The requirement for nebulization provides a logistical hurdle to the common use of these agents. Prospective controlled trials are necessary to evaluate the potential role of inhaled anaesthetics in the management of cough.

## Acute cough

Fortunately, acute cough, which is most commonly associated with a URTI, is usually transient and self-limited. However, if cough is severe, interferes with sleep or persists, patients will consult their physician or pharmacist. Indeed, cough is the most common complaint for which outpatient medical attention is sought in the US [78].

Despite the significance of the problem, very few adequate clinical trials have been performed to evaluate treatments for acute cough [4]. Of those, only a minority have clearly demonstrated the efficacy of pharmacological therapy. Among non-specific antitussive agents, the narcotic opioid codeine, as discussed above, has been shown to be ineffective against acute cough associated with the common cold [33]. Although a meta-analysis demonstrated antitussive efficacy of the non-narcotic opioid dextromethorphan in acute cough due to URTI [54], two other studies showed little or no benefit compared to placebo [79,80]. Moguisteine, the peripherally acting non-specific antitussive agent, likewise demonstrated little if any benefit in patients with acute cough [81]. The combination of a first-generation antihistamine and decongestant, considered the most effective therapy for PNDS-induced chronic cough [8], should theoretically be of some benefit in acute cough as well, by attenuating the postnasal drip which may accompany a URTI. This concept is supported by one study [82], but, interestingly, not by a subsequent trial that employed a newer-generation, non-sedating antihistamine in combination with a decongestant [12].

Further complicating the situation is the lack of consensus among clinicians regarding the optimal therapeutic strategy for acute cough [5]. Some physicians maintain that antitussive therapy should be avoided in cough associated with acute URTI because of a concern that excessive respiratory secretions may accumulate within the airways. Although this concept may be relevant in conditions associated with copious sputum production, such as bronchiectasis or cystic fibrosis, acute cough due to URTI is rarely associated with significant sputum production. Clearly, adequately performed clinical trials aimed at evaluating currently available therapeutic agents, and determining optimal management of acute cough, are required.

Agents other than antitussives are marketed worldwide for the treatment of cough, usually as non-prescription preparations. Often these formulations contain combinations of agents. As with antitussives, few adequately performed clinical trials are available to evaluate these products [4].

Expectorants presumably act by decreasing the viscosity of respiratory secretions, thereby facilitating their expulsion and decreasing the intensity of cough with its associated physical discomfort. Guaifenesin, the only expectorant considered 'safe and effective' by the US Food and Drug Administration [83], is a component of numerous cough and cold preparations. Studies (performed over two decades ago) evaluating the effect of guaifenesin on sputum characteristics [84], rate of mucociliary clearance [85] and cough suppression [86,87] have yielded contradictory results.

Demulcents such as sugar often comprise a significant proportion of many cough products. These agents are thought to suppress cough by coating the inflamed oral mucosa [62].

## Future antitussive therapies

Since antitussive therapy aimed at a specific aetiology of cough is highly successful [1–3], the greatest current need is for more effective non-specific antitussive medications. Presently available non-specific therapy is severely limited by lack of effective agents and/or their unacceptable side-effects. A huge unmet need exists for safe and more effective non-specific cough inhibition, especially for patients with chronic idiopathic cough; cough due to irreversible causes such as inoperable lung cancer; severe acute or persistent postinfectious cough associated with URTI; and severe cough requiring transient relief while specific antitussive therapy takes effect.

Below is a brief overview of several areas of current scientific inquiry that may eventually result in the

**Table 24.3** Potential future antitussive agents.*

Delta-opioid receptor antagonists
Opioid-like orphan (NOP) receptor antagonists
Tachykinin receptor (NK$_1$, NK$_2$, NK$_3$) antagonists
Vanilloid (VR1) receptor antagonists
Endogenous cannabinoids
Antiallergic agents/eosinophil antagonists
GABA$_B$ agonists
5-Hydroxytryptamine (5-HT) receptor agonists
Large conductance calcium-activated potassium channel
   openers

* See text for discussion; most agents listed have only been
evaluated in animal studies.

development of novel antitussive therapeutic agents
(Table 24.3).

### Opioid receptor subtypes and opioid-like receptor antagonists

Agonists of the μ-opioid receptor (including codeine
and hydrocodone) achieve antitussive effect at the
expense of side-effects, which may include sedation,
respiratory depression, nausea, constipation and
potential for abuse. A compound that could inhibit
cough without these associated adverse effects
would offer a significant advantage over currently
available narcotic antitussives. To that end, selective
agonists of the δ-opioid receptor have been developed,
and have demonstrated antitussive activity in animal
trials [88].

Opioid-like orphan (NOP) receptors are present
throughout the mammalian central and peripheral
nervous system, including within the lung. Nociceptin/orphanin FQ (N/OFQ) is an endogenous ligand
for the NOP receptor. Intravenously administered
N/OFQ has been shown to inhibit mechanically stimulated cough in cats [89] and, when given by either a central or peripheral route, inhibited capsaicin-induced
cough in guinea-pigs [90]. Subsequent studies demonstrated the ability of N/OFQ to block capsaicin-induced tachykinin release and bronchoconstriction
through a mechanism involving the activation of an
inward-rectifier potassium channel [91].

### Tachykinin receptor antagonists

The tachykinins include various neuropeptide transmitters such as substance P, neurokinin (NK) A, NKB,
and calcitonin gene-related peptide (CGRP). Animal
studies have implicated that tachykinins, through
stimulation of three receptor subtypes (NK$_1$, NK$_2$ and
NK$_3$), induce bronchial hyperresponsiveness, neurogenic inflammation and cough [92]. In human airways, inflammatory cells appear to be the major source
of tachykinins [93]. Antagonists of the three NK
receptor subtypes have been isolated, and are being
actively investigated for potential therapeutic effect.
Although clinical trials in asthma and chronic obstructive pulmonary disease have been disappointing
[93], antagonists of all three receptor subtypes have
demonstrated antitussive activity in animal studies
[92–95].

### Vanilloid (VR1) receptor

Capsaicin, the pungent extract of red peppers, has
achieved common usage in clinical research because it
induces cough in a reproducible and dose-dependent
manner [96]. Recently, the target receptor of capsaicin, the type 1 vanilloid (VR1) receptor, was discovered on peripheral pain-sensing neurones [97], as
well as throughout the central nervous system [98].
The isolation of the VR1 receptor now provides the
opportunity for the development of potentially useful
antagonists.

### Endogenous cannabinoids

Anandamide is an endogenous cannabinoid that has
been shown in rodents to inhibit capsaicin-induced
cough and bronchospasm, while inducing bronchospasm in animals devoid of vagal tone [99]. These
contrasting effects are both mediated through peripheral CB1 cannabinoid receptors present in airway
nerves. The development of more selective cannabinoid
receptor agonists provides a potential source of future
antitussive agents.

### Eosinophil antagonists

Recent studies have demonstrated that eosinophilic airway inflammation is an important cause of chronic
non-asthmatic cough [16]. The antiallergic agent, su-

platast tosilate, is a T-helper (Th) 2-cytokine inhibitor that inhibits interleukin (IL)-4, IL-5 and immunoglobulin E production, as well as local eosinophil accumulation [100]. In guinea-pigs, suplatast tosilate inhibited antigen-induced cough hypersensitivity and airway eosinophilia [100]. Agents that prevent eosinophilic airway inflammation may offer therapeutic benefit to a particular subgroup of patients suffering from chronic cough.

## GABA$_B$ agonists

As discussed above, the central inhibitory neurotransmitter baclofen, an agonist of the GABA$_B$ receptor, has demonstrated antitussive activity against induced as well as pathological cough [45,59–61]. A common side-effect of baclofen, especially at high doses, is sedation. The discovery of potent GABA$_B$ agonists with less sedative properties than baclofen may provide clinically useful antitussives.

## 5-Hydroxytryptamine (5-HT) receptor agonists

5-HT has been shown to suppress induced cough in healthy volunteers [101]. Furthermore, pretreatment with pizotifen, a 5-HT receptor antagonist, attenuated the inhibitory effect of morphine against capsaicin-induced cough, thereby suggesting a role for 5-HT receptors in the antitussive, but not sedative, effect of opiates [102]. Further insights into 5-HT receptor pharmacology may yield effective antitussive agents that lack the undesirable side-effects of opiates.

## Large conductance calcium-activated potassium channel openers

Animal studies have provided evidence that modulation of potassium channels can attenuate experimentally induced cough. In guinea-pigs, the benzimidazolone compound NS1619, an opener of large conductance calcium-activated potassium (BK$_{Ca}$) channels, inhibited airway sensory nerve activity (as measured by single-fibre recording experiments) as well as citric acid-induced cough [103]. Pinacidil, an ATP-sensitive potassium channel opener, has been shown to inhibit cough in guinea-pigs. The antitussive effect of pinacidil, as well as that of moguisteine, were attenuated by glibenclamide, an ATP-sensitive potassium channel blocker, thus suggesting a role for ATP-sensitive potassium channels in the mechanism of action of both agents [71].

## References

1 Irwin RS, Curley FJ, French CL. Chronic cough. The spectrum and frequency of causes, key components of the diagnostic evaluation, and outcome of specific therapy. *Am Rev Respir Dis* 1990; **141**: 640–7.

2 Pratter MR, Bartter T, Akers S, Dubois J. An algorithmic approach to chronic cough. *Ann Intern Med* 1993; **119**: 977–83.

3 McGarvey LPA, Heaney LG, Lawson JT *et al.* Evaluation and outcome of patients with chronic nonproductive cough using a comprehensive diagnostic protocol. *Thorax* 1998; **53**: 738–43.

4 Schroeder K, Fahey T. Systematic review of randomised controlled trials of over the counter cough medicines for acute cough in adults. *Br Med J* 2002; **324**: 329–31.

5 Morice AH, Widdicombe J, Dicpinigaitis P, Groenke L. Understanding cough. *Eur Respir J* 2002; **19**: 6–7.

6 Smyrnios NA, Irwin RS, Curley FJ, French CL. From a prospective study of chronic cough. Diagnostic and therapeutic aspects in older adults. *Arch Intern Med* 1998; **158**: 1222–8.

7 Marchesani F, Cecarini L, Pela R, Sanguinetti CM. Causes of chronic persistent cough in adult patients: the results of a systematic management protocol. *Monaldi Arch Chest Dis* 1998; **53**: 510–14.

8 Irwin RS, Boulet LP, Cloutier MM *et al.* Managing cough as a defense mechanism and as a symptom: a consensus panel report of the American College of Chest Physicians. *Chest* 1998; **114** (Suppl.): 133S–81S.

9 Smyrnios NA, Irwin RS, Curley FJ. Chronic cough with a history of excessive sputum production: the spectrum and frequency of causes and key components of the diagnostic evaluation, and outcome of specific therapy. *Chest* 1995; **108**: 991–7.

10 Gaffey MJ, Kaiser DL, Hayden FG. Ineffectiveness of oral terfenadine in natural colds: evidence against histamine as a mediator of common cold symptoms. *Pediatr Infect Dis J* 1988; **7**: 223–8.

11 Berkowitz RB, Tinkelman DG. Evaluation of oral terfenadine for the treatment of the common cold. *Ann Allergy* 1991; **67**: 593–7.

12 Berkowitz RB, Connell JT, Dietz AJ, Greenstein SM, Tinkelman DG. The effectiveness of the nonsedating antihistamine loratadine plus pseudoephedrine in the symptomatic management of the common cold. *Ann Allergy* 1989; **63**: 336–9.

13 Corrao WM, Braman SS, Irwin RS. Chronic cough as the

# 25 Placebo effects of antitussive treatments on cough associated with acute upper respiratory tract infection

*Ronald Eccles*

## Introduction

Treatment of cough associated with acute respiratory tract infection (URTI) is mainly based on the treatment of cough as a symptom rather than treating the underlying viral infection. Many cough medicines for the treatment of cough associated with URTI contain codeine or dextromethorphan, which are believed to act by inhibiting the central control of cough [1]. However, studies on the antitussive effects of codeine and dextromethorphan in patients with cough associated with URTI have often failed to demonstrate that these medicines have any greater effect on cough than placebo treatment [2–4].

The very large effect of placebo treatment on cough in clinical trials on antitussive medicines has usually been perceived as a problem in clinical trial design and there has been little interest in trying to understand the nature of this antitussive placebo response.

This chapter will discuss the various factors that influence the severity of cough when a patient is treated with a cough medicine, and in particular will focus on the nature of the placebo response on cough associated with URTI.

## Factors that influence changes in cough severity in a clinical trial

Since the introduction of the double-blind placebo-controlled clinical trial as a standard tool of clinical research, any placebo component of treatment has been considered more of a nuisance to the investigator than a benefit to the patient. Clinical trials are designed to test the superiority of the pharmacological component of the treatment compared with any placebo component, and there is little interest in trying to understand or quantify the placebo effect in clinical trials.

The results of a representative clinical trial to investigate the effects of an antitussive medicine on cough associated with URTI are illustrated in Fig. 25.1 [4]. In this study the reduction in cough frequency following treatment with a single dose of 30 mg dextromethorphan in capsule form appears impressive, until it is compared with the reduction in cough frequency associated with treatment with an identical capsule containing only lactose (placebo). The magnitude and time course of the changes in cough frequency associated with placebo treatment are almost identical to those associated with treatment with the active medicine. The importance of including a placebo control in clinical trials on antitussive medicines can be clearly seen from the results of the trial illustrated in Fig. 25.1. Without a placebo control it would be impossible to determine the antitussive effect of the dextromethorphan.

The changes in cough frequency associated with treatment with an antitussive medicine, such as a cough syrup containing dextromethorphan, can be attributed to at least four different effects: a pharmacological effect, a physiological effect, a true placebo effect, and a non-specific effect as illustrated in Fig. 25.2. These four effects of treatment are discussed below.

### Pharmacological effect

The pharmacological effect of treatment with a cough medicine is related to the active ingredient of the medicine, such as codeine or dextromethorphan. The phar-

**259**

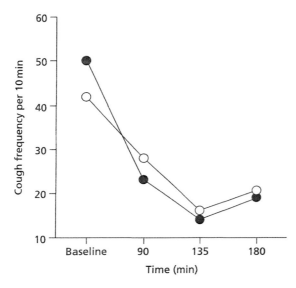

Fig. 25.1 Median cough frequency for patients with cough associated with upper respiratory tract infection. A single dose of 30 mg dextromethorphan powder in a hard gelatin capsule or matched placebo containing lactose powder was ingested by the patient with a small amount of water. Treatment groups: placebo (○), n=22; dextromethorphan (●), n=21 [4].

macologically active ingredient has a high affinity for a specific pharmacological receptor, such as the interaction of codeine with opioid receptors. Slight changes in the molecular structure of the active ingredient may have marked effects on its affinity with the receptor and its biological activity.

In clinical trials on cough medicines, it is the pharmacological effect of the medicine that is under investigation, and any other effects of the treatment are controlled by comparison with the effects of a placebo medication that is identical in appearance, colour, taste, etc. with the active medication.

## Physiological effect

The physiological effects of treatment are the non-pharmacological effects of the treatment such as taste, smell and colour. Physical and chemical properties of the medicine such as viscosity, pH and temperature may also be important. These properties can influence the magnitude of the placebo effect as they provide sensory information about the nature of the treatment.

The physiological component of treatment is usually included as part of the placebo effect, as it is difficult to separate some of the physiological effects of treatment from the placebo effect. However, a case can be made that some aspects of the physiological effect are quite separate from the placebo effect of treatment. Since the majority of cough medicines are sugar-based syrups there has been some speculation that a demulcent effect of the sugar may make a major contribution to the antitussive activity of the medicine [5]. Such a demulcent effect would be in addition to any pharmacological and placebo effects of the medicine.

The demulcent action of the syrup has been proposed to exert its antitussive effect by at least three mechanisms according to Fuller [5].
1 The sugar content of the cough mixture encourages saliva production and swallowing; the act of swallowing may interfere with the cough reflex.
2 The sugar solution may coat sensory nerve endings in the epipharynx and cause their stimulation; this stimulation may suppress cough by a 'gating' process.
3 The sugar solution may act as a protective barrier to sensory receptors that can either produce cough or heighten the cough reflex.

The demulcent effect of antitussive medicines is exploited to the maximum in cough syrups that contain sapid substances such as sugar and honey, and bitter-tasting substances such as lemon and citric acid. These sapid substances promote salivation and may also promote secretion of airway mucus. Gustatory rhinorrhoea has been shown to occur after eating spicy foods, and this observation demonstrates a link between gustation and airway secretion of mucus [6]. Many cough medicines contain capiscum which is a potent gustatory stimulus and which may also promote airway secretions. The fact that almost all cough medicines are formulated as a sapid syrup indicates that the demulcent action of the syrup may contribute to the antitussive activity of the treatment or make the medicine more palatable.

Cooling and warming agents are often added to give extra sensations to the treatment and these agents may influence the activity of cold and warm receptors. Cooling agents such as menthol are sometimes included as flavouring agents in cough medicines, although menthol may also have pharmacological activity as a local anaesthetic [7]. The cooling properties of menthol and other cooling agents could also be considered as a phar-

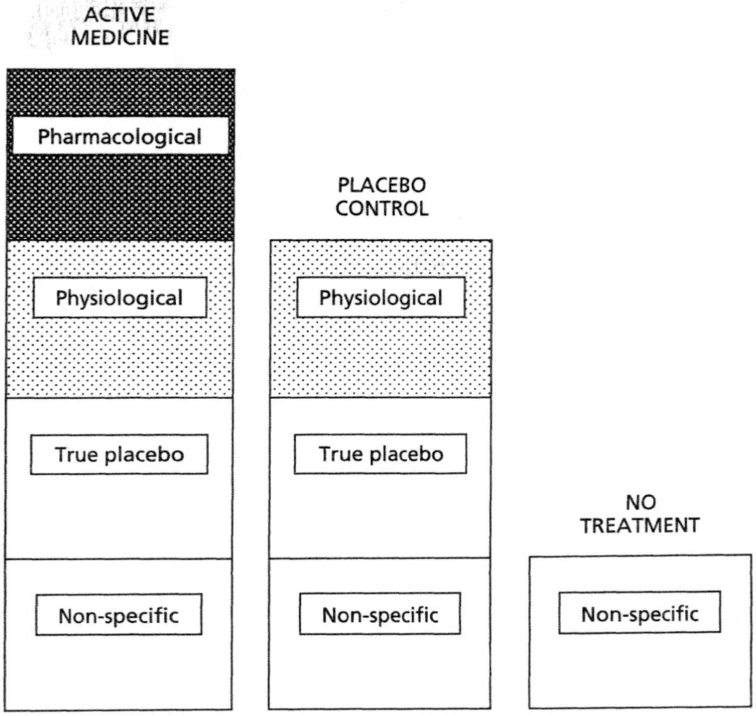

**Fig. 25.2** Components of a cough medicine. The reduction in cough severity in a clinical trial may be explained by four different effects: pharmacological (related to the active ingredient); physiological (related to a demulcent effect, salivation and swallowing); true placebo (related to the sensory impact of the treatment and belief about the efficacy of the treatment); and non-specific (related to natural recovery of patients). The figure illustrates the components in three treatments: active medicine, placebo control and 'no treatment'.

macological component of treatment, as there is some evidence that cooling properties are determined by interaction with a menthol type of pharmacological receptor on sensory nerves [7]. Although menthol is usually declared as a flavouring agent in cough medicines there is some evidence that it may have specific antitussive activity [8].

Other medicines apart from cough medicines may have a physiological effect that can be distinguished from a pharmacological or placebo effect. The efficacy of throat lozenges for the treatment of sore throat is mainly related to the stimulation of salivation, and in this respect there is some similarity between the effects of throat lozenges and cough syrups. Many treatments for common cold are taken as a hot tasty drink, and this mode of treatment may have a physiological effect by stimulating salivation and airway secretions.

The physiological effect of a cough syrup may exhibit similar characteristics to a pharmacological effect, with a time course of action, peak effect, cumulative effect and carry-over effect, but at present there is no information on the pharmacodynamics of any physiological effect of treatment on cough. In the case of cough

medicines, there is likely to be a large physiological effect with a cough syrup, but little, if any, physiological effect with a tablet or capsule formulation.

## Placebo effect

A major problem in defining the placebo effect of a cough treatment is that the effects attributed to placebo treatment often include those effects that could also be attributed to natural recovery from the disease. Some definitions of the placebo effect of treatment refer to all those effects of treatment apart from the pharmacological effects [9]. But this definition is too broad as it includes any changes associated with natural recovery from the disease, and any physiological effects of the medicine.

The placebo effect (as measured in a clinical trial) has been divided into a perceived placebo effect and a true placebo effect by Ernst and Resch [10]. This division will be used in the present discussion.

The perceived placebo effect is defined as the total effect of the placebo medicine, which includes the true placebo effect and other effects such as any physiologi-

**261**

cal effect, and non-specific effects such as natural recovery from the disease. The perceived placebo effect is normally measured in a placebo-controlled clinical trial, but it is not possible to estimate the contribution of the true placebo effect to any changes in cough severity from this parameter, as the perceived placebo effect also includes the physiological effect and non-specific effect of treatment as shown in Fig. 25.2.

In clinical trials where a 'no treatment' group is included in the design, it is possible to control for any non-specific effects of treatment by subtracting any changes in the no treatment group from those changes observed in the placebo treatment group. This leaves us with a measure of any true placebo effect plus any physiological effect. In the case of cough treatments that use a tablet or capsule formulation, any physiological effect of treatment will be minimal and the use of a no treatment group will allow determination of the true placebo effect. But in the case of a cough syrup there could be a large physiological effect and it will not be possible to separate this from any true placebo effect.

The true placebo effect refers to a psychological therapeutic effect of the treatment, and this will depend on many factors such as the belief in the effectiveness of the treatment, the attitude of the patient towards the therapist, and what the therapist says to the patient.

The psychological therapeutic effect attributed to the true placebo effect of treatment with a cough medicine is related to the patient's belief about the efficacy of the medicine [11]. The degree of belief in the treatment will depend on many factors, such as the healer–patient interaction, cultural beliefs about traditional treatments, the environment in which the medicine is administered, the properties of the medicine such as taste, colour and smell, advertising and claims made about the efficacy of the medicine, the brand name of the medicine, and side-effects associated with treatment that may reinforce the belief of efficacy. This list of factors that may influence the efficacy of a placebo is not exhaustive, and it illustrates how difficult it is to properly control and standardize studies on the true placebo effect.

### Non-specific effect

'Sick people often get better'. In an acute illness natural recovery may occur and this is not due to any effect of the treatment [10].

Patients recruited to a clinical trial to determine the efficacy of an antitussive medicine are screened to determine the severity of cough, as only those patients with a high subjective score and/or objective measure of cough are recruited for the study. By recruiting only those patients with a severe or troublesome cough and excluding those patients with a mild cough, the population of patients on the trial is skewed towards those with a severe cough. In these circumstances the cough severity of the patients on trial is unlikely to increase during the course of the study and it is more likely that the cough severity will decrease due to the process of natural recovery. The mean measure of cough severity is likely to decline during the course of the clinical trial and this statistical effect is often referred to as 'regression to mean' [9]. The changes in cough frequency illustrated in Fig. 25.1 could be explained by regression to mean since the patients were recruited with high cough frequency and this declined in both treatment groups during the course of the study.

It is not possible to control for the effects of rest and spontaneous recovery in controlled clinical trials that involve only placebo and active treatment groups, as both these treatment groups will be affected by rest and recovery. However, if a 'no treatment' group is included in the trial design then this will allow direct comparison with the placebo treatment group [10]. If the 'no treatment' group does not show any great change in cough severity during the course of the study then any change in the placebo group must be due to a true placebo effect (plus a physiological effect if the treatment is a syrup). In a study on patients with cough associated with URTI comparing the antitussive effects of 'no treatment' vs. placebo treatment, the 'no treatment' group had a 7% decrease in cough frequency compared to a 50% decrease in the placebo treatment group [12]. In this study the placebo medicine was a capsule, rather than a syrup, so the placebo effect cannot be explained by a demulcent effect of the treatment, or by rest, and it may be reasonably defined as a true placebo effect.

### Magnitude of the perceived placebo response

A literature survey found eight placebo-controlled clinical trials on antitussive medicines used in the treatment of cough associated with URTI [2–4,13–15], and the results of these studies are given in Fig. 25.3 and Table 25.1. The formulation of the placebo medication was a syrup in two of the studies [2,13] and a capsule or

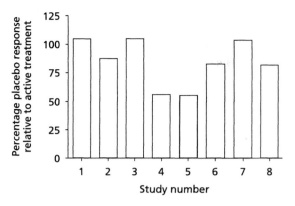

**Fig. 25.3** Magnitude of perceived placebo response relative to active medication in clinical trials on cough associated with upper respiratory tract infection. The perceived placebo response is calculated as a percentage relative to the change in cough observed with the active medication. Therefore a perceived placebo response of 100% means that the change in cough severity on placebo treatment is equal to that observed with treatment with the active medicine. The study numbers refer to those given in Table 25.1 which gives further details of the studies.

tablet in the remaining studies. Only subjective scores were used in the early studies [13,14], whereas both subjective and objective measures of cough were used in the later studies [2–4,15].

The studies are presented in order to assess the magnitude of the perceived placebo effect rather than debate the efficacy of the antitussive medications. The perceived placebo effect is calculated as a percentage relative to the change in cough observed with the active medication. Thus in the study by Tukiainen *et al.* [13] a perceived placebo effect of 105% indicates that the placebo treatment was actually more effective than the active medicine in treating cough. Theoretically, one would expect the maximum perceived placebo effect to be equal to or less than 100% of the active treatment effect as all aspects of the placebo treatment should be present in the active treatment. A perceived placebo effect above 100% may be explained by variance in the measures of cough.

The perceived placebo effect varied from a minimum of 56% up to a maximum of 105% with a mean of 85%. Six of the eight studies had a perceived placebo effect of over 80%. The three studies by Parvez *et al.* [15] had the lowest perceived placebo effects. This may be because of the relatively greater pharmacological effect

of dextromethorphan in their study population of Indian patients compared to a European or American population. The Indian patients had an average body weight of around 50 kg, with some patients having a body weight as low as 27 kg. The greater antitussive activity of dextromethorphan demonstrated in the Indian patients may indicate that higher doses of dextromethorphan will have a similar antitussive efficacy in the heavier patients in the other studies. However, the greater efficacy in the Indian patients may also be explained by side-effects that perhaps reinforce and increase the magnitude of the placebo effect of the active treatment.

The mean perceived placebo effect of 85% can be attributed to a true placebo effect plus other non-specific factors such as natural recovery and, in the case of a cough syrup, a physiological effect.

## Mechanism of the true placebo effect

Science and medicine have debated the relevance of mind and body interactions for over 2000 years and there has been much debate about the role of the mind in the onset and treatment of disease. There is very good evidence which indicates that the mind does influence many bodily functions. Voluntary control of skeletal muscle and voluntary control of cough are well-established examples of mind–body interactions. The 'flight or fight response' with activation of the sympathetic nervous system when a real or imaginary threat is perceived is an example of a mind–body interaction that is not under voluntary control [16].

Studies on patients with cough associated with URTI have demonstrated that cough can be voluntarily suppressed and that there is an inverse relationship between the duration of cough suppression and the baseline frequency of cough [17]. In general, one would expect that any therapeutic effect of treatment would be greatest in those patients with the most severe illness. Similarly the magnitude of any placebo effect may be related to the severity of the illness.

The fact that cough can be initiated and inhibited voluntarily demonstrates a link between the mind and the control of cough. However, discussion on mind–body interactions is limited by the problem that there is no real understanding of what exactly constitutes the mind. If one accepts that the basis of mind depends on complex neurophysiological activity, then at

**Table 25.1** Magnitude of placebo response relative to active medication in clinical trials on cough associated with upper respiratory tract infection (URTI). The placebo response is calculated as a percentage relative to the change in cough observed with the active medication. Therefore a placebo response of 100% means that the change in cough severity is equal to that observed with treatment with the active medication.

| Study no. | Investigator | Medication | Dosing | Duration of study | Cough measure | Placebo response (%) | Patients |
|---|---|---|---|---|---|---|---|
| 1 | Tukiainen et al. (1986) | Dextromethorphan syrup? | 30 mg 3 times daily | 4 days | Subjective cough frequency on day 4 of treatment | 105 P>0.05 n.s.* | 108 patients with acute cough |
| 2 | Adams et al. (1993) | Moguisteine tablets | 200 mg twice a day | 3.5 days | Subjective cough severity on day 3 of treatment | 88 P>0.05 n.s.† | 108 patients with acute cough |
| 3 | Eccles et al. (1992) | Codeine syrup | 30 mg single dose | Laboratory study on 1 day | Cough frequency at 150 min after treatment | 105 P>0.05 n.s. | 91 patients with cough associated with URTI |
| 4 | Parvez et al. (1996) Study 1 | Dextromethorphan capsules | 30 mg single dose | Laboratory study on 1 day | Cough bouts at 120–150 min after treatment | 56 P>0.05 n.s. | 108 patients with cough associated with URTI |
| 5 | Parvez et al. (1996) Study 2 | Dextromethorphan capsules | 30 mg single dose | Laboratory study on 1 day | Cough bouts at 120–150 min after treatment | 55 P<0.05 | 134 patients with cough associated with URTI |
| 6 | Parvez et al. (1996) Study 3 | Dextromethorphan capsules | 30 mg single dose | Laboratory study on 1 day | Cough bouts at 150–180 min after treatment | 83 P>0.05 n.s. | 209 patients with cough associated with URTI |
| 7 | Freestone et al. (1997) | Codeine capsule | 50 mg single dose | Laboratory study on 1 day | Cough frequency at 90 min after treatment | 104 P>0.05 n.s. | 82 patients with cough associated with URTI |
| 8 | Lee et al. (2000) | Dextromethorphan capsules | 30 mg single dose | Laboratory study on 1 day | Cough frequency at 180 min after treatment | 82 P>0.05 n.s. | 43 patients with cough associated with URTI |

The probability values (P) refer to the difference between the active treatment and placebo.
n.s., not significant.
* Not significant on any day.
† Main group analysis not significant on any day but some subgroups with high cough scores did show a significant difference on some days.

some point this neurophysiological activity must link up via distinct nervous pathways with the area of the brain that controls cough. It is at this point that we move from the realms of mind into the more easily understood realms of neuroscience. If the belief that one is exposed to danger can bring about a range of autonomic nervous responses, then it is reasonable to assume that belief about the effects of treatment may also influence bodily functions such as the control of cough. This interaction can be termed a psychoneuropharmacological response that implies that a mind response has triggered a distinct nervous pathway with its own neurotransmitters that can be influenced by pharmacological intervention.

The placebo response associated with the treatment of pain has been explained on the basis that the belief in treatment in some way activates nervous pathways that cause the release of endogenous opioid substances [18]. Treatment with exogenous opioids such as codeine and morphine may inhibit pain by mimicking the effects of endogenous opioids. Thus administration of a placebo may inhibit pain by a placebo effect that causes the release of endogenous opioids. The analgesic effect of placebo treatment can be inhibited by administration of opioid antagonists such as naloxone [19], and this supports the theory that endogenous opioids are involved in the placebo response to pain.

There are many similarities between the pharmacology of analgesics and the pharmacology of antitussives, as codeine and morphine are potent analgesics and antitussives. The hypothesis that the placebo analgesia is mediated by endogenous opioids may also be relevant to cough, as the true placebo antitussive response may also be mediated by endogenous opioids.

## Kinetics and dynamics of true placebo effect

'In a literal sense, there can be no such thing as the pharmacokinetics of a placebo because there is nothing to be absorbed, distributed, metabolized, excreted or sought at specific tissue sites' [16]. However, 'placebo-generated perceptions can result in the production or release of endogenous active materials that may indeed have a kinetic fate analogous to that of administered active exogenous drugs' [16]. A review by Lasagna et al. [20] on the 'pharmacology' of placebo medicines discusses time–effect curves, peak effects, cumulative effects and

'carry-over' effects. All of these properties of the true placebo effect support the concept that placebo treatment can be studied in terms of pharmacokinetics and pharmacodynamics. This implies that treatment with a placebo in some way influences neurotransmitter systems in the brain and that the pharmacology of the true placebo effect is related to the pharmacology of the neurotransmitters [21]. The release and actions of the central neurotransmitters associated with the true placebo effect is not an 'on and off' effect, but an effect with a definite time course and peak effect, similar to that obtained by administration of a pharmacologically active medicine.

## Cough model

A model illustrating the true placebo effect of cough treatment is illustrated in Fig. 25.4. The model proposes that cough may be initiated by two separate mechanisms, reflex cough and voluntary cough.

Reflex cough is initiated by airway irritation mediated by the vagus nerve that relays with the cough control centre in the respiratory area of the brainstem. When airway irritation reaches a sufficient level, cough is initiated via a descending pathway from the brainstem to the respiratory muscles. The descending pathway controlling cough may be different from that controlling spontaneous breathing [22]. Reflex cough can also be initiated by the entry of food and fluid into the airway.

Voluntary cough can be initiated by a sensation of airway irritation mediated by the vagus nerve, with central pathways ascending from the cough control centre in the brainstem to the cerebral cortex. Cough is initiated from the cortex by descending pathways to the cough control centre in the brainstem. The pathway from the cerebral cortex to the cough centre may induce or inhibit cough, as experimental studies in humans have shown that cough associated with URTI can be voluntarily inhibited [17]. The term 'voluntary cough' does not necessarily mean a cough that is 'willed' or 'desired', but a cough that can be voluntarily inhibited, whereas reflex cough cannot be suppressed. It is possible that all types of human cough involve a sensation of irritation and involve both cortical and brainstem mechanisms, but that the relative involvement of cortical control varies from complete control to almost no influence on the cough response.

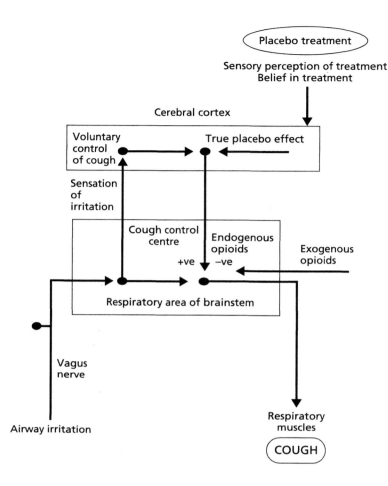

Fig. 25.4 Model to illustrate the control of cough, and the mechanism of the true placebo effect. Airway irritation causes cough via a reflex pathway in the respiratory area of the brainstem and may also initiate voluntary cough via a sensation of irritation and the cerebral cortex. The cerebral cortex may induce or inhibit cough via a pathway that influences the activity of the cough control centre in the brainstem. The act of taking a placebo cough medicine initiates a true placebo response that influences cough via a pathway from the cerebral cortex to the cough control centre. This pathway may involve endogenous opioid neurotransmitters. Exogenous opioids such as morphine and codeine may mimic the inhibitory effects of endogenous opioids.

Cough can be thought of as varying from a reflex cough that cannot be inhibited, such as cough in response to food or fluid entering the airway, to a voluntary cough that is used as a signal or means of communicating. In these cases the reflex cough may be initiated via the brainstem pathway, and the voluntary cough initiated via the cerebral cortex. Cough associated with URTI may be a mix of reflex and voluntary cough, as some of the cough can be suppressed by voluntary control [17].

The cough control model illustrated in Fig. 25.4 indicates that placebo treatment causes a true placebo effect via sensory perception of the placebo treatment. This assumes that treatment with a placebo medicine must be perceived by the patient via sensory cues, such as sight, taste and smell, if the placebo treatment is to have any true placebo effect. If the patient is not aware that they are being treated then it is not possible for the treatment to exert any psychological effect. The belief by the patient that they are being treated with an effective medicine may be related to previous experience and belief in the system of medicine in their culture. If the patient has little belief in the efficacy of the treatment then the true placebo effect may be limited.

The true placebo effect represents the interface between mind and body interactions and can be discussed in terms of psychoneuropharmacology as described above. At some point the neurophysiological activity associated with the true placebo effect must link up via distinct nervous pathways with the area of the brain that controls cough, and modify cough via a descending pathway from the cerebral cortex to the brainstem cough centre. Inhibition of cough via a true placebo effect need not enter consciousness as the true placebo effect could operate outside of consciousness. Although both voluntary control of cough and the true placebo effect on cough may share a common final pathway to influence cough, the sites initiating these responses may be in different parts of the brain.

The descending pathway from the cerebral cortex that inhibits cough may do so by the release of endogenous opioid neurotransmitters [21]. This would explain why opioids such as morphine and codeine when administered exogenously act as antitussives.

## Discussion

One definition of the placebo nicely fits in with its effects on cough, and states that the placebo is the 'most effective medication known to science, subjected to more clinical trials than any other medicament yet nearly always does better than anticipated' [23]. The majority of published studies on the effects of antitussive medicines on cough associated with URTI have demonstrated that placebo treatment is just as effective as the active medicine, and there must be a large number of clinical studies on file that have never been published in the public domain that support the antitussive efficacy of placebo treatment. One could criticize some of the studies on their design, population size, etc., but the overall impression is that there is little difference in antitussive activity between placebo treatments and active pharmacological treatments such as codeine and dextromethorphan when administered in the over-the-counter dose range for treatment of cough associated with URTI. The present review has concentrated on the antitussive effect of placebo treatments in clinical trials on cough associated with URTI, and the results and discussion may not be relevant to other types of cough such as chronic cough [24,25] and induced cough in healthy volunteers [26] where antitussives such as codeine and dextromethorphan appear to have significantly greater efficacy than placebo treatment.

The fact that placebo treatment is often as effective as treatment with codeine and dextromethorphan for cough associated with URTI can be interpreted in several ways. It may indicate that codeine and dextromethorphan are relatively ineffective in treating cough associated with URTI. A meta-analysis of studies on dextromethorphan indicates that the average superiority of dextromethorphan above placebo ranges from 12 to 17% [27]. This indicates that placebo treatment is responsible for 83–88% of the reduction in cough. In other studies the perceived placebo effect has been responsible for 100% of the reduction in cough [2–4]. These results could be interpreted as supporting a very powerful antitussive placebo effect, but since there is no comparison with a 'no treatment' control group in these studies, it is also possible that nonspecific effects such as natural recovery have a great contribution to the perceived placebo effect.

More cough clinical trials are needed that use a 'no treatment' group in order to determine the true placebo effect and control for factors such as natural recovery. The vehicle syrup used in many cough medicines for the treatment of cough associated with URTI has both physiological and true placebo effects that are likely to produce a very effective antitussive action. Pharmaceutical companies have developed cough syrups with powerful physiological and placebo effects. The additional antitussive benefit of the active ingredient such as codeine or dextromethorphan is only a minor factor in the antitussive efficacy of the syrup medicine. In a safety vs. benefit analysis, the small extra benefit provided by dextromethorphan and codeine over that provided by placebo must be weighed against the risks incurred by their inclusion in cough medicines, especially when considering the potential for recreational abuse [28] and side-effects in children [29].

## References

1 Widdicombe JG. Advances in understanding and treatment of cough. *Monaldi Arch Chest Dis* 1999; **54**: 275–9.

2 Eccles R, Morris S, Jawad M. Lack of effect of codeine in the treatment of cough associated with acute upper respiratory tract infection. *J Clin Pharm Ther* 1992; **17**: 175–80.

3 Freestone C, Eccles R. Assessment of the antitussive efficacy of codeine in cough associated with common cold. *J Pharm Pharmacol* 1997; **49**: 1045–9.

4 Lee PCL, Jawad MSM, Eccles R. Antitussive efficacy of dextromethorphan in cough associated with acute upper respiratory tract infection. *J Pharm Pharmacol* 2000; **52**: 1137–42.

5 Fuller RW, Jackson DM. Physiology and treatment of cough. *Thorax* 1990; **45**: 425–30.

6 Choudry NB, Harrison AJ, Fuller RW. Inhibition of gustatory rhinorrhea by intranasal ipratropium bromide. *Eur J Clin Pharmacol* 1992; **42**: 561–2.

7 Eccles R. Menthol and related cooling compounds. *J Pharm Pharmacol* 1994; **46**: 618–30.

8 Morice AH, Marshall AE, Higgins KS *et al*. Effect of inhaled menthol on citric acid induced cough in normal subjects. *Thorax* 1994; **49**: 1024–6.

9 Kienle G, Kiene H. Placebo effect and placebo concept: a critical methodological and conceptual analysis of reports on the magnitude of the placebo effect. *Altern Ther* 1996; **2**: 39–54.

10 Ernst E, Resch KL. Concept of true and perceived placebo effects. *Br Med J* 1995; **311**: 551–3.

11 Morris D. Placebo, pain and belief: a biocultural model. In: Harrington A, ed. *The Placebo Effect. An Interdisciplinary Approach*. Cambridge, MA: Harvard University Press, 1999: 187–207.

12 Lee PCL, Jawad MSM, Hull JD *et al*. The effect of placebo treatment on cough associated with common cold. *Br J Clin Pharmacol* 2001; **51**: 373P.

13 Tukiainen H, Karttunen P, Silvasti M *et al*. The treatment of acute transient cough—a placebo-controlled comparison of dextromethorphan and dextromethorphan-beta$_2$-sympathomimetic combination. *Eur J Respir Dis* 1986; **69**: 95–9.

14 Adams R, Hosie J, James I *et al*. Antitussive activity and tolerability of moguisteine in patients with acute cough: a randomized, double blind, placebo-controlled study. *Adv Ther* 1993; **10**: 263–71.

15 Parvez L, Vaidya M, Sakhardande A *et al*. Evaluation of antitussive agents in man. *Pulm Pharmacol* 1996; **9**: 299–308.

16 Weiner M, Weiner GJ. The kinetics and dynamics of responses to placebo. *Clin Pharmacol Ther* 1996; **60**: 247–54.

17 Hutchings HA, Eccles R, Smith AP *et al*. Voluntary cough suppression as an indication of symptom severity in upper respiratory tract infections. *Eur Respir J* 1993; **6**: 1449–54.

18 ter Riet G, de Craen AJM, de Boer A *et al*. Is placebo analgesia mediated by endogenous opioids? A systematic review. *Pain* 1998; **76**: 273–5.

19 Benedetti FAM. The neurobiology of placebo analgesia: from endogenous opioids to cholecystokinin. *Prog Neurobiol* 1997; **52**: 109.

20 Lasagna L, Laties V, Dohan J. Further studies on the 'pharmacology' of placebo administration. *J Clin Invest* 1958; **37**: 533–7.

21 Sher L. The placebo effect on mood and behavior: the role of the endogenous opioid system. *Med Hypotheses* 1997; **48**: 347.

22 Newsom Davis J, Plum F. Separation of descending spinal pathways to respiratory motoneurons. *Exp Neurol* 1972; **34**: 78–94.

23 O'Donnell M. Our oath is hypocritical. *Monitor Weekly* 1995; March 1: 44.

24 Aylward M, Maddock J, Davies DE, Protheroe DA, Leidman T. Dextromethorphan and codeine: comparison of plasma kinetics and antitussive effects. *Eur J Respir Dis* 1984; **65**: 283–91.

25 Matthys H. Dextromethorphan and codeine: objective assessment of antitussive activity in patients with chronic cough. *J Int Med Res* 1983; **11**: 92–100.

26 Morice AH, Kastelik JA, Thompson R. Cough challenge in the assessment of cough reflex. *Clin Pharmacol* 2001; **52**: 365–75.

27 Pavesi L, Subburaj S, Porter-Shaw K. Application and validation of a computerized cough acquisition system for objective monitoring of acute cough—a meta-analysis. *Chest* 2001; **120**: 1121–8.

28 Noonan WC, Miller WR, Feeney DM. Dextromethorphan abuse among youth. *Arch Fam Med* 2001; **9**: 791–2.

29 Taylor JA, Novack AH, Almquist JR *et al*. Efficacy of cough suppressants in children. *J Pediatrics* 1993; **122**: 799–802.

# 26 Mucoactive agents for the treatment of cough

*Bruce K. Rubin*

## Introduction

Medications that are used to treat cough or to enhance cough clearance fall into three broad classes [1]. The first of these, the cough suppressants, are discussed elsewhere in this book. They are mentioned here only to note that there are many medications available without prescription in the US and Canada that contain a combination of a 'cough suppressant' and a secretagogue 'expectorant'. This counterproductive combination would be potentially harmful to the patient if both of these medications were effective. Perhaps it is fortunate for the patient that nearly always either one or both of the medications in these combination products is ineffective, at least at the dosage provided.

The second and largest class of mucoactive medications used as cough therapy are those agents that are meant to improve the ability to expectorate secretions. These, in turn, fall into several subgroups. Expectorants are medications that increase the volume of airway secretion either by inducing mucus secretion or by increasing the transport of water into the airway. They are meant to 'loosen' secretions and thus make them easier to expectorate. Medications that are proposed to add water to the airway can be as simple as fluid ingestion or as complex as gene transfer to enhance the expression of epithelial proteins that control airway ion and water transport. A second group of mucokinetic medications are those that alter the biophysical properties of airway secretions making them easier to expectorate. This would include the mucolytic agents that degrade the mucin polymer network (classic mucolytics) or the DNA and F-actin polymer network derived from inflammatory cell necrosis (peptide mucolytics).

Mucoactive drugs that reduce the adhesivity of secretions and thus their binding to the epithelium will make sputum easier to expectorate. Such medications include surfactant preparations. Medications that enhance expiratory airflow can also be considered as mucokinetic drugs, as cough clearance is dependent not only on the properties of the mucus but also on expiratory air volume and velocity (flow). Thus in patients who have increased airflow following the use of bronchodilators, the bronchodilator medication might be considered to be mucokinetic.

The third class of medications effecting cough clearance are those that are meant to reduce the quantity of airway secretions. Because airway inflammation leads to mucus hypersecretion, and chronic infection and inflammation often lead to mucous gland hypertrophy and hyperplasia of goblet cells, it is assumed that patients with chronic bronchitis, cystic fibrosis (CF), diffuse panbronchiolitis (DPB), bronchiectasis and perhaps asthma have an increased airway secretion burden [2]. Mucoregulatory medications are meant to reduce mucus hypersecretion without affecting constitutive or basal secretion. Examples of these medications are anti-inflammatory drugs, anticholinergics and some of the macrolide antibiotics.

An overview of these agents and proposed mechanism of action is listed in Table 26.1.

## Mucoactive medications

'Mucoactive' is a general term used to indicate a medication that is used to reduce mucus secretion or to promote mucus clearance. This would include mucolytic,

**Table 26.11** Classification of mucoactive medications by proposed mechanisms of action.

| Mucoactive agent | Potential mechanisms of action |
|---|---|
| *Classical mucolytics* | |
| N-acetylcysteine, nacystelyn | Severs disulphide bonds in proteins, antioxidant |
| *Peptide mucolytics* | |
| Dornase alfa | Hydrolyses DNA molecules with reduction in DNA length |
| Gelsolin | Depolymerizes F-actin |
| Thymosin $\beta_4$ | Depolymerizes F-actin |
| *Non-destructive mucolytics* | |
| Dextran, low molecular weight heparin | Break hydrogen and ionic bonds |
| *Expectorants* | |
| P2Y$_2$ agents | Increase epithelial mucus and chloride secretion |
| Hypertonic saline, mannitol | Reduce ionic bonds and increases secretion hydration |
| Gene therapy, aquaporin activators | Normalize secretory cell function (may increase airway water) |
| *Mucoregulatory agents* | |
| Anticholinergic agents | Decrease volume of stimulated secretions |
| Glucocorticoids | Decrease airway inflammation and mucin secretion |
| Indometacin | Decreases airway inflammation |
| Macrolide antibiotics | Decrease airway inflammation and mucin secretion |
| *Mucokinetic agents* | |
| Bronchodilators | Can improve cough clearance by increasing expiratory flow |
| Surfactants | Decrease sputum adhesiveness (abhesive) |

mucokinetic, mucospissic, mucoregulatory and expectorant medications but not cough suppressants [3].

## Expectorants

Expectorants are meant to increase the volume of airway secretions in order to improve their bulk mobilization, or medications that add water to airway secretions and presumably free mucus from attachments to the epithelium.

Oral and intravenous hydration have been studied as a simple method to increase the hydration of airway secretions. In animal models of airway hypersecretion induced by allergy, Wanner and colleagues showed that intravenous fluids were of no benefit in altering the volume or biophysical properties of airway secretions and that when hyperhydration was provided intravenously, there was deterioration in pulmonary function and gas exchange [4]. In another study, patients with chronic bronchitis were encouraged to drink large amounts of water under direct supervision over a specific period of time. This did not improve expectoration, pulmonary function or clinical well-being in these patients [5].

Hyperosmolar aerosol inhalation has been used to draw fluid into the airway and induce mucus secretion. This has been shown to assist expectoration acutely in patients with asthma, chronic bronchitis and CF [6].

This technique has primarily been used either to obtain secretions for diagnostic purposes for the bacteriological diagnosis of tuberculosis or *Pneumocystis carinii*, or to obtain airway secretions from patients with asthma or CF for research evaluation [7]. There have been several short-term clinical trials evaluating the use of inhaled hyperosmolar saline for the treatment of CF or chronic bronchitis that have demonstrated increased radioaerosol clearance and improved pulmonary function [8]. Similar short-term benefits have been demonstrated with the inhalation of dry powder mannitol [9]. The long-term clinical benefit of this therapeutic intervention is uncertain.

Transepithelial water flux is primarily regulated by paracellular epithelial ion and water channels [10]. In health, there is probably a smaller contribution from transcellular pathways. Luminal chloride secretion through the cystic fibrosis ion transport regulator (CFTR) protein and the calcium-dependent chloride channels will tend to draw water into the airway while sodium resorption through the epithelial sodium channel (ENaC) draws water from the airway into the cell. Patients with CF have impaired chloride secretion through the CFTR channel and increased sodium resorption through the ENaC. Early attempts to block sodium resorption in order to normalize water transport across the CF airway involved the inhalation of an aerosol of amiloride, a diuretic that blocks sodium resorption. These trials produced promising acute results but long-term trials did not demonstrate a benefit in pulmonary function or mucus clearance [11]. While tricyclic nucleotides such as UTP have been used to acutely increase calcium-dependent chloride secretion via the purinergic $P2Y_2$ receptors, the half-life of inhaled UTP is extremely short so current studies are focusing on similar compounds with a longer half-life [12].

Water transport across epithelial surfaces is also modulated by selective water channels called aquaporins. Initially identified in the renal tubules, there are several aquaporins expressed in airway epithelium, in particular, aquaporin 5 (AQP5) [13,14]. Because these channels selectively transport water, they may be an attractive target for manipulating airway water content.

It has been demonstrated, both in cell culture and in airway and nasal tissue, that it is possible to temporarily replace the abnormal CF gene protein product in airway cells by means of gene transfer using viral or liposomal vectors. While gene transfer has successfully corrected the ion transport defect in transfected cells, at this time transfer is fairly inefficient and temporary, and there have been problems with increased inflammation and immune response directed against the gene transfer vector [15].

Although theoretically adding water to the airway lumen can potentially 'unstick' secretions from the epithelium making them easier to expectorate, with the exception of short-term improvements in pulmonary function and sputum expectoration using hyperosmolar aerosol inhalation, there are no medications in this class of mucoactive drugs that have been proven to be clinically effective.

### Medications that alter the properties of secretions

Airway mucus is an inhomogeneous, adhesive gel that has properties both of a liquid (viscosity) and of a solid (elasticity) (Fig. 26.1). When subjected to an applied stress, mucus initially stores energy, it then begins to

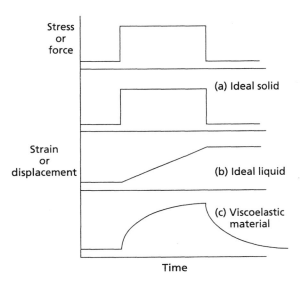

**Fig. 26.1** Viscoelasticity measures the stress/strain response of a material. (a) An ideal or Hookian solid responds to a stress by energy storage or elasticity. This energy is released when the strain is removed. (b) An ideal or Newtonian liquid responds to stress by deforming continuously with no energy storage. This rate of deformation or energy loss is viscosity. (c) A viscoelastic gel initially stores energy like a solid and, with continued strain, will then deform more like a liquid.

deform, and finally it flows. Energy storage or elasticity is critical for the efficient transmission of energy from beating cilia to the mucus layer in order to propel the mucus by ciliary clearance. Mucus flow is essential for it to be extruded from submucosal glands and transported up the airway. Mucus with increased viscosity is more difficult to clear, especially by the ciliary elevator. It has not been demonstrated that increased viscoelasticity alone will impair cough clearance [16].

*Mucolytic medications*

Mucolytic medications non-selectively decrease both the viscosity and elasticity of airway secretions by degrading the polymer networks that give mucus or sputum its gel-like structure. Classic mucolytics disrupt mucin polymers either by severing the disulphide bonds that covalently link mucin monomers into elongated and stiff oligomers, or by dispersing the tangled mucin network by disrupting hydrogen ion bonding or van der Waals forces through mechanisms such as charge shielding.

With chronic airway infection and inflammation there is recruitment of inflammatory cells, predominantly neutrophils, into the airway. These cells release proinflammatory cytokines and chemokines, serine proteases such as neutrophil elastase, and reactive oxygen species all of which further damage the airway epithelium and recruit more inflammatory cells. Inflammatory cell necrosis also releases cell wall-associated F-actin and nuclear DNA which copolymerize into a stiff secondary polymer network increasing secretion viscoelasticity and adhesivity. Peptide mucolytics degrade the secondary network by acting primarily on DNA (dornase alfa) or by acting on the actin network and secondarily the DNA polymer (gelsolin, thymosin $\beta_4$) [17,18].

The only mucolytic approved for use in the United States and Canada is dornase alfa, marketed by Genentech as Pulmozyme®. This is administered as an inhalation aerosol at a dosage of 2.5 mg/day. Studies have demonstrated that dornase alfa decreases viscosity and substantially decreases the adhesivity of airway secretions in patients with CF, and that long-term use in many patients improves pulmonary function, reduces the rate of deterioration of pulmonary function, and reduces the need for hospitalization and antibiotic therapy [19]. Dornase alfa is administered by jet nebulization and is not mixed with other medications, although often patients will inhale a bronchodilator

first. Although it is generally administered before chest physical therapy, there are data to suggest greater deposition and perhaps increased efficacy if it is administered simultaneously with external high-frequency chest wall oscillation [20]. *In vitro* studies suggest an additive effect when dornase alfa is combined with either gelsolin or thymosin $\beta_4$ [21].

A vexing problem has been trying to determine *a priori* which patients are most likely to clinically respond to dornase alfa Therapeutic response appears to be unrelated to sputum concentration of DNA. Although there was initially a concern that dornase alfa might overliquefy secretions, making them more difficult to expectorate, especially in patients with severe disease and compromised airflow, many patients with severe pulmonary compromise appear to benefit from dornase alfa. Studies suggest that dornase alfa may also be beneficial when initiated very early in life, before there are overt signs of pulmonary infection [22]. Nevertheless many patients fail to improve pulmonary function even after several months of therapy and a small number have worsening of pulmonary function. Anecdotal reports suggest that the most severely affected patients (those with $FEV_1 < 30\%$ predicted) may obtain benefit but are also at greatest risk for pulmonary function compromise with the use of this medication.

Dornase alfa can also interact with other medications. For this reason it is always administered alone. There are *in vitro* data to suggest that azithromycin may inactivate dornase alfa [23]. On the other hand, mucolysis may also allow greater penetration of drugs into airway secretions [24]. This may be of particular importance when the patient is using aerosolized antibiotics.

Side-effects with the use of dornase alfa have generally been mild. Hoarseness and occasional sore throat have been reported. These will usually disappear when the medication is stopped and often will not recur when restarted. Although low levels of anti-DNase antibodies have been reported in some patients, these do not appear to lead to adverse outcomes nor does this appear to reduce the efficacy of inhaled dornase alfa.

Dornase alfa has also been studied for the treatment of chronic bronchitis, non-CF bronchiectasis and plastic bronchitis [25–27]. A small study in patients with severe chronic obstructive pulmonary disease (COPD) suggested that dornase alfa inhalation may reduce mortality but a much larger study showed no benefit. There are several small studies that suggest that some patients with less severe chronic bronchitis may benefit from dornase alfa inhalation. Studies of patients with non-CF bronchiectasis have generally, and surprisingly, proved disappointing in that no clinical or pulmonary function benefit has been demonstrated. In a subset of these patients, those with primary ciliary dyskinesia, there have been a few case reports that suggest benefit from dornase alfa inhalation [28].

Patients with respiratory syncytial virus (RSV) bronchiolitis have high concentrations of DNA in their bronchial lavage fluid. In a small study conducted evaluating infants admitted to hospital for severe RSV bronchiolitis a small improvement in X-ray scores, but not in hospital length of stay, was seen in those who were administered dornase alfa [29]. Anecdotal reports have consistently failed to show benefit in patients with plastic bronchitis (bronchial casts, often in association with congenital heart disease) who used dornase alfa. Pilot studies (unpublished) from our laboratory suggest that these casts are largely comprised of mucin and are not affected by *in vitro* exposure to dornase alfa.

### Clinical use of classic mucolytics

Although N-acetyl-L-cysteine (NAC) is available as a nebulizer solution in North America it is not on formulary as an approved mucolytic drug. Outside of North America, NAC is the most commonly prescribed mucolytic drug for the treatment of lung diseases and it is available in both oral and inhalation forms. The free sulphydryl group in NAC can dissociate the disulphide bond between adjacent cysteine residues linking mucin monomers. However, aerosolized NAC has a pH of 2.2 and an unpleasant odour, and both of these can make inhalation difficult for patients who are sensitive to odours or who have airway hyperresponsiveness. Airway irritation, bronchospasm and coughing paroxysms have been reported frequently in patients inhaling NAC. NAC cannot be detected in plasma or bronchial lavage even after 2 weeks of oral dosing [30]. Glutathione is an important oxygen scavenger and its synthesis requires cysteine. Orally administered NAC has very low bioavailability and is rapidly deacetylated to cysteine. Therefore NAC has antioxidant properties. Side-effects of oral acetylcysteine are nausea and diarrhoea.

There have been many studies over the last 40 years that evaluate the use of NAC in patients with chronic bronchitis but few of these have been rigorously conducted, randomized and placebo controlled with a long enough duration of treatment to determine changes in primary outcomes of clinical relevance such as lung function. Convincing demonstration of the effectiveness of either inhaled or orally administered NAC in improving lung function, sputum properties or clinical morbidity in patients with chronic bronchitis is lacking.

Preliminary studies in patients with CF who inhaled the lysine salt of NAC (called nacystelyn) suggest that there may be an acute improvement in pulmonary function following the inhalation of 16 actuations from the pressurized metered dose inhaler (pMDI) [31]. Lysine is a basic amino acid with mucolytic properties and the lysine salt of NAC has a pseudoneutral pH making it better tolerated when administered by aerosol. Long-term trials of this medication for the treatment of CF presumably await the development of a more convenient dosage form.

A fairly large number of derivatives of NAC with blocked sulphydryl groups have been developed. These include carbocysteine (S-carboxymethylcysteine), erdosteine (N-carboxymethylthilacetyl) the lysine salt of carbocysteine (carbocysteine-LYS), L-ethylsysteine and stepronin. None of these medications has direct mucolytic activity but they may act as scavengers for reactive oxygen species and may also be metabolized to active drugs with thiol groups capable of severing disulphide bonds [32].

### Polymer dispersion and charge shielding

The elongated mucus oligomers are loosely held together in what has been termed a tangled network gel structure by relatively weak hydrogen ion bonding and van der Waals forces. Low molecular weight dextran or heparin can reduce the viscosity of both mucus and sputum *in vitro* [33] presumably by charge shielding and disrupting these weak forces. This allows increased hydration or disentanglement of the mucin network. Clinical trials of these types of agents have not yet been reported.

## Medications that affect the interaction between mucus and epithelium

Experimental data strongly suggest that the cough clearability of mucus or sputum (in other words the ability for airflow to move secretions) is more strongly influenced by the adhesive interaction between the secretions and the epithelium than by the bulk viscosity of the mucus [34]. In fact, viscous mucus would be beneficial for cough clearance as it would present a greater profile to the propelling air column.

Adhesion is the attractive interaction between two different substances, generally a liquid and a solid. Important to this interaction is the ability of the liquid to wet the solid surface. This is generally measured as the contact angle, $\theta$, at the liquid–solid–vapour interface. One of the best known of the commercial applications of this phenomenon is the use of Teflon™ to coat surfaces so that substances will not adhere. Teflon™ is very poorly wettable and this is the reason for its non-stick properties. The other important factor determining this interaction is the interfacial force between the liquid and the solid. Between liquid and vapour phases this is referred to as surface tension, and between two liquid phases or between a liquid and a solid it is called the interfacial tension. The Neumann equation for a sessile drop allows us to calculate the work of adhesion as $\gamma(1+\cos\theta)$ where gamma ($\gamma$) is the interfacial tension and theta ($\theta$) is the vapour–liquid–solid contact angle [35].

The force of tenacity is the product of adhesivity (defined above) and cohesivity or the ability of a substance to 'stick to itself'. An approximation of cohesivity can be measured using the Filancemeter which evaluates the stringiness of a substance as the maximal length that a set volume of a liquid can be stretched before it breaks. Initially developed to measure the *spinnbarkeit* of cervical mucus, the application of these

measurements to airway secretions has shown that high cohesivity significantly impairs both ciliary and cough clearability by increasing the tethering of secretions [36]. This tethering has also been demonstrated histologically, and is particularly prominent in the CF airway and in patients with severe asthma. Thus tenacity can be imagined as similar to sticky chewing gum spread across the bottom of a shoe and on the flooring surface, with both the stickiness and the stringiness contributing to the difficulty in breaking free. *In vitro* studies have shown that tenacity is the strongest determinant of secretion cough clearability and that medications that have the ability to reduce adhesivity (abhesives) or cohesivity will improve cough clearability of secretions in a simulated cough machine *in vitro* [37] (Fig. 26.2).

Surfactants are critical to airway stability and the free flow of mucus. In the alveolus, surfactant prevents alveolar collapse and reduces the pressure needed to expand the airway with each breath. In small airways surfactant permits free and unidirectional mucus flow, thus preventing airway obstruction. A thin surfactant layer between the mucus gel and the periciliary fluid facilitates mucus spreading after it is extruded from submucosal glands, and allows the efficient transfer of kinetic energy from beating cilia to the mucus layer preventing ciliary entanglement in the mucus. This airway surfactant is thought to be derived both from the alveolar type II cells and from submucosal glands.

Airway inflammation can degrade surfactant

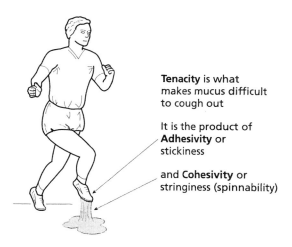

**Tenacity** is what makes mucus difficult to cough out

It is the product of **Adhesivity** or stickiness

and **Cohesivity** or stringiness (spinnability)

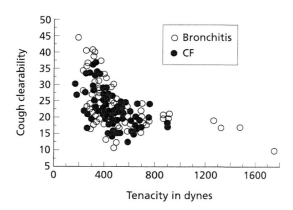

Fig. 26.2 Tenacity, the product of adhesivity and cohesivity, is the strongest determinant of sputum cough clearability as measured in the simulated cough machine.

through several different mechanisms. Transudate of proteins such as albumen, the presence of products of inflammation and cellular necrosis such as DNA, and hydrolysis of surfactant phospholipids—in particular dipalmitoyl phosphatidylcholine (DPPC) and phosphatidylglycerol (PG)—by secretory phospholipases A2 (sPLA2) can all produce surfactant dysfunction. The lysophospholipids products of surfactant hydrolysis not only lack surfactant function but further impair proper functioning of airway surfactant [38]. Cell wall-associated phospholipids such as sphingomyelin may have a similar effect.

There are increased amounts of sPLA2 in bronchial lavage from patients with asthma and these phospholipases readily hydrolyse surfactant phospholipids. Sputum from patients with chronic bronchitis or CF have greater quantities of cell wall-associated phospholipids and lower amounts of surfactant phospholipids than mucus from healthy individuals. Theoretically, surfactant administration should reconstitute the airway surfactant and enhance mucus clearance. Such an effect has been well demonstrated in clinical trials of aerosolized surfactant in patients with stable CF or chronic bronchitis. There is a dose-dependent improvement in pulmonary function, a decrease in the volume of trapped thoracic gas as measured by the ratio of residual volume to total lung capacity (RV/TLC), and an increase in the sputum cough clearability in bronchitis patients inhaling a surfactant aerosol [39]. One of the difficulties in the aerosolization of surfactant is its low surface tension and therefore its propensity to foam. Further clinical trials await the development of more efficient means for generating surfactant aerosols.

Mucolytic agents may also work, in part, as abhesives but through a different mechanism than by altering surface tension. With airway inflammation the mucus has a greater tendency to entangle in airway cilia and bind to the airway epithelium. Mucolysis may dissolve some of this mucus surface entanglement, making it easier for airflow to expel secretions as sputum.

## Medications that increase airflow

Cough clearance depends on the biophysical properties of the airway secretions, the interaction between the mucus and the airway epithelium, and the force and volume of expiratory airflow. Any manoeuvre that increases expiratory airflow would thus be expected to

improve cough clearance. This is the basis behind most chest physical therapy manoeuvres and devices that are currently in use. The medications most commonly used to increase the expiratory airflow are inhaled bronchodilators. These agents are effective in enhancing secretion clearance in those patients with bronchial hyperresponsiveness who have demonstrable improvement in expiratory flow following their use. Although the β-agonist bronchodilators have a small stimulatory effect on ciliary beat frequency, this has a trivial effect on mucus clearance [40]. A warning is in order, because bronchodilator medications, by virtue of their ability to relax airway smooth muscle, may increase the collapsibility of the airway, particularly in patients with bronchomalacia or bronchiectasis [41]. This collapse can lead to gas trapping and paradoxical decrease in flow. Therefore if these medications are to be used to assist with cough it is imperative that the patient first be tested for bronchodilator responsiveness.

## Medications that reduce mucus hypersecretion (mucoregulatory medications)

Chronic airway inflammation leads to the release of mediators that damage the epithelium and, presumably as a protective mechanism, lead to hypertrophy and hyperplasia of surface goblet (mucous) cells and submucosal glands. The increased volume of airway submucosal glands is a characteristic of chronic bronchitis reflected in the Reid index. Hypertrophy and hyperplasia of the secretory apparatus is also characteristic of asthma, CF, bronchiectasis and other inflammatory airway diseases. This increased number and volume of secretory cells coupled with an increased responsiveness to secretagogues, the elaboration of mucus secretagogues during inflammation (e.g. serine proteases such as neutrophil elastase), and destruction of the airway epithelium which impairs mucociliary clearance, all lead to airway mucus retention. Although in health, mucus secretion is beneficial, the hypersecretion of chronic airway disease leads to entrapment of bacteria, airflow obstruction, and deterioration in lung function and quality of life. Mucoregulatory agents are meant to reduce hypersecretion usually by modifying the inflammatory response.

Anti-inflammatory agents are probably the most commonly used immunomodulatory agents. Adrenal corticosteroids can reduce airway inflammation and are the most effective medications currently used to treat chronic asthma. Oral corticosteroids have also been shown to be beneficial to patients with CF. There is less clear evidence of benefit for these medications in patients with chronic bronchitis or bronchiectasis; nevertheless, inhaled corticosteroids are commonly used to 'treat' these conditions. Other medications such as ibuprofen or indometacin have been used to treat airway inflammation. Trials of oral ibuprofen have demonstrated a slower decline in pulmonary function and improvement in weight gain in young patients with CF [42]. Indometacin aerosol has been shown to decrease the hypersecretion commonly seen in patients who have DPB [43].

Atropine and its derivatives decrease cholinergic-mediated secretion through a blockade of the M3 receptor interaction. Atropine has not been demonstrated to decrease the normal or baseline level of airway secretions *in vitro*, and in animals it does not appear to increase the viscosity of airway secretions [44]. Atropine is extremely effective at blocking cholinergic-mediated hypersecretion *in vivo*. It is less clear whether there is or is not an effect on secretion viscosity in healthy individuals who are administered atropine perioperatively.

Derivatives of atropine with greater specificity include glycopyrrolate and quaternary ammonium derivatives of atropine, ipratropium bromide and oxitropium bromide. Clinical studies have shown that these latter medications neither reduce mucociliary clearance nor alter the biophysical properties of secretions, but they decrease mucus hypersecretion in patients with chronic bronchitis when given over an extended period of time [45].

Bacterial killing and prevention of airway infection are effective ways to reduce inflammation and hypersecretion. Because of this, antibiotics can be considered 'mucoregulatory medications' when used to treat infection. Of great recent interest is the non-antibacterial actions of some antibiotics. The 14- and 15-member macrolactam ring macrolide antibiotics have profound immunomodulatory and mucoregulatory activity as detailed below. There is evidence that some of the quinolone antibiotics may also have immunomodulatory effects.

The macrolide derivatives of erythromycin A have significant anti-inflammatory and immunomodulatory effects and decrease the hyperimmune state associated with chronic airway inflammation. These effects were first suspected when it was demonstrated that trolean-domycin was an effective 'steroid-sparing' medication when given to patients with prednisolone-dependent asthma [46]. Although initially it was suspected that this was due to decreased steroid metabolism [47], many patients who received troleandomycin were able to completely discontinue steroids while retaining control of their asthma. Steroid-associated side-effects were generally decreased in patients receiving the macrolide without any decline in pulmonary function, suggesting a secondary effect on the inflammatory response unrelated to steroid metabolism.

Evidence has since accumulated demonstrating the immunomodulatory effects of the macrolide antibiotics [48]. In the early 1980s it was shown that low-dose and long-term therapy with erythromycin or clarithromycin made a dramatic difference in morbidity and mortality in patients with DPB [49]. DPB is a form of chronic sinobronchitis that occurs primarily in adult non-smokers in Japan and Korea. DPB is generally associated with chronic *Pseudomonas* infection, mucus hypersecretion and severe sinusitis. The cause of this disease is unknown but it has been associated with HLA haplotypes that differ in Japan, Korea and China. Before 1985, most patients with DPB died within 5 years of diagnosis, even with antibiotic and corticosteroid therapy. Therapy with erythromycin, clarithromycin or azithromycin, but not the 16-member macrolides, dramatically improves survival and often leads to complete resolution of the disease. More recently, studies show similar dramatic improvements in mucus hypersecretion and airway inflammation in patients with CF given oral macrolide therapy [50]. *In vitro* the macrolides have a profound effect on neutrophil migration, cytokine production and the oxidative burst [51]. They also appear to have direct effects on the development of bacterial biofilm, preventing planktonic organisms from producing the necessary quorum-sensing peptides to develop a biofilm and thus rendering them more sensitive to antibiotics and more susceptible to host defences. The 14- and 15-member macrolides and ketolides also have direct and specific effects on mucus hypersecretion [52].

## Indications for the use of mucoactive drugs

Expectorants and mucolytics are widely used in

Europe, South America and Asia although there are few data that demonstrate efficacy [32]. For the most part, these drugs are not available in North America as prescription medications (which requires documentation of efficacy) but many 'expectorant' cough medications are sold over the counter as non-prescription therapy for respiratory tract infections. Iodinated expectorants such as domiodol, iodinated glycerol or supersaturated potassium iodide (SSKI) provide little benefit for acute or chronic airway diseases and pose a risk of iodide toxicity including skin rash, gastrointestinal upset and thyroid suppression. There is a similar lack of proven efficacy for guaifenesin, glycerol guaiacolate [53] or the thiol-containing mucolytics such as N-acetylcysteine (NAC). A recent meta-analysis of published studies evaluating the efficacy of NAC in patients with chronic bronchitis suggests a small decrease in the frequency of pulmonary exacerbations of disease for those patients taking NAC [54]. Publication bias for positive studies was acknowledged and the small benefit was thought to be primarily due to the antioxidant properties of NAC. Because of the paucity of established data, European and North American guidelines for the treatment of chronic bronchitis do not recommend the routine use of expectorants or mucolytic agents. There is a similar lack of data supporting the use of expectorants and, except for dornase alfa, mucolytics in the treatment of asthma or CF. The most likely reason for this lack of demonstrated efficacy for these drugs is the paucity of well-controlled clinical studies.

Clinical practice guidelines suggest that dornase alfa should be used for CF patients who are documented to have pulmonary function improvement after a 2–3 month trial with this medication [55]. Although this may exclude some patients with intervening concomitant illness who do not appear to respond or may include other patients who are recovering from illness but would otherwise have limited response to this medication, these guidelines are probably a useful way to initially identify patients likely to receive benefit. There is ongoing research into specific markers that may predict which patients are more likely to benefit from mucoactive medication therapy. The use of dornase alfa in infants and children with CF who are too young to perform pulmonary function manoeuvres is somewhat more controversial. Guidelines for the use of dornase alfa in this age group will require the evaluation of more longitudinal data.

The indication for dornase alfa use in other diseases is not as clearly established. Although it is frequently used in patients with non-CF-associated bronchiectasis, it appears that most patients with bronchiectasis will not respond to dornase alfa therapy with improved pulmonary function. There are few data to suggest efficacy in patients with asthma, chronic bronchitis or other chronic airway diseases because of the lack of well-controlled clinical trials [25].

Although in vitro data and limited clinical data suggest a significant benefit for aerosol surfactant therapy in chronic bronchitis and perhaps in asthma and CF, these medications are quite expensive. Long-term studies with a greater number of subjects await the development of more easily and consistently administered formulations.

β-Agonist bronchodilators are indicated for patients with bronchial hyperresponsiveness who demonstrate improved airflow following their inhalation. Given the risk of decreased airflow with airway collapse in patients with bronchiectasis or bronchomalacia [56], it is strongly recommended that patients have spirometry to assess bronchodilator response before these medications are administered on a routine basis. Ipratropium and oxitropium bromide are used long term for the treatment of chronic bronchitis, principally as bronchodilator medications. Some of their efficacy may be rooted in their ability to suppress cholinergic-mediated hypersecretion. Glycopyrrolate is occasionally given for long periods to patients who have an artificial airway and mucus hypersecretion, but there are few data to critically support this use. This class of medication may become more useful in the future with the development of specific M3 antagonists.

Long-term and low-dose macrolide therapy is clearly indicated for the treatment of patients with DPB. There is tremendous interest in and enthusiasm for this therapy in patients with CF. There are several ongoing studies evaluating not only the clinical effectiveness but also potential mechanisms of action of macrolide antibiotics as immunomodulatory medications.

There is a theoretical risk of using medications that thin secretions or loosen them in patients with profoundly compromised expiratory airflow (generally those with an $FEV_1$ of less than 20% predicted) as this could potentially lead to retrograde flow of secretions in a patient unable to expectorate because of muscle weakness and diminished expiratory flow.

**277**

## Assessment of therapeutic efficacy

There is a great deal of controversy regarding the most appropriate therapeutic outcomes to use for the evaluation of mucoactive therapy both in large clinical trials and in the individual patient [57]. Although measurement of expiratory airflow such as $FEV_1$ is reliable, reproducible and easily obtainable for most patients, it is generally insensitive for determining the therapeutic efficacy of mucoactive medications with the exception being the assessment of bronchodilator therapy and perhaps the use of dornase alfa in patients with CF. The measurement of gas trapping such as the ratio of residual volume to total lung capacity (RV/TLC) may be more sensitive to recruitment of volume in association with unplugging small airways as secretions are mobilized and expectorated [58]. Theoretically other measurements of small airway function (e.g. inspiratory and expiratory high-resolution computed tomographic scanning for evidence of gas trapping) may be useful for the assessment of mucus mobilization in some patients.

It seems simple and thus attractive to measure the volume of expectorated sputum to assess the efficacy of mucoactive medications. Unfortunately, expectorated sputum volume bears no relationship to changes in pulmonary function or objective measurements of patient well-being. There is extraordinary day-to-day and patient-to-patient variability in sputum expectoration which may be related to diurnal variability in salivary volume, variability in secretion swallowing and variability in sputum production, leading to differences in secretion and expectoration volumes that are unrelated to the medication being given. There are also cultural and gender differences in the willingness to expectorate sputum that will influence this measurement. Even in patients with CF who have a clear improvement in pulmonary function with inhaled dornase alfa, there is no difference in expectorated sputum volume when compared with patients who have no response or even a decline in pulmonary function. Similar observations have been made for other mucoactive medications. The 'normalization' of sputum volume by drying in an attempt to eliminate the effect of salivary contamination does not improve the accuracy of this measurement as an assessment for sputum clearance [57].

Quality of life scores have been used in an attempt to evaluate the efficacy of mucoactive medications. However, existing scoring systems lack objective validation for this use and tend to be insensitive to other measurements of clinical improvement such as pulmonary function changes or functional exercise capacity [59].

For patients with severe chronic lung disease who have limitation in their activities of daily living, a potentially useful efficacy measurement is functional exercise capacity by means of a 6-min walking test or a shuttle test. Patient and caregiver training is essential to obtain the most consistent results for this type of testing, and practice is needed to ensure that the test is valid and reproducible [60]. However, when this test is conducted under controlled circumstances and in a laboratory that is familiar with functional exercise testing, it appears to reflect fairly well the subjective feeling of clinical improvement with medications used to treat decreased sputum clearance.

## Summary

Airway mucus is a mixture of water, mucous glycoproteins, low molecular weight ions, proteins and lipids, whose properties are important for airway defence. The factors that contribute to the physical properties of mucus are complex, and there are various pharmacological strategies that can potentially improve the clearability of airway mucus. Although there are a very large number of drugs used as mucoactive medications to assist cough clearance and to suppress mucus hypersecretion, with few exceptions unequivocal clinical data supporting their use are lacking. For this reason, most guidelines for the management of asthma, chronic bronchitis, bronchiectasis and CF do not routinely recommend the use of mucoactive medications. This is not to say that these medications are ineffective, but rather that carefully designed and well-powered randomized clinical trials with appropriate controls and well-selected outcome measurements and of sufficient duration must be conducted before determining which groups of patients are most likely to benefit.

## References

1 Rubin BK, Tomkiewicz RP, King M. Mucoactive agents: old and new. In: Wilmott RW, ed. *The Pediatric Lung*. Basel, Switzerland: Birkhäuser Publishing Ltd, 1997: 155–79.

2 Wanner A, Salathé M, O'Riordan TG. Mucociliary clearance in the airways. *Am J Respir Crit Care Med* 1996; **154**: 1868–902.

3 Rubin BK. Frontiers in mucus clearance. In: Goldstein AL, ed. *Frontiers in Biomedicine*. New York: Kluwer Academic/Plenum Publishers, 2000: 237–50.

4 Wanner A, Rao A. Clinical indications for and effects of bland, mucolytic, and antimicrobial aerosols. *Am Rev Respir Dis* 1980; **122**: 79–87.

5 Shim C, King M, Williams MH Jr. Lack of effect of hydration on sputum production in chronic bronchitis. *Chest* 1987; **92**: 679–82.

6 Eng PA, Morton J, Douglass JA, Riedler J, Wilson J, Robertson CF. Short-term efficacy of ultrasonically nebulized hypertonic saline in cystic fibrosis. *Pediatr Pulmon* 1996; **21**: 77–83.

7 Pin I, Freitag AP, O'Byrne PM, Girgis-Gabardo A, Watson RM, Dolovich J, Denburg JA, Hargreave FE. Changes in the cellular profile of induced sputum after allergen-induced asthmatic responses. *Am Rev Respir Dis* 1992; **145**: 1265–9.

8 Robinson M, Hemming AL, Regnis JA *et al*. Effect of increasing doses of hypertonic saline on mucociliary clearance in patients with cystic fibrosis. *Thorax* 1997; **52**: 900–3.

9 Daviskas E, Anderson SD, Brannan JD, Chan HK, Eberl S, Bautovich G. Inhalation of dry-powder mannitol increases mucociliary clearance. *Eur Respir J* 1997; **10**: 2449–54.

10 Boucher RC. State of the art: human airway ion transport. *Am J Respir Crit Care Med* 1994; **150**: 581–93.

11 Graham A, Hashani A, Alton EW, Martin GP, Marriott C, Hodson ME, Clarke SW, Geddes DM. No added benefit from nebulized amiloride in patients with cystic fibrosis. *Eur Respir J* 1993; **6**: 1243–8.

12 Noone PG, Bennett WD, Regnis JA, Zeman KL, Carson JL, King M, Boucher RC, Knowles MR. Effect of aerosolized uridine-5′-triphosphate (UTP) on cough clearance in patients with primary ciliary dyskinesia. *Am J Respir Crit Care Med* 1999; **160**: 144–9.

13 King LS. Surprises from the airway epithelium. *Proc Natl Acad Sci USA* 2001; **98**: 14192–4.

14 Song Y, Verkman AS. Aquaporin-5 dependent fluid secretion in airway submucosal glands. *J Biol Chem* 2001; **276**: 41288–92.

15 Rubin BK. Emerging therapies for cystic fibrosis lung disease. *Chest* 1999; **115**: 1120–6.

16 King M, Rubin BK. Mucus rheology, relationship with transport. In: Takishima T, ed. *Airway Secretion: Physiological Bases for the Control of Mucus Hypersecretion*. New York: Marcel Dekker, Inc., 1994: 283–314.

17 Shak S, Capon DJ, Hellmiss R, Marsters SA, Baker CL. Recombinant human DNase I reduces the viscosity of cystic fibrosis sputum. *Proc Natl Acad Sci USA* 1990; **87**: 9188–92.

18 Vasconcellos CA, Allen PG, Wohl M, Drazen JM, Janmey PA. Reduction in sputum viscosity of cystic fibrosis sputum *in vitro* by gelsolin. *Science* 1994; **263**: 969–71.

19 Fuchs HJ, Borowitz DS, Christiansen DH, Morris EM, Nash ML, Ramsey BW, Rosenstein BJ, Smith AL, Wohl ME. Effect of aerosolized recombinant human DNase on exacerbations of respiratory symptoms and on pulmonary function in patients with cystic fibrosis. *N Engl J Med* 1994; **331**: 637–42.

20 Dasgupta B, Tomkiewicz RP, Boyd WA, Brown NE, King M. Effects of combined treatment with rhDNase and airflow oscillations on spinnability of cystic fibrosis sputum *in vitro*. *Pediatr Pulmonol* 1995; **20**: 78–82.

21 Tomkiewicz RP, Kishioka C, Freeman J, Rubin BK. DNA and actin filament ultrastructure in cystic fibrosis sputum. In: Baum G, ed. *Cilia, Mucus and Mucociliary Interactions*. New York: Marcel Dekker, 1998: 333–41.

22 Quan JM, Tiddens HA, Sy JP, McKenzie SG, Montgomery MD, Robinson PJ, Wohl ME, Konstan MW, The Pulmozyme Early Intervention Trial Study Group. A two-year randomized, placebo-controlled trial of dornase alfa in young patients with cystic fibrosis with mild lung function abnormalities. *J Pediatrics* 2001; **139**: 813–20.

23 Ripoll L, Reinert P, Pepin LF, Lagrange PH. Interaction of macrolides with alfa dornase during DNA hydrolysis. *J Antimicrob Chemother* 1996; **37**: 987–91.

24 Stern M, Caplen NJ, Browning JE, Griesenbach U, Sorgi F, Huang L, Gruenert DC, Marriot C, Crystal RG, Geddes DM, Alton EW. The effect of mucolytic agents on gene transfer across a CF sputum barrier *in vitro*. *Gene Ther* 1998; **5**: 91–8.

25 Rubin BK. Who will benefit from DNase? *Pediatric Pulmonol* 1999; **27**: 3–4.

26 Crockett AJ, Cranston JM, Latimer KM, Alpers JH. Mucolytics for bronchiectasis (Cochrane Review). *Cochrane Database Syst Rev* 2001; **1**.

27 Wills PJ, Wodehouse T, Corkery K, Mallon K, Wilson R, Cole PJ. Short-term recombinant human DNase in bronchiectasis. Effect on clinical state and *in vitro* sputum transportability. *Am J Respir Crit Care Med* 1996; **154**: 413–7.

28 Desai M, Weller PH, Spencer DA. Clinical benefit from nebulized human recombinant DNase in Kartagener's syndrome. *Pediatric Pulmonol* 1995; **20**: 307–8.

29 Nasr SZ, Strouse PJ, Soskolne E, Maxvold NJ, Garver KA, Rubin BK, Moler FW. Efficacy of recombinant human DNase I in the hospital management of RSV bronchiolitis. *Chest* 2001; **120**: 203–8.

30 Cotgreave IA, Eklund A, Larsson K, Moldeus PW.

No penetration of orally administered N-acetylcysteine into bronchoalveolar lavage fluid. *Eur J Respir Dis* 1987; **70**: 73–7.

31 Dasgupta B, King M. Reduction in viscoelasticity in cystic fibrosis sputum *in vitro* using combined treatment with nacystelyn and rhDNase. *Pediatr Pulmonol* 1996; **22**: 161–6.

32 Rogers DF. Mucolytic and mucoactive drugs for asthma and COPD. Any place in therapy? *Expert Opin Investig Drugs* 2002; **11**: 15–35.

33 Feng W, Garrett H, Speert DP, King M. Improved clearability of cystic fibrosis sputum with dextran treatment *in vitro*. *Am J Respir Crit Care Med* 1998; **157**: 710–4.

34 Rubin BK. Surface properties of respiratory secretions: relationship to mucus transport. In: Baum G, ed. *Cilia, Mucus and Mucociliary Interactions*. New York: Marcel Dekker, 1998: 317–24.

35 Neumann AW, Good RJ, Hope CJ, Sejpal M. An equation-of-state approach to determine surface tensions of low-energy solids from contact angles. *J Colloid Interfac Sci* 1974; **49**: 291–304.

36 King M, Zahm JM, Pierrot D, Vaquez-Girod S, Puchelle E. The role of mucus gel viscosity, spinnability, and adhesive properties in clearance by simulated cough. *Biorheology* 1989; **26**: 737–45.

37 Albers GM, Tomkiewicz RP, May MK, Ramirez OE, Rubin BK. Ring distraction technique for measuring the surface tension of sputum and relationship of the work of adhesion to clearability. *J Appl Physiol* 1996; **81**: 2690–5.

38 Lema G, Enhorning G. Surface properties after a simulated PLA2 hydrolysis of pulmonary surfactant's main component, DPPC. *Biochim Biophys Acta* 1997; **1345**: 86–92.

39 Anzueto A, Jubran A, Ohar JA, Piquette CA, Rennard SI, Colice G, Pattishall EN, Barret J, Engle M, Perret K, Rubin BK. Effects of aerosolized surfactant in patients with stable chronic bronchitis. A prospective randomized controlled trial. *JAMA* 1997; **278**: 1426–31.

40 Isawa T, Teshima T, Hirano T, Ebina A, Konno K. Effect of oral salbutamol on mucociliary clearance mechanisms in the lungs. *Tohoku J Exp Med* 1986; **150**: 51–61.

41 Rubin BK. Tracheomalacia as a cause of respiratory compromise in infants. *Clin Pulm Med* 1999; **6**: 195–7.

42 Konstan MW, Byard PJ, Hoppel CL, Davis PB. Effect of high-dose ibuprofen in patients with cystic fibrosis. *N Engl J Med* 1995; **332**: 848–54.

43 Tamaoki J, Chiyotani A, Kobayashi K, Sakai N, Kanemura T, Takizawa T. Effect of indomethacin on bronchorrhea in patients with chronic bronchitis, diffuse panbronchiolitis, or bronchiectasis. *Am Rev Respir Dis* 1992; **145**: 548–52.

44 King M, Viires N. Effect of methacholine chloride on rheology and transport of canine tracheal mucus. *J Appl Physiol* 1979; **47**: 26–31.

45 Tamaoki J, Chiyotani A, Tagaya E, Sakai N, Konno K. Effect of long term treatment with oxitropium bromide on airway secretion in chronic bronchitis and diffuse panbronchiolitis. *Thorax* 1994; **49**: 545–8.

46 Zeiger RS, Schatz M, Sperling W, Simon RA, Stevenson DD. Efficacy of troleandomycin in outpatients with severe, corticosteroid-dependent asthma. *J Allerg Clin Immunol* 1980; **66**: 438–46.

47 Szefler SJ, Rose JQ, Ellis EF, Spector SL, Green AW, Jusko WJ. The effect of troleandomycin on methylprednisolone elimination. *J Allerg Clin Immunol* 1980; **66**: 447–51.

48 Jaffé A, Bush A. Anti-inflammatory effects of macrolides in lung disease. *Pediatric Pulmonol* 2001; **31**: 464–73.

49 Kudoh S, Uetake T, Hagiwara K, Hirayama M, Hus LH, Kimura H, Sugiyama Y. Clinical effects of low-dose long-term erythromycin chemotherapy on diffuse panbronchiolitis. *Jap J Thorac Dis* 1987; **25**: 632–42.

50 Jaffe A, Francis J, Rosenthal M, Bush A. Long-term azithromycin may improve lung function in children with cystic fibrosis. *Lancet* 1998; **351**: 420.

51 Çulic O, Erakovic V, Parnham MJ. Anti-inflammatory effects of macrolide antibiotics. *Eur J Pharmacol* 2001; **429**: 209–29.

52 Rubin BK, Tamaoki J. Macrolides as biologic response modifiers. *Curr Opin Invest Drugs* 2000; **1**: 169–72.

53 Jager EG. Double-blind, placebo-controlled clinical evaluation of guaimesal in outpatients. *Clin Ther* 1989; **11**: 341–62.

54 Grandjean EM, Berthet P, Ruffmann R, Leuenberger P. Efficacy of oral long-term N-acetylcysteine in chronic bronchopulmonary disease: a meta-analysis of published double-blind, placebo-controlled clinical trials. *Clin Ther* 2000; **22**: 209–21.

55 Davis PB, Drumm M, Konstan MW. State of the art: cystic fibrosis. *Am J Respir Crit Care Med* 1996; **154**: 1229–56.

56 Panitch HB, Keklikian EN, Motley RA, Wolfson MR, Schidlow DV. Effect of altering smooth muscle tone on maximal expiratory flows in patients with tracheomalacia. *Pediatr Pulmonol* 1990; **9**: 170–6.

57 Rubin BK, van der Schans CP. Determinants of mucociliary and cough clearance and outcome measures for clinical trials. In: Rubin BK, van der Schans CP, eds. *Therapy for Mucus Clearance Disorders*. New York: Marcel Dekker, Inc., 2003 (in press).

58 Regnis JA, Robinson M, Bailey DL, Cook P, Hooper P, Chan HK, Gonda I, Bautovich G, Bye PT. Mucociliary clearance in patients with cystic fibrosis and in

normal subjects. *Am J Respir Crit Care Med* 1994; **150:** 66–71.

59 Piquette C, Clarkson L, Okamoto K, Kim JS, Rubin BK. Respiratory related quality of life: relationship with pulmonary function, functional exercise capacity, and sputum biophysical properties. *J Aerosol Med* 2000; **13:** 263–72.

60 Nixon PA, Orenstein DM, Kelsey SF, Doershuk CF. The prognostic value of exercise testing in patients with cystic fibrosis. *N Engl J Med* 1992; **327:** 1785–8.

# 27 Management of cough

*Kian Fan Chung*

Most aspects of the management of cough have been dealt with in this book in separate chapters. This final chapter presents a resumé of the overall management of the patient presenting with a cough, and more detailed aspects can be obtained by referring to the appropriate chapter. Previous reviews on the management of cough have been published [1–3]. Much of the clinical practice surrounding the management of cough depends on best current practice according to expert opinion, and there is a relative lack of good placebo-controlled studies particularly when it comes to the management of cough.

## Approach to the patient with cough

The major aim of the management of a patient presenting with cough is to identify the cause of the cough, and then to treat the cause. Antitussive therapy that suppresses cough by inhibiting the cough pathway without treating the cause ('symptomatic' antitussives) is needed if the cough is very severe, or if treatment of the cause does not lead to sufficient cough suppression or is not possible or successful.

Cough may be indicative of trivial to very serious airway or lung pathology. The differential diagnosis of cough is extensive and includes infections, inflammatory and neoplastic conditions, and many pulmonary conditions (Table 27.1). The protocol for investigating cough, particularly for a cough that has persisted for more than 1 month, takes into account several factors pertaining to the pathophysiology of cough and the most common causes of cough. Persistent cough may be due to the presence of excessive secretions, or to air-

way damage and infection, or to the establishment of a sensitive cough reflex.

The foremost consideration for the clinician at the first visit is to (i) assess the cause of the cough and (ii) determine the severity. Various indicators in the history and examination of the patient will provide clues to the diagnosis.

A period of 3 weeks has been taken as a cut-off point for an acute cough usually due to an upper respiratory virus infection, although some postviral cough may persist for many weeks or months. The only caveat to this is that sometimes such a cough may last for more than 3 weeks and many patients with an 'idiopathic' cough often state that their cough was a postinfectious cough that never recovered. A cough that has lasted for more than 2–3 months is less likely to be due to an upper respiratory tract infection, and further investigations in terms of other associated causes must be looked for.

The separation of the diagnostic categories into a productive or non-productive cough may be clinically helpful. Cough with sputum production usually points towards conditions such as chronic bronchitis and bronchiectasis or other causes of bronchorrhoea. There is limited information on the diagnostic value of knowing that the cough is productive. One study indicates that similar causes are often found for both productive and dry cough [4]. Against this background, the assessment of the volume of sputum produced is usually inaccurate, and coughing itself leads to sputum production. The concept of a dry vs. a productive cough as delineating a cough secondary to an increased cough reflex for the former, and a cough secondary to excessive mucus production for the latter is not entirely cor-

**Table 27.1** Common causes of cough.

*Acute infections*
Tracheobronchitis
Bronchopneumonia
Viral pneumonia
Acute-on-chronic bronchitis
Pertussis

*Chronic infections*
Bronchiectasis
Tuberculosis
Cystic fibrosis

*Airway disease*
Asthma
Chronic bronchitis
Chronic postnasal drip

*Parenchymal disease*
Chronic interstitial lung fibrosis
Emphysema
Sarcoidosis

*Tumours*
Bronchogenic carcinoma
Alveolar cell carcinoma
Benign airway tumours
Mediastinal tumours

*Foreign body*

*Middle ear pathology*

*Cardiovascular*
Left ventricular failure
Pulmonary infarction
Aortic aneurysm

*Other disease*
Reflux oesophagitis
Recurrent aspiration
Endobronchial sutures

*Drugs*
Angiotensin-converting enzyme inhibitors

**Table 27.2** Potential complications from excessive cough.

*Respiratory*
Pneumothorax
Subcutaneous emphysema
Pneumomediastinum
Pneumoperitoneum
Laryngeal damage

*Cardiovascular*
Cardiac dysrhythmias
Loss of consciousness
Subconjunctival haemorrhage

*Central nervous system*
Syncope
Headaches
Cerebral air embolism

*Musculoskeletal*
Intercostal muscle pain
Rupture of rectus abdominis muscle
Increase in serum creatine phosphokinase
Cervical disc prolapse

*Gastrointestinal*
Oesophageal perforation

*Other*
Social embarrassment
Depression
Urinary incontinence
Disruption of surgical wounds
Petechiae
Purpura

they expect that the irritant effect of cigarette smoke is causing their cough. A change in the pattern of their cough such as an increase in intensity (usually after an upper respiratory tract infection), or accompanying haemoptysis may force a smoker to seek medical attention. A chest radiograph is mandatory in this situation.

## Measuring cough severity

Assessment of cough severity traditionally rests on asking the patient for his or her perception of the symptom. In very severe cough, complications arising from cough may be experienced (Table 27.2), and the presence of these indicate that the intensity of the cough is severe.

rect. An increased cough reflex may be present in both productive and non-productive cough. However, there are features that are associated with an increased cough reflex such as cough triggered by taking a deep breath, laughing, inhalation of cold air and prolonged talking.

Many cigarette smokers have a chronic cough, but rarely seek medical advice regarding their cough as

Measurement of the cough reflex can be done by counting the cough responses to inhalation of tussive agents such as capsaicin, the hot extract of peppers, acid or low-chloride content solutions. Although cough can be induced directly by airway secretions and irritants, persistent cough may also result from an increase in the sensitivity of the cough receptor. Most patients with a non-productive persistent cough due to a range of causes have an enhanced cough reflex to capsaicin when compared to healthy non-coughing subjects [5]. Successful treatment of the primary condition underlying the chronic cough often leads to a normalization of the cough reflex. The degree of the cough responsiveness to inhaled capsaicin may be a reflection of the severity of the cough, but this has not been examined yet. Of relevance to the evaluation and treatment strategies for persistent dry cough is the fact that the cough response can be augmented by various mediators of inflammation such as the prostaglandins $PGE_2$ and $PGF_{2\alpha}$ and bradykinin through a process of sensitization [6,7].

Direct measurement of the number of coughs as a measure of severity has not been extensively assessed. A significant correlation between daytime cough numbers and daytime cough symptom scores has been shown for a group of chronic dry coughers [8]. In patients with cough both of unknown cause and associated with asthma, the number of coughs counted were highest during the daytime, and very few coughs were observed at night during sleep. Both ambulatory monitoring of cough and measurement of the cough reflex are not routinely used in the clinical setting. A quality of life questionnaire specific for the evaluation of the impact of chronic cough has been devised but the sensitivity of the instrument is not known [9].

## Causes of acute and chronic cough

There is a very wide range of respiratory and non-respiratory causes of cough (Table 27.1). A useful clinical classification is to consider whether the cough is acute or chronic.

### Acute cough

Acute cough is usually due to a viral or bacterial upper respiratory tract infection. The cough of the common cold is usually self-limiting and accompanies the cold in the majority of sufferers within the first 48 h [10]. Other symptoms of postnasal drip, throat-clearing, irritation of the throat, sore throat, nasal obstruction and nasal discharge also accompany the cough which usually resolves within 2 weeks, although it can be sometimes prolonged. Pertussis should be considered in the differential diagnosis, particularly with a whooping characteristic of the cough and often associated with vomiting. Other causes of acute cough that should be considered are pneumonia, congestive cardiac failure, exacerbation of chronic obstructive pulmonary disease (COPD), aspiration or pulmonary embolism. These conditions are usually accompanied by other symptoms such as shortness of breath and fever, but cough may be the predominant or rarely the only symptom.

Many patients with the common cold usually self-medicate with various antitussive over-the-counter preparations if they have a problem with their cough. However, there are few effective preparations on the market. Codeine appears to be ineffective compared with placebo against the acute cough of the common cold [11], while dextromethorphan has been shown to have some effect in a meta-analysis [12], but not in two smaller studies [13,14]. A first-generation antihistamine and decongestant has been proposed for the treatment of cough associated with a postnasal drip in acute cough [10], but a study using a newer-generation antihistamine, loratidine, in combination with a decongestant showed no effect [15]. Sometimes, the rhinitis associated with the common cold may become mucopurulent, but this is not an indication for antibiotic therapy unless this persists for more than 10–14 days.

### Chronic cough

Chronic cough (cough that persists for more than 3 weeks) can be caused by many diseases, but it is most commonly due to asthma, gastro-oesophageal reflux (GOR), postnasal drip, chronic bronchitis and bronchiectasis [16–18].

#### Postnasal drip (rhinosinusitis)

The strong association between postnasal drip (rhinosinusitis) and chronic persistent cough is based on epidemiological evidence, and on a prospective study in adults. In acute cough of the common cold, postnasal drip is likely to play an important role [10]. In some studies, postnasal drip has been shown to be the most common cause of a chronic cough [16,19]. Post-nasal drip ('nasal catarrh') is characterized by a sensation of nasal secretions or of a 'drip' at the back of the throat, accompanied very often by frequent need to clear the throat ('throat-clearing'). There may be a nasal quality to the voice due to concomitant nasal blockage and congestion, and there may be hoarseness. Physical examination of the pharynx is often unremarkable, although infrequently a 'cobblestoning' appearance of the mucosa and draining secretions are observed, but these appearances are non-specific. The diagnosis of rhinosinusitis is made usually on a combination of symptoms, physical examination, radiographic findings, and response to specific therapy. Computed tomography of the sinuses may reveal mucosal thickening or sinus opacification and air–fluid levels, and is the best investigation compared to sinus radiography. Extrathoracic variable upper airway obstruction has been described, presumably arising from upper airway inflammation but this is not invariably present [20]. Testing for allergens may be helpful and presence of allergy to pollens support the presence of seasonal allergic rhinitis. The presence of house dust mite allergy may be of value if perennial allergic rhinitis is being considered.

Topical administration of corticosteroid drops in the head-down position is the best treatment, sometimes with the concomitant use of antihistamines. Topical steroids offer the minimum local effect with the minimum of side-effects. Occasionally, severe symptoms may be controlled initially by a short course of oral steroids, followed by topical therapy. Betamethasone drops have the best penetrance into the nose and have to be administered in the head-back or dependent position, and are particularly useful in gaining control of symptoms in the initial phase. It is better to avoid long-term use of betamethasone, and to follow 1–2 months of treatment with betamethasone by other topical nasal sprays currently available such as beclometasone dipropionate, fluticasone, flunisolide, mometasone or budesonide.

Older-generation antihistamines, probably due to concomitant anticholinergic effects, may be preferable to newer-generation antihistamines in treating acute cough due to upper respiratory tract viral infections. This beneficial effect has been shown in one study [10]. However, the beneficial effects of older antihistamines in chronic cough has not been demonstrated, and the newer antihistamines combined with a topical anti-cholinergic spray to the nose (such as ipratropium bromide) to dry excessive nasal secretions may provide benefit.

Topical decongestant vasoconstrictor sprays may be useful adjunct therapy for a few days, but rebound nasal obstruction may occur after prolonged use. Antibiotic therapy is advisable and necessary in the presence of acute sinusitis involving bacterial infection with the presence of mucopurulent secretions that has persisted for at least 10 days.

### Asthma and associated eosinophilic conditions

Chronic cough may occur in asthma under different clinical settings. Asthma may present predominantly with cough, often nocturnal, and the diagnosis is supported by the presence of reversible airflow limitation and bronchial hyperresponsiveness [21]. This condition of 'cough-variant' asthma is a common type of asthma in children. Elderly asthmatics may also give a history of chronic cough prior to a diagnosis of asthma made on the basis of episodic wheeze. Some studies have reported that cough has been the only symptom of asthma from 6.5 to 57% of the time. Cough is often the most prominent symptom complained of by patients with chronic asthma [22]. More recently, a condition of eosinophilic bronchitis characterized by cough without asthma symptoms or bronchial hyperresponsiveness but with eosinophilia in sputum has been described [23]. Cough may also occur as a first sign of worsening of asthma, usually presenting first at night, associated with other symptoms such as wheeze and shortness of breath with falls in early morning peak flows. Some patients with asthma on the other hand develop a persistent dry cough despite good control of their asthma with antiasthma therapy.

Patients with asthma do not usually have an enhanced cough reflex, although a subgroup with a persistent cough may do so [24]. In these latter patients, cough receptors may be sensitized by inflammatory mediators such as bradykinin, tachykinins and prostaglandins. Another cause of cough in asthma may be due to the presence of bronchial smooth muscle constriction, which may activate cough receptors through physical deformation. Indeed, in some patients with cough-variant asthma, β-adrenergic bronchodilators are effective antitussives [25]. Induction of sputum by inhalation of hypertonic saline often reveals a predominance of eosinophils, and bronchial hyperresponsiveness is invariably present. Interestingly, in eosinophilic bronchitis, cough responsiveness to capsaicin is increased without bronchial hyperresponsiveness [26]. When asthma is suspected as being a cause of cough, the following investigations should be considered: baseline spirometry, recording of peak flow measurements morning and evening, airway responsiveness to methacholine or histamine, and bronchodilator response to salbutamol. Measurement of capsaicin cough response and of eosinophil counts in induced sputum are investigations that should now be considered to diagnose eosinophilic bronchitis. Indeed, these conditions would come under the umbrella of airway eosinophilic conditions causing cough, which invariably responds well to inhaled corticosteroid therapy.

Cough associated with asthma should be treated with antiasthma medication including inhaled corticosteroid therapy and bronchodilators such as $\beta_2$-adrenergic agonists. It is well to remember that the particles from the inhaler may in some patients induce cough, and in such a situation, the side-effect may disappear by changing to an alternative form of delivery. Usually, such treatment may need to be given over a prolonged period of time (3–6 months) at a minimum dose that controls the cough. Often, a trial of oral corticosteroids (e.g. prednisolone 40 mg/day for 2 weeks) may be recommended, particularly in those asthmatics who have had a cough despite being on adequate antiasthma medication. More recently, the use of a combination of inhaled corticosteroids and a long-acting $\beta$-agonist has become established as being the best available maintenance treatment for moderate to severe asthma, but the effect of this combination on cough alone has not been studied. However, it is likely that such combination has additive benefits on cough suppression, as it does on other measures of asthma control. Treatment with nedocromil sodium can be a useful addition. Leukotriene receptor antagonists may control cough-variant asthma in patients in whom inhaled steroids have not been helpful.

*Gastro-oesophageal reflux*
GOR, the movement of acid and other components of gastric contents from the oesophagus into the larynx and trachea, is one of the most common associated cause of chronic cough in all age groups. GOR may lead to symptoms or physical complications such as heartburn, chest pain, a sour taste or regurgitation, and also a chronic persistent cough. Not infrequently, there may be no symptoms associated with GOR or

impaired clearance of oesophageal acid. Prolonged exposure of the lower oesophagus to acid may lead to oesophagitis, Barrett's oesophagus, oesophageal ulceration and stricture and bleeding. An oesophageal–tracheobronchial cough reflex mechanism has been proposed on the basis of studies in which distal oesophageal acid perfusion induced coughing episodes in such patients [27]. Local distal oesophageal perfusion of lidocaine suppressed the acid-induced cough in patients with chronic cough, and the inhaled anticholinergic agent, ipratropium bromide, was also effective. Over 90% of the cough episodes have been shown to be temporally related to reflux episodes. Significant reflux occurs in both supine and upright positions. A high proportion of patients with GOR also appear to have gastrohypopharyngeal reflux, and there may be a direct effect of acid reflux on cough receptors in the larynx and trachea. Coughing itself may precipitate reflux, creating a vicious circle of acid-inducing cough which in turn induces acid reflux. Continuous monitoring of tracheal and oesophageal pH in patients with symptomatic GOR has demonstrated significant increases in tracheal acidity with pHs falling down to 4 during episodes of reflux [28]. Other components of the refluxate, apart from acid, such as the content of pepsin or other enzymes may also contribute to stimulating cough, but this is not known.

There is no particular pattern of the cough of GOR, although one small study indicated that the cough occurred predominantly during the day and in the upright posture, with minimal nocturnal symptoms. The cough may have been longstanding, and may or may not be productive. In the presence of reflux and microaspiration, laryngeal symptoms may be present with dysphonia, hoarseness and sore throat; often posterior vocal cord laryngeal inflammation is visible. There may be associated oesophageal dysmotility characterized by heartburn, waterbrash and oral regurgitation, worse in the supine position.

The most specific test to diagnose GOR is a 24-h ambulatory oesophageal pH monitoring. Episodes of pH below 4 in the oesophagus are usually looked for and the temporal relationship between cough and falls in pH msut be looked for. However, there is a low frequency of acid reflux episodes associated in time with cough, with up to 13% of coughs occurring shortly after an acid reflux episode [29]. Twenty-four-hour pH testing does not predict which patients with atypical symptoms have GOR disease-related complaints.

Other tests that may be used are oesophageal manometry to measure dysmotility particularly associated with reflux episodes, upper gastrointestinal contrast series to detect reflux of barium into the oesophagus, or endoscopy. A trial of antireflux treatment may be used in patients as a diagnostic measure where ambulatory 24-h pH oesophageal monitoring is not available. This is also indicated in patients with chronic cough that remains unexplained after diagnostic work-up or exclusion of other associated causes.

The aim of treatment of GOR is to decrease the frequency and duration of the events. Conservative measures should be advocated for all patients with significant GOR events diagnosed on a 24-h pH monitoring of the oesophagus. Weight reduction, high-protein, low-fat diet, elimination of food and drinks of low pH, elevation of the head of the bed, avoidance of coffee and smoking should be advised. Reduction of acid production by stomach can be achieved with either $H_2$-histamine blockers or proton pump inhibitors, but there has been no comparative studies between the two classes of acid inhibitors. Given the increasing use of proton pump inhibitors and their superior effect in acid suppression and in treating GOR, these drugs will remain more popular. In a placebo-controlled study, of 17 patients with a positive pH test, six had improvement or resolution of cough with omeprazole treatment for 12 weeks, within the first 2 weeks of treatment [30]. In another double-blind, placebo-controlled trial, omeprazole 40 mg/day for 8 weeks relieved GOR-related cough, and this improvement continued after the treatment period [31]. A duration of 3 months' treatment at the highest recommended dose of proton pump inhibitor is recommended. One of the reasons for medical failure of therapy is the effect of persistent non-acid refluxate. Antireflux surgery such as open or laparoscopic fundoplication may be considered for patients with proven GOR disease who have failed to respond to medical therapy [32].

### Chronic bronchitis/chronic obstructive pulmonary disease (COPD)
Given that up to 30–40% of the community smokes, it may be surprising that chronic bronchitis is only reported in 5% of patients seeking medical attention for cough. Chronic bronchitis should be considered in a patient who produces sputum on most days over at least 3 consecutive months, particularly during the winter months, over at least 2 consecutive years. In a

smoker, the presence of chronic bronchitis may be predictive of progressive irreversible airflow obstruction, but there is no evidence for this [33]. The cough of chronic bronchitis may result from excessive sputum production associated with mucus cell hyperplasia and bronchiolar inflammation. The presence of airflow obstruction diagnosed on the basis of a ratio of $FEV_1$/FVC of less than 70% or of an $FEV_1$ of less than 70% of the predicted value would indicate the diagnosis of COPD [34].

The productive cough in chronic bronchitis is exacerbated by upper respiratory infections with common viruses, or by exposure to irritating dusts. Other causes of productive cough should be excluded such as bronchiectasis or postnasal drip. It is important to exclude also the presence of an endobronchial tumour. Cessation of cigarette smoking is usually successful in reducing the cough, occurring most often within 4–5 weeks of smoking cessation [35]. Various adjuncts such as nicotine replacement or buprorion tablets may help smoking cessation [36]. Treatment of any associated chronic airflow obstruction with short-acting and/or long-acting $\beta_2$-adrenergic agonists and anticholinergic agents may be tried. Suppression of the inflammatory process in the small airways may be tried with inhaled corticosteroids, but the inflammation may not be responsive to steroids. However, corticosteroids are more effective in the treatment of exacerbations of COPD. Use of indirect antitussive therapies is not recommended in the treatment of COPD and the role of mucolytic therapy at present is not clear.

### Bronchiectasis
The cough of bronchiectasis is associated with excessive secretions from overproduction together with reduced clearance of airway secretions. Usually, the patient produces 30 mL or more of mucoid or mucopurulent sputum per day, sometimes accompanied by fever, haemoptysis and weight loss. In early cases of bronchiectasis, the condition may only present with a persistent productive cough. Bronchiectasis may be associated with postnasal drip and rhinosinusitis, asthma, GOR disease and chronic bronchitis. Common pathogens cultured from sputum include *Haemophilus influenzae*, *Staphyloccocus aureus* and *Pseudomonas aeruginosa*. The chest radiograph may show increased bronchial wall thickening particularly in the lower lobes in advanced cases, but thin-section computed axial tomography of the chest can reveal

early changes of intrapulmonary airway wall thickening, dilatation and distortion, with mucus plugging and evidence of bronchiolitis [37].

The cough of bronchiectasis serves as a useful function in facilitating clearance of excessive mucus. In fact, it is the most effective mechanism for clearing airway secretions. The cough during infective exacerbations of bronchiectasis may become a tiring symptom, but treatment of the exacerbation will lead to a curbing of cough. The cough due to bronchiectasis may be successfully controlled with inhaled $\beta_2$-agonist which improves mucociliary clearance and reverses any associated bronchoconstriction, postural drainage of airway secretions, and the use of intermittent antibiotic therapy.

### Angiotensin-converting enzyme inhibitor cough

Angiotensin-converting enzyme (ACE) inhibitors are often prescribed for the treatment of hypertension and heart failure, and cough has been observed in 2–33% of patients [38,39]. The cough is typically described as dry, associated with a tickly irritating sensation in the throat. It may appear within a few hours of taking the drug, but may also only become apparent after weeks or even months. The cough disappears within days or weeks following withdrawal of drug. Patients with ACE inhibitor cough demonstrate an enhanced response to capsaicin inhalation challenge. The mechanisms underlying ACE inhibitor cough are not clear but accumulation of bradykinin and prostaglandins which sensitize cough receptors directly has been implicated. The best treatment for ACE inhibitor cough is to discontinue the treatment and to replace it with alternative therapies such as an angiotensin II receptor antagonist which does not cause cough. However, sulindac, indomethacin, nifedipine, picotamide or inhaled sodium cromoglycate can be beneficial in ACE inhibitor-induced cough [40–43].

### Postinfectious cough

Postinfectious cough has been reported in 11–25% of patients with chronic cough [44,45]. A persistent cough occurs in 25–50% of patients following *Mycoplasma* or *Bordetella pertussis* infection [46]. *B. pertussis* infection has now been increasingly recognized as a cause of both acute and chronic cough [47,48]. In children, respiratory viruses (respiratory syncytial virus and parainfluenzae), *Mycoplasma*, *Chlamydia* and *B. pertussis* have been implicated [49].

The cough of *B. pertussis* usually lasts for only 4–6 weeks and is spasmodic with a typical whoop, but can last for a longer period of time. In most patients with a postinfectious cough, the initial trigger is usually an upper respiratory tract infection, and cough that is expected to have lasted for only a week at most persists for many months, often severe. Such patients are often referred to the cough clinic and are usually investigated for the more common associated causes of cough. It is assumed that there may have been persistent damage to the cough receptor, or persistent airway inflammation induced initially by the virus. Bronchial epithelial inflammation and damage is present in children with chronic cough following lower respiratory tract illness. Irritants may penetrate more readily through the damaged epithelium. This may represent a vicious circle of events of coughing-induced damage that maintains and triggers further cough. Inhaled corticosteroids are often prescribed, but with variable success. There has been no controlled trial. Oral steroids may be successful [44]. Inhaled ipratropium bromide has been shown to be effective in a small study [50].

### Other conditions

Other conditions causing cough include bronchogenic carcinoma, metastatic carcinoma, sarcoidosis, chronic aspiration, interstitial lung disease or left ventricular failure, conditions that can be excluded by performing a chest radiograph. Psychogenic or habit cough is not uncommon, particularly in children, and is usually a diagnosis arrived at after exclusion of other causes. Habit cough is a throat-clearing noise made by a person who is nervous and self-conscious. Cough may be associated with a depressive illness and long-standing cough may cause depression. In the paediatric population, other cough aetiologies specific for this age group need to be considered such as congenital abnormalities, e.g. vascular rings, tracheobronchomalacia, pulmonary sequestration or mediastinal tumours, foreign bodies in the airway or oesophagus, aspiration due to poor coordination of swallowing or oesophageal dysmotility, and heart disease.

## Chronic persistent cough of unknown cause

Identification of a potential cause of cough has been reported in 78–99% of patients presenting at a specialized cough clinic [16,51]. Treatment of identifiable causes may also not be successful; in one study, 31% of patients did not improve with treatment of the associated cause. These patients with a persistent cough of unknown cause or not responding to treatment of associated causes present in a similar way as others in terms of their cough symptoms where a cause has been identified. An enhanced cough reflex is usually found, and this usually improves when the associated cause has been successfully treated. Patients often complain of a persistent tickling sensation in the throat that often leads to paroxysms of coughing. This sensation can be triggered by factors such as changes in ambient temperature, taking a deep breath, cigarette smoke or other irritants such as aerosol sprays or perfumes. These symptoms are typical of a sensitized cough reflex. Mucosal biopsies taken from a group of non-asthmatic patients with chronic dry cough showed evidence of epithelial desquamation and inflammatory cells, particularly mononuclear cells [52]. These changes could represent the sequelae of chronic trauma to the airway wall following intractable cough, and could also lead to sensitization of the cough reflex. It is likely that many patients with postinfectious cough end up being classified as having cough of unknown cause. Because relatively few effective and safe antitussives are available, the control of persistent cough without associated cause remains difficult. Indirect antitussive therapy should be tried and may be reserved for severe paroxysms of the cough.

## Diagnosis and investigations of chronic cough

The history and examination will often indicate likely associated diagnosis or diagnoses, and the timing of various investigations may vary according to presentation. Table 27.3 shows the range of possible investigations. Initial investigation may be limited to a chest radiograph, particularly if there is a high suspicion of a tumour in a cigarette smoker. There is no indication as to how good the yield of a diagnosis of a bronchial tumour is by routinely performing a chest radiograph in all patient presenting with a cough that has been persistent for more than a few weeks. Abnormalities have been reported in 10–30% of chest radiographs, although the yield of tumours is likely to be lower. If there is high degree of suspicion of a lung tumour, further in-

**Table 27.3** Investigations of chronic cough.

1 Chest radiograph.
2 Spirometry and peak expiratory flow measurements over several days.
3 Bronchoprovocation testing with methacholine or histamine.
4 Rhinosinus imaging (radiography or computed tomography).
5 Direct examination of nasal passages and upper airways.
6 24-h oesophageal pH monitoring and oesophageal manometry.
7 Computed tomography of the lungs.
8 Fibreoptic bronchoscopy and mucosal biopsies.
9 Induced sputum for examination of eosinophils.

vestigations (e.g. computed tomography or fibreoptic bronchoscopy) must be pursued despite a 'normal' chest radiograph.

A period of observation of 3–4 weeks in a patient who provides a good history of an upper respiratory tract infection prior to further investigation or therapeutic trial is adequate, although institution of an anti-inflammatory therapy such as inhaled corticosteroids can be useful in controlling this type of cough.

Postnasal drip ('nasal catarrh'), asthma and GOR are the three most common conditions associated with a chronic dry cough. It would be sensible in the diagnostic approach to exclude these conditions first. Examination of the nose and sinuses with a computed axial tomograph of the sinuses may be indicated with a history of postnasal drip or rhinosinusitis, and ambulatory oesophageal pH monitoring to exclude the possibility of GOR. The diagnosis of asthma is supported by the presence of diurnal variation in peak flow measurements, bronchial hyperresponsiveness to histamine or methacholine challenge and the presence of eosinophils in sputum. Under the umbrella of 'asthma' would also be included cough-variant asthma and eosinophilic bronchitis. However, a therapeutic trial may be the best initial approach, particularly when the history and examination provide supportive clues. It is important that effective doses of medication over a sufficient period of time is given. Often a longer than usual period of treatment is necessary to control the cough. Postnasal drip is a frequently overlooked condition, and aggressive treatment should consist of corticosteroid nasal drops with an antihistamine, with the possibility of adding antibiotic therapy and a short period of treatment with a nasal decongestant. Often more than one of these conditions may coexist and cough may only respond with concomitant treatment of these. For example, inhaled steroid therapy and acid suppression with $H_2$-histamine blockers or a proton pump inhibitor would be indicated for the coexistence of asthma and GOR. There continues to be some debate as to whether investigations are necessary, or whether one should proceed to a therapeutic trial once a diagnosis of the associated cause has been made from the history and examination.

Bearing in mind that there are a myriad of other less common causes of a chronic cough, investigations must proceed further if the above causes have been excluded. Full lung function tests to include lung volumes and gas transfer factor, and a computed axial tomograph of the lungs should be considered in case of bronchiolar or parenchymal disease or unsuspected bronchiectasis. Fibreoptic bronchoscopy should be considered, and

apart from excluding small central tumours provides mucosal biopsies for histological examination. A simple algorithm for investigating patients with chronic cough is presented in Table 27.4.

## Therapies aimed towards cough suppression ('symptomatic' therapies)

An outline of the treatment approach for specific underlying causes of cough is presented in Table 27.5. When the treatment of the cause of cough is not effective or not available, therapies directed at eliminating the symptom of cough irrespective of the cause of the cough should be tried. These therapies are also termed symptomatic. Drugs that affect the complex mechanism of the cough reflex may act in several ways (Fig. 27.1). They may act by inhibition of central mechanisms within the cough centre, or by reducing the response of cough receptors in the airways. Opiates,

**Table 27.4** Diagnostic evaluation of chronic cough.

1 History and physical examination.

2 Chest radiograph, particularly in smokers.

3 Initial evaluation may lead to diagnosis of chronic bronchitis in cigarette smokers, and of angiotensin-converting enzyme inhibitor cough. Discontinue cigarette smoking and offending drug.

4 Further diagnostic evaluation on basis of initial evaluation:
 (i) If suggestive of postnasal drip, order a computed tomographic scan of sinuses, and allergy tests.
 (ii) If suggestive of asthma, request a record of peak expiratory flow measurements at home for 2 weeks and a bronchoprovocation test with histamine or methacholine, and/or a trial of antiasthma treatment.
 (iii) If suggestive of gastro-oesophageal reflux disease, request 24-h pH monitoring, and if necessary, an endoscopic examination of the oesophagus, or a barium swallow series.
 (iv) If the chest radiograph is abnormal, consider examination of sputum and a fibreoptic bronchoscopy. A computed tomographic scan of the thorax and further lung function evaluation may be necessary.

5 Treat specifically for associated conditions. The cause(s) of cough is (are) determined when specific therapies eliminate or improve the cough. There may be more than one associated cause for the cough.

**Table 27.5** Treatments for cough.

| | |
|---|---|
| **1** *Treating the specific underlying cause(s)* | |
| Asthma, cough-variant asthma | Bronchodilators and inhaled corticosteroids |
| Eosinophilic bronchitis | Inhaled corticosteroids; leukotriene inhibitors |
| Allergic rhinitis and postnasal drip | Topical nasal steroids and antihistamines |
| | Topical nasal anticholinergics (with antibiotics, if indicated) |
| Gastro-oesophageal reflux | Conservative measures |
| | Histamine $H_2$-antagonist or proton pump inhibitor |
| Angiotensin-converting enzyme inhibitor | Discontinue and replace with alternative drug such as angiotensin II receptor antagonist |
| Chronic bronchitis/chronic obstructive pulmonary disease (COPD) | Smoking cessation |
| | Treat for COPD |
| Bronchiectasis | Postural drainage. Treat infective exacerbation and airflow obstruction |
| Infective tracheobronchitis | Appropriate antibiotic therapy |
| | Treat any postnasal drip |
| **2** *Symptomatic treatment (only after consideration of cause of cough)* | |
| Acute cough likely to be transient, e.g. upper respiratory viral infection | Simple linctus |
| Persistent cough, particularly nocturnal | Opiates (codeine or pholcodeine) |
| Persistent intractable cough due to terminal incurable disease | Opiates (morphine or diamorphine) |
| | Local anaesthetic aerosol |
| Cough in children | Simple linctus (paediatric) |

demulcents, expectorants, local anaesthetics and antiasthma drugs have been used as antitussive agents with varying degrees of success. More effective antitussive therapies are urgently needed [53].

The use of 'indirect' antitussive agents is particularly relevant for patients with lung cancer. Persistent cough is experienced in up to 79% of patients with a non-small cell carcinoma, of whom 50% rated their cough as moderate to severe [54]. Lung cancer itself, or its complications and treatment may be the cause of the cough, and persistent cough can cause headaches, insomnia, rib fractures and syncope [55].

### Narcotic and non-narcotic antitussives

Opiates including morphine, diamorphine and codeine are the most effective antitussive agents. At their effective doses they cause physical dependence, respiratory depression and gastrointestinal colic. Morphine and diamorphine are reserved for the control of cough and pain of terminal bronchial cancer patients, but codeine, dihydrocodeine and pholcodeine can be tried in other cases of chronic cough.

Codeine is the methylether of morphine and has long been the standard centrally acting antitussive drug against which the pharmacological and clinical effects of newer drugs have been measured. Codeine is probably the most commonly prescribed antitussive. It has good analgesic and antitussive activity when given orally. Codeine has been shown to possess antitussive activity against pathological cough [56,57] and against induced cough in normal volunteers [58]. On the other hand, it appears to be ineffective against acute cough of the common cold [11].

It should be used cautiously in patients with reduced hepatic function, but it can be used without dose modi-

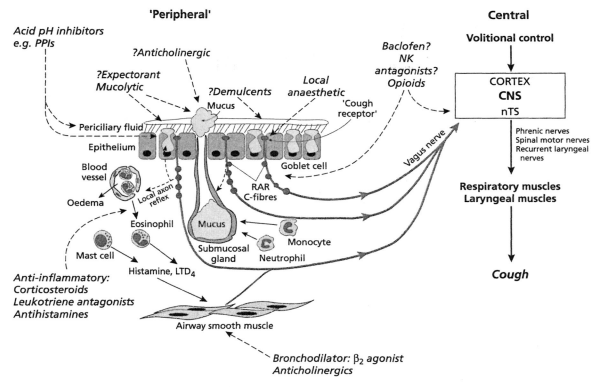

**'Peripheral'**

**Central**

*Acid pH inhibitors
e.g. PPIs*

**Volitional control**

*?Anticholinergic*

*Baclofen?
NK
antagonists?
Opioids*

*?Expectorant
Mucolytic*

*Local
anaesthetic*

CORTEX
**CNS**
nTS

Mucus

*?Demulcents*

'Cough
receptor'

Periciliary fluid

Phrenic nerves
Spinal motor nerves
Recurrent laryngeal
nerves

Epithelium

Goblet cell

Blood
vessel

Local axon
reflex

RAR
C-fibres

Vagus nerve

**Respiratory muscles
Laryngeal muscles**

Oedema

Eosinophil

Mucus

Mast cell

Submucosal
gland

Monocyte

Neutrophil

**Cough**

Histamine, LTD₄

*Anti-inflammatory:
Corticosteroids
Leukotriene antagonists
Antihistamines*

Airway smooth muscle

*Bronchodilator: β₂ agonist
Anticholinergics*

**Fig. 27.1** Afferent pathways of the cough reflex and some potential sites of action of direct and indirect antitussive drugs. Drugs may be divided according to their peripheral effects on airways or their central effects on the central nervous system (CNS). nTS, nucleus tractus solitarius; $LTD_4$, leukotriene $D_4$; NK, neurokinin; RAR, rapidly adapting receptor; PPI, proton pump inhibitor.

fication in patients with renal failure. Drowsiness may be an incapacitating side-effect, together with nausea, vomiting and constipation. Rarely allergic cutaneous reactions such as erythema multiforme have been described. Codeine can cause physical dependence, but on a smaller scale than morphine. Dihydrocodeine has no particular advantage over codeine and may cause more addiction than codeine. Pholcodeine is also as effective as codeine but has little or no analgesic effect. There seems little to choose between codeine and pholcodeine.

Morphine and diamorphine should only be used for severe distressing cough which cannot be relieved by other less potent antitussives, and are therefore usually confined to patients with terminal illness such as bronchial carcinoma. These opioids also relieve anxiety and pain. They cause sedation, respiratory depression and constipation. Opioids can exacerbate wheezing through the release of histamine, but this is rare. Diamorphine may be preferred to morphine because of its lower incidence of nausea and vomiting. Morphine may be given by mouth every 4 h, and also by suppository. Diamorphine is preferably given by injection.

Non-narcotic antitussives include dextromethorphan which is a synthetic derivative of morphine with no analgesic or sedative properties and which is usually included as a constituent of many compound cough preparations sold over the counter. Dextromethorphan is a synthetic derivative of morphine with no analgesic or sedative properties. It is as effective as codeine in suppressing acute and chronic cough when given orally [57,59], with one study showing its superiority over codeine [60]. Antitussive efficacy of a single 30-mg dose has been demonstrated against cough associated with upper respiratory tract infections [12]. It is commonly used as a constituent of many compound cough preparations which are sold over the counter. Side-effects are few with the usual dose, but at higher doses dizziness, nausea and vomiting, and headaches may occur. It should be avoided in patients with hepatic insufficiency as it undergoes metabolic degradation in the liver. Dextromethorphan should be used with caution also in patients on monoamine oxidase inhibitors as cases of central nervous depression and death have occurred.

Other non-narcotic preparations include noscapine and levopropoxyphene, although their antitussive efficacy has not been proven. Levodropropizine, a non-opioid antitussive with peripheral inhibition of sensory cough receptors, has a favourable benefit–risk profile compared to dextromethorphan [61]; this is currently available in several European countries. Other drugs acting on cough receptors include benzonatate which inhibits vagal stretch lung receptors, with a possible central effect. Baclofen, an agonist of γ-aminobutyric acid, an inhibitory neurotransmitter, had demonstrable inhibitory effects in two patients with chronic cough [62], and against ACE inhibitor cough [63].

## Expectorants and mucolytics

The basis for using these agents as antitussives lies in the belief that altering the volume of secretions or their composition will lead to suppression of the cough reflex. Despite the lack of proof, mucolytic agents such as acetylcysteine, carbocisteine, bromhexine and methylcysteine are often used to facilitate expectoration by reducing sputum viscosity in patients with chronic bronchitis. A small reduction in the exacerbation of bronchitis has ben reported with oral acetylcysteine, accompanied by small improvement in cough, a decrease in volume of sputum and some ease of expectoration. Aromatic agents such as eucalyptus and menthol have decongestant effects in the nose and can be useful in short-term relief of cough. Menthol inhibits capsaicin-induced cough in normal volunteers [64], and acts on a cold-sensitive receptor. Demulcents also form an important component of many proprietary cough preparations and may be useful because the thick sugary preparation may act as a protective layer on the mucosal surface.

## Local anaesthetics

Lidocaine aerosol inhaled from a nebulizer has been administered in cases of intractable cough with variable results, and should be reserved for such individual cases [65]. Local anaesthetics work by inhibiting sensory neural activity, but also remove reflexes that protect the lung from noxious substances. Their effects are transient and they should be avoided in patients with asthma or a past history of asthma because they can induce severe bronchoconstriction. There has been no controlled trials of local anaesthetics, but their efficacy in controlling cough is not ideal because of the short duration of effect of these agents. In the author's experience, this treatment is not very effective. It may be that we have not understood the best way of targeting the larynx and large airways with this agent.

## Antiasthma therapy

Often antiasthma therapy ($\beta_2$-agonist and anticholinergic therapy or corticosteroid therapy) may be tried, even in the absence of symptoms or tests supporting asthma. Cough may be accompanied by bronchoconstriction, which in turn could worsen cough, an effect that could be prevented by an inhaled $\beta_2$-agonist. In addition, airway inflammation may be present in the airways as a contributory factor, and could be controlled by an inhaled corticosteroid. However, apart from eosinophilic airway inflammation, it may not respond to corticosteroids. Such treatment should be instituted as a trial after diagnostic evaluation has excluded most causes associated with the cough.

## References

1 Chung KF, Lalloo UG. Diagnosis and management of chronic persistent dry cough. *Postgrad Med J* 1996; **72**: 594–8.
2 Irwin RS, Madison JM. The diagnosis and treatment of cough. *N Engl J Med* 2000; **343**: 1715–21.
3 Irwin RS, Boulet LP, Cloutier MM, Fuller R, Gold PM, Hoffstein V et al. Managing cough as a defense mechanism and as a symptom. A consensus panel report of the American College of Chest Physicians. *Chest* 1998; **114**: 133S–81S.
4 Smyrnios NA, Irwin RS, Curley FJ. Chronic cough with a history of excessive sputum production. The spectrum and frequency of causes, key components of the diagnostic evaluation, and outcome of specific therapy. *Chest* 1995; **108**: 991–7.
5 Choudry NB, Fuller RW. Sensitivity of the cough reflex in

patients with chronic cough. *Eur Respir J* 1992; **5**: 296–300.

6 Nichol GM, Nix A, Barnes PJ, Chung KF. Prostaglandin F2 alpha enhancement of capsaicin-induced cough in man: modulation by beta-adrenergic agonist and anticholinergic agent. *Thorax* 1990; **45**: 694–8.

7 Myers AC, Kajekar R, Undem BJ. Allergic inflammation-induced neuropeptide production in rapidly adapting afferent nerves in guinea pig airways. *Am J Physiol Lung Cell Mol Physiol* 2002; **282**: L775–L781.

8 Hsu J-Y, Stone RA, Logan-Sinclair R, Worsdell M, Busst C, Chung KF. Coughing frequency in patients with persistent cough using a 24-hour ambulatory recorder. *Eur Respir J* 1994; **7**: 1246–53.

9 French CL, Irwin RS, Curley FJ, Krikorian CJ. Impact of chronic cough on quality of life. *Arch Intern Med* 1998; **158**: 1657–61.

10 Curley FJ, Irwin RS, Pratter MR, Tivers DH, Doern GV, Vernaglia PA *et al.* Cough and the common cold. *Am Rev Respir Dis* 1988; **138**: 305–11.

11 Freestone C, Eccles R. Assessment of the antitussive efficacy of codeine in cough associated with common cold. *J Pharm Pharmacol* 1997; **49**: 1045–9.

12 Pavesi L, Subburaj S, Porter-Shaw K. Application and validation of a computerized cough acquisition system for objective monitoring of acute cough: a meta-analysis. *Chest* 2001; **120**: 1121–8.

13 Tukiainen H, Karttunen P, Silvasti M, Flygare U, Korhonen R, Korhonen T *et al.* The treatment of acute transient cough: a placebo-controlled comparison of dextromethorphan and dextromethorphan-beta 2-sympathomimetic combination. *Eur J Respir Dis* 1986; **69**: 95–9.

14 Lee PCL, Jawad MS, Eccles R. Antitussive efficacy of dextromethorphan in cough associated with acute upper respiratory tract infection. *J Pharm Pharmacol* 2000; **52**: 1137–42.

15 Berkowitz RB, Connell JT, Dietz AJ, Greenstein SM, Tinkelman DG. The effectiveness of the nonsedating antihistamine loratadine plus pseudoephedrine in the symptomatic management of the common cold. *Ann Allergy* 1989; **63**: 336–9.

16 Irwin RS, Curley FJ, French CL. Chronic cough: the spectrum and frequency of causes, key components of the diagnostic evaluation, and outcome of specific therapy. *Am Rev Respir Dis* 1990; **141**: 640–7.

17 O'Connell F, Thomas VE, Pride NB, Fuller RW. Capsaicin cough sensitivity decreases with successful treatment of chronic cough. *Am J Respir Crit Care Med* 1994; **150**: 374–80.

18 McGarvey LP, Heaney LG, Lawson JT, Johnston BT, Scally CM, Ennis M *et al.* Evaluation and outcome of patients with chronic non-productive cough using a comprehensive diagnostic protocol. *Thorax* 1998; **53**: 738–43.

19 Mello CJ, Irwin RS, Curley FJ. Predictive values of the character, timing, and complications of chronic cough in diagnosing its cause. *Arch Intern Med* 1996; **156**: 997–1003.

20 Irwin RS, Pratter MR, Holland PS, Corwin RW, Hughes JP. Postnasal drip causes cough and is associated with reversible upper airway obstruction. *Chest* 1984; **85**: 346–52.

21 Carrao WM, Braman SS, Irwin RS. Chronic cough as the sole presenting manifestation of bronchial asthma. *N Engl J Med* 1979; **300**: 633–7.

22 Osman LM, McKenzie L, Cairns J, Friend JA, Godden DJ, Legge JS *et al.* Patient weighting of importance of asthma symptoms. *Thorax* 2001; **56**: 138–42.

23 Gibson PG, Dolovich J, Denburgh J, Ramsdale EH, Hargreave FE. Chronic cough: eosinophilic bronchitis without asthma. *Lancet* 1989; **1**: 1246–7.

24 Doherty MJ, Mister R, Pearson MG, Calverley PM. Capsaicin responsiveness and cough in asthma and chronic obstructive pulmonary disease. *Thorax* 2000; **55**: 643–9.

25 Fujimura M, Kamio Y, Hashimoto T, Matsuda T. Cough receptor sensitivity and bronchial responsiveness in patients with only chronic non-productive cough: effect of bronchodilator therapy. *J Asthma* 1994; **31**: 463–72.

26 Brightling CE, Ward R, Wardlaw AJ, Pavord ID. Airway inflammation, airway responsiveness and cough before and after inhaled budesonide in patients with eosinophilic bronchitis. *Eur Respir J* 2000; **15**: 682–6.

27 Ing AJ, Ngu MC, Breslin AB. Pathogenesis of chronic persistent cough associated with gastroesophageal reflux. *Am J Respir Crit Care Med* 1994; **149**: 160–7.

28 Jack CIA, Calverley PMA, Donnelly RJ, Tran J, Russell G, Hind CRK *et al.* Simultaneous tracheal and oesophageal pH measurements in asthmatic patients with gastro-esophageal reflux. *Thorax* 1995; **50**: 201–4.

29 Paterson WG, Murat BW. Combined ambulatory esophageal manometry and dual-probe pH-metry in evaluation of patients with chronic unexplained cough. *Dig Dis Sci* 1994; **39**: 1117–25.

30 Ours TM, Kavuru MS, Schilz RJ, Richter JE. A prospective evaluation of esophageal testing and a double-blind, randomized study of omeprazole in a diagnostic and therapeutic algorithm for chronic cough. *Am J Gastroenterol* 1999; **94**: 3131–8.

31 Kiljander TO, Salomaa ER, Hietanen EK, Terho EO. Chronic cough and gastro-oesophageal reflux: a double-blind placebo-controlled study with omeprazole. *Eur Respir J* 2000; **16**: 633–8.

32 Novitsky YW, Zawacki JK, Irwin RS, French CT, Hussey VM, Callery MP. Chronic cough due to gastroesophageal reflux disease: efficacy of antireflux surgery. *Surg Endosc* 2002; **16**: 567–71.

33 Vestbo J, Lange P. Can GOLD Stage 0 provide information of prognostic value in chronic obstructive pulmonary disease? *Am J Respir Crit Care Med* 2002; **166**: 329–32.

34 Pauwels RA, Buist AS, Calverley PM, Jenkins CR, Hurd SS. Global strategy for the diagnosis, management, and prevention of chronic obstructive pulmonary disease. NHLBI/WHO Global Initiative for Chronic Obstructive Lung Disease (GOLD) Workshop summary. *Am J Respir Crit Care Med* 2001; **163**: 1256–76.

35 Wynder EL, Kaufman PL, Lesser RL. A short-term follow-up study on ex-cigarette smokers. With special emphasis on persistent cough and weight gain. *Am Rev Respir Dis* 1967; **96**: 645–55.

36 Jorenby DE, Leischow SJ, Nides MA, Rennard SI, Johnston JA, Hughes AR et al. A controlled trial of sustained-release bupropion, a nicotine patch, or both for smoking cessation. *N Engl J Med* 1999; **340**: 685–91.

37 Roberts HR, Wells AU, Milne DG, Rubens MB, Kolbe J, Cole PJ et al. Airflow obstruction in bronchiectasis: correlation between computed tomography features and pulmonary function tests. *Thorax* 2000; **55**: 198–204.

38 Israili ZH, Hall WD. Cough and angioneurotic edema associated with angiotensin-converting enzyme inhibitor therapy. A review of the literature and pathophysiology. *Ann Intern Med* 1992; **117**: 234–42.

39 Berkin KE, Ball SG. Cough and angiotensin converting enzyme inhibition. *Br Med (Clin Res Ed)* 1988; **296**: 1279.

40 Fogari R, Zoppi A, Tettamanti F, Malamani GD, Tinelli C, Salvetti A. Effects of nifedipine and indomethacin on cough induced by angiotensin-converting enzyme inhibitors: a double-blind, randomized, cross-over study. *J Cardiovasc Pharmacol* 1992; **19**: 670–3.

41 McEwan JR, Choudry NB, Fuller RW. The effect of sulindac on the abnormal cough reflex associated with dry cough. *J Pharmacol Exp Ther* 1990; **255**: 161–4.

42 Malini PL, Strocchi E, Zanardi M, Milani M, Ambrosioni E. Thromboxane antagonism and cough induced by angiotensin-converting-enzyme inhibitor. *Lancet* 1997; **350**: 15–8.

43 Hargreaves MR, Benson MK. Inhaled sodium cromoglycate in angiotensin-converting enzyme inhibitor cough. *Lancet* 1995; **345**: 13–6.

44 Poe RH, Harder RV, Israel RH, Kallay MC. Chronic persistent cough. Experience in diagnosis and outcome using an anatomic diagnostic protocol. *Chest* 1989; **95**: 723–8.

45 Hoffstein V. Persistent cough in nonsmoker. *Can Respir J* 1994; **1**: 40–7.

46 Davis SF, Sutter RW, Strebel PM, Orton C, Alexander V, Sanden GN et al. Concurrent outbreaks of pertussis and *Mycoplasma pneumoniae* infection: clinical and epidemiological characteristics of illnesses manifested by cough. *Clin Infect Dis* 1995; **20**: 621–8.

47 Gilberg S, Du Njamkepo ECI, Partouche H, Gueirard P, Ghasarossian C et al. Evidence of *Bordetella pertussis* infection in adults presenting with persistent cough in a French area with very high whole-cell vaccine coverage. *J Infect Dis* 2002; **186**: 415–8.

48 Birkebaek NH, Kristiansen M, Seefeldt T, Degn J, Moller A, Heron I et al. *Bordetella pertussis* and chronic cough in adults. *Clin Infect Dis* 1999; **29**: 1239–42.

49 Kamei RK. Chronic cough in children. *Pediatr Clin North Am* 1991; **38**: 593–605.

50 Holmes PW, Barter CE, Pierce RJ. Chronic persistent cough: use of ipratropium bromide in undiagnosed cases following upper respiratory tract infection. *Respir Med* 1992; **86**: 425–9.

51 O'Connell F, Thomas VE, Pride NB, Fuller RW. Capsaicin cough sensitivity decreases with successful treatment of chronic cough. *Am J Respir Crit Care Med* 1994; **150**: 374–80.

52 Boulet LP, Milot J, Boutet M, St Georges F, Laviolette M. Airway inflammation in non-asthmatic subjects with chronic cough. *Am J Respir Crit Care Med* 1994; **149**: 482–9.

53 Chung KF. Cough: potential pharmacological developments. *Expert Opin Invest Drugs* 2002; **11**: 955–63.

54 Muers MF, Round CE. Palliation of symptoms in non-small cell lung cancer: a study by the Yorkshire Regional Cancer Organisation Thoracic Group. *Thorax* 1993; **48**: 339–43.

55 Dudgeon DJ, Rosenthal S. Management of dyspnea and cough in patients with cancer. *Hematol Oncol Clin North Am* 1996; **10**: 157–71.

56 Eddy NB, Friebel H, Hahn KJ, Halbach H. Codeine and its alternates for pain and cough relief. 3. The antitussive action of codeine—mechanism, methodology and evaluation. *Bull World Health Organ* 1969; **40**: 425–54.

57 Aylward M, Maddock J, Davies DE, Protheroe DA, Leideman T. Dextromethorphan and codeine: comparison of plasma kinetics and antitussive effects. *Eur J Respir Dis* 1984; **65**: 283–91.

58 Empey DW, Laitinen LA, Young GA, Bye CE, Hughes DT. Comparison of the antitussive effects of codeine phosphate 20 mg, dextromethorphan 30 mg and noscapine 30 mg using citric acid-induced cough in normal subjects. *Eur J Clin Pharmacol* 1979; **16**: 393–7.

59 Eddy NB, Friebel H, Hahn KJ, Halbach H. Codeine and its alternates for pain and cough relief. 4. Potential alternates for cough relief. *Bull World Health Organ* 1969; **40**: 639–719.

60 Matthys H, Bleicher B, Bleicher U. Dextromethorphan and codeine: objective assessment of antitussive activity in patients with chronic cough. *J Intern Med* 1983; **11**: 92–100.